*Epidemic Disease*
*in*
*Fifteenth Century England*

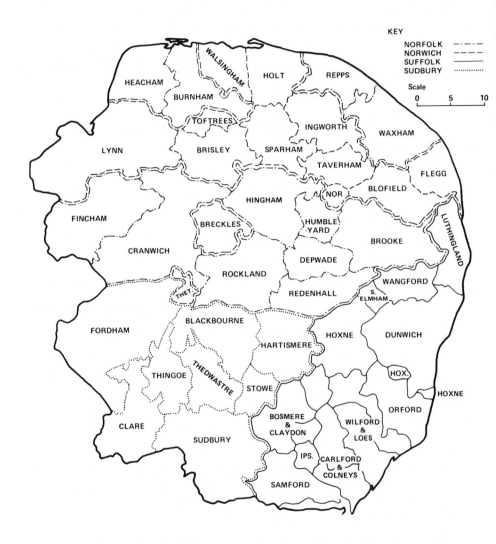

*Map 1.* Consistory Court of Norwich, Jurisdiction of the Deaneries and Archdeaconries

# *Epidemic Disease*
## *in*
# *Fifteenth Century England*

## The Medical Response
## and the
## Demographic Consequences

Robert S. Gottfried

**Rutgers University Press**
New Brunswick, New Jersey

**Library of Congress Cataloging in Publication Data**

Gottfried, Robert S., 1949–
    Epidemic disease in fifteenth century England.

    Bibliography: p.
    Includes index.
    1. Epidemics—England—History.   2. England—Social
conditions—Medieval period, 1066–1485.   3. Medicine—
England—History.   4. England—Population—Statistics.
5. England—Statistics, Vital.   I. Title.
RA650.6.G6G67        614.4′9′42        78-1122
ISBN 0-8135-0861-4

For
Jane

# CONTENTS

# LIST OF TABLES

# LIST OF MAPS

# LIST OF ABBREVIATIONS

| | |
|---|---|
| Amundesham | Johannes Amundesham, *Annales Monasterii S. Albani*, 2 vols., ed. H. T. Riley (London: Longmans, 1870–71) |
| Arnold | Richard Arnold, *Customs of the City of London* (London: F. C. and J. Rivington, 1811) |
| B.M. | British Museum |
| Brut | *The Brut: Chronicles of England*, 2 vols., F. W. D. Brie (London: Oxford Univ. Press, 1960) |
| B.S.E. | Bury St. Edmunds |
| C.C.P. | Canterbury Cathedral Priory, MS d 12F |
| C.L. | *Chronicle of London, 1089–1483*, ed. N. H. Nicolas (London: Longmans, 1827) |
| Croyland | *Ingulph's Chronicle of the Abbey of Croyland*, ed. H. T. Riley (London: H. G. Bohn, 1854) |
| E | Exchequer |
| Ec. H.R. | *Economic History Review* |
| Fabyan | Robert Fabyan, *New Chronicles of England and France*, ed. H. Ellis (London: F. C. and J. Rivington, 1811) |
| G.C.L. | *Great Chronicle of London*, ed. A. H. Thomas (London: G. W. Jones, 1938) |
| Gregory | *Historical Collections of a Citizen of London in the Fifteenth Century*, ed. James Gairdner (London: Camden Society, n.s., XVII, 1876) |
| Grey Friars | *Chronicles of the Grey Friars of London*, ed. J. G. Nichols (London: Camden Society, LIII, 1852) |
| Herryson | John Herryson, *Abbreviata Chronica ab Anno 1377 Usque ad Annum 1469*, Caius College, Cambridge Ms. |
| H | Hertfordshire |

| | |
|---|---|
| *Lacy* | *Register of Edmund Lacy, Bishop of Exeter, 1420–55,* 5 vols., ed. G. R. Dunstan (Torquay: Canterbury and York Society and Devon and Cornwall Society Publications, n.s. 7, 1967) |
| *Milan* | *Calendar of State Papers Relating to Milan,* ed. A. B. Hinds (London: H. M. Stationery Office, 1912) |
| N | Norfolk |
| N.C.C. | Norwich Consistory Court |
| *Papal Registers* | *Calendar of Papal Registers,* Vols. VII–XIII, ed. J. A. Tremlow (London: H. M. Stationery Office, 1906–55) |
| *Paston* | *Paston Letters,* Vols. I–III, ed. James Gairdner (London: Chatto and Windus, 1904) |
| P.C.C. | Prerogative Court of Canterbury |
| *Privy Proc.* | *Proceedings and Ordinances of the Privy Council of England,* Vol. IV, ed. N. Harris Nicholas (London: Eyre and Spottiswoode, 1835) |
| P.R.O. | Public Record Office, London |
| *Rot. Parl.* | *Rotuli parliamentorum ut et petitiones* (London, 1767–77) |
| S | Suffolk |
| *T.R.H.S.* | *Transactions of the Royal Historical Society* |
| *Three Chronicles* | *Three Fifteenth Century Chronicles,* ed. James Gairdner (Westminster: Camden Society, n.s. XXVIII, 1880) |
| *Venice* | *Calendar of State Papers and Manuscripts Relating to English Affairs: Venice,* ed. Rawdon Brown (London: H. M. Stationery Office, 1864) |
| *V.C.H.* | *Victoria History of the Counties of England* |
| *Visitations* | *Visitations and Memorials of Southwell Minster,* ed. A. F. Leach (Westminster: Camden Society, n.s. XLVIII, 1891) |
| Warkworth | *A Chronicle of the First Thirteen Years of the Reign of King Edward the Fourth,* ed. J. O. Halliwell (London: Camden Society, X, 1839) |
| Worcestre | William of Worcestre, *Itineraries,* ed. John Harvey (Oxford: Clarendon Press, 1969) |

# ACKNOWLEDGMENTS

In preparing this book, I have received help from many quarters. I would like to thank the librarians at the University Library, Cambridge University, the University of London Library, the Graduate Library of the University of Michigan, and the librarians and archivists of the British Museum, the Public Record Office in London, and the county record offices in Norwich, Ipswich, and Bury St. Edmunds. Dorothy Foster and Shirley Meinkoth typed my manuscript, Nancy Lynn Simpson proofread the galleys, and John Illingworth of the Computer Centre of University College, the University of London, spent many hours helping me write and rewrite my computer program.

Many scholars kindly read all or part of the book in manuscript form. They include Marvin Becker, David Bien, the late E.M. Carus-Wilson, R.R. Davies, David Herlihy, Maurice Lee, Jr., Ronald Lee, Kenneth Lockridge, Katherine Olstein, Jacob Price, Roger Schofield, Daniel Scott Smith, Charles Tilly, Jeffrey Williamson and E.A. Wrigley. Above all, I would like to thank my mentor, Sylvia L. Thrupp, who read my manuscript through innumerable drafts and without whose guidance the book could not have been written. Finally, thanks are due Saul Rudes, whose special skills made publication of the manuscript possible.

*Epidemic Disease*
*in*
*Fifteenth Century England*

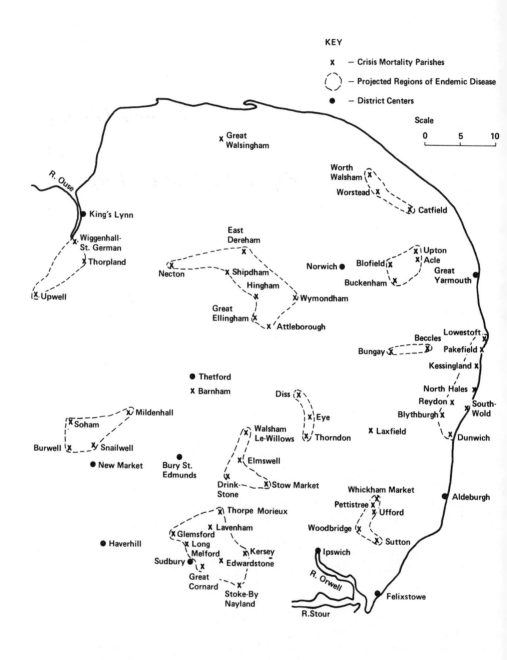

*Map 2.* Regions of Endemic Disease in East Anglia

2

# Introduction

Fifteenth century England remains in many respects an historical enigma, and, until quite recently, has received a bad press. It is still very much an epoch in which popular and to some extent professional historical conceptions have been formed by William Shakespeare's histories, and reinforced by Johan Huizinga's *Waning of the Middle Ages*. It is a period in which many historians, even medievalists, care not to tread—and it is small wonder, given the popular perceptions, which one recent authority has described as the "dark looking glass of the fifteenth century".[1]

This notion of decline pervades all aspects of fifteenth century history.[2] The century has been labeled as backward and isolated, in contrast with an earlier age, when English scholars and merchants regularly crossed the Channel to the continent. We have been handed a well-formed image of a country cursed by an overlong minority and years of weak kings saddled with avaricious and scheming uncles, always ready to manipulate and even murder their charges. The event which triggered the disputes was the usurpation of 1399, an act accompanied by that most heinous of crimes to the medieval mind, regicide, a flagrant violation of God's will. Richard II was deposed and then murdered by his cousin, the Duke of Lancaster, to become Henry IV. This Henry in turn was forced to spend much of his reign defending his crown against rebels who felt that their royal pretensions were as sound as those of a regicide; and there were those contemporaries and later observers who felt that Henry's reign of frustration and the woes of the fifteenth century were divine retribution for the usurpation. Popular conceptions hold that that dissent was hushed during the reign of the second Lancastrian, the great hero-king Henry V, but that dissatisfaction again flared up in the reign of his heir, Henry VI. During the latter's tenure, England was plunged to its later medieval nadir. A new

3

element in the political drama was introduced in the form of a wicked, scheming, dowerless, and—perhaps worst of all—French queen; and she, along with corrupt councillors and the ever-warlike aristocracy began to move England toward chaos. Before the reign of Henry VI was over, the long efforts to restore the Norman-Angevin empire of William the Conqueror and Henry II had failed. And worst of all, with France eliminated from their martial focus, the English aristocracy along with their retinues took to fighting one another, and plunged England into the Wars of the Roses.

This portrait of ineptitude and chaos was initially fostered by the ultimate victors of the Wars of the Roses, the Tudors. Having dubious legal claim to the English throne, they went about propounding and expanding the myth of fifteenth century decline and decay. Henry VII and his heirs sought to portray a war-weary England welcoming the firm but just imposition of Tudor rule. Using new and refined "Renaissance" techniques in history and propaganda, the Tudor image of fifteenth century decline was eloquently formed first by Polydore Vergil and Thomas More, then reinforced by the mid-sixteenth century historians Edward Hall and Ralph Holinshed, and finally and firmly implanted in the imaginations of the English reading world by the plays of Shakespeare.[3]

The image of fifteenth century decline was thus consciously propagated by the Tudors, and despite occasional dissent, passed on to the nineteenth century. And as historians became more thorough, exacting and professional in their studies, and as they expanded their focus from political and diplomatic questions to other fields of inquiry, so the Tudor portrait of fifteenth century decline was extended into social, economic, religious, cultural and constitutional questions. In constitutional and institutional terms, the fifteenth century was seen as barren and sterile. Earlier developments in royal justice and administration were perceived as having come to an abrupt halt. Parliament ceased to "develop," and even feudalism as it had existed in its purest high medieval form gave way to a system of retainers appropriately called "bastard feudalism." Once again, historians portrayed England in 1485 as a kingdom ready and willing to accept Tudor absolutism, good if firm government over chaos.

The interpretation of decline permeated religious and cultural history. The church was said to have slipped into ignorance, barbarity, superstition and witchcraft, a sharp contrast with the glories of the twelfth and thirteenth centuries. The fifteenth century produced not even a great reformer like John Wyclif, and its clergy were depicted as worldly and corrupt, licentious and gluttonous, more interested in hunting and wenching than in ministering to the needs of their flocks. That charge of the church, education, was likewise seen in terms of decline. Oxford University became moribund, settling down to a stale and unrewarding form of scholasticism. No Robert Grosseteste, Roger Bacon, Duns Scotus or William of Ockham would emerge from fifteenth century universities. The decline was alleged to have affected even secular and vernacular culture. There were also no Chaucers or Langlands in the fifteenth century.

But perhaps the most persuasive and pervasive of the detractors of the fifteenth century were those historians who argued for decline from an economic point of view.[4] They pointed to a fall in trade, diminished customs revenues and a collapsing wool trade. They pointed to the shrinking amount of land under active cultivation, the fall in rents and the newly impoverished landlords. They pointed to a crown which had to borrow money from foreign sources to remain solvent, and to once booming provincial towns like York and Lincoln, which in the fifteenth century plunged into decline. Most telling of all, they pointed to population decline and plague, to an England caught in the grip of the second pandemic of plague, with a population falling to a three-century low by 1450. What better evidence of decline could there be than falling population?

Historians' unwillingness to investigate such a seemingly unrewarding epoch was furthered by the real hardships involved in doing research for fifteenth century England. A great deal of this reluctance comes from the nature of the evidence. In a recent survey of historical sources from the thirteenth to the mid-seventeenth centuries, one of our most distinguished contemporary historians described the fifteenth century's narrative records as "real dearth."[5] In fact, there are few continuous descriptive sources, and those which survive tend to be of abysmal quality, both in the literary and the historical senses. A good collection of official state and ecclesiastical materials exist, but they are often difficult to deal with, due to a marked deterioration of calligraphic standards and the use of poor writing and vellum materials. More important, they exist in large and, at times, seemingly unmanageable masses. All in all, until quite recently, scholars have been lured into studying the more accessible, and on the surface, more attractive periods, which precede and follow the fifteenth century.[6]

Within the last generation, fifteenth century studies have gone through something of a revival. The period has now attracted many scholars and, through their extensive research and publications, our knowledge of this era has improved sufficiently to erase many of the Tudor misconceptions.[7] No longer is the fifteenth century condemned outright as an epoch of fruitless civil wars and economic decline; rather, it is seen by many as a period of dynamism and change from medieval to modern. It has been pointed out several times that most of the Tudor innovations, governmental and otherwise, were built on earlier Lancastrian and Yorkist foundations. The Wars of the Roses have been reduced to a series of aristocratic vendettas, a last fling of private warfare, as well as an occasional dynastic battle between Lancaster and York. It has been demonstrated that at no time did the so-called civil wars involve more than a tiny fraction of the total English population, and that some of the "battles" were little more than street brawls between a few dozen men. We have been shown that although the organized church was in decline, popular religious sentiment and piety were on the rise, that Cambridge developed as Oxford declined, and that the new culture of humanism began in the last years of the fifteenth century to supplement the older scholastic culture. Recent research has even established a mixed economic picture. Arrayed against those who argue for unmitigated depression are those who propose a per capita gain accompanying depopulation.[8] Against those who argue for a decline in trade are those who point to developing industry, and show that England moved from raw wool to finished cloth. And to those historians who point to moribund York and Lincoln, others point to dynamic and growing Exeter and Southampton, and to a general change in the economic life and direction of the kingdom. But with all the recent research, comparatively little has been done on the crucial subject of demography.

* * *

The goals of this book include an attempt to add to the corpus of the existing knowledge about fifteenth century England by studying its population trends and movements. Strictly speaking, it is not an attempt to enter into the more general historiographical socio-economic debate as to whether the fifteenth century was a wasteland and a period of decline, or a period of per capita prosperity and transition, though these topics will necessarily be touched upon at various times. Rather, it will try to lay a quantitative and objective framework for one crucial aspect of society, population, in one particular region, East Anglia. It will try to show that one crucial socio-economic factor in fifteenth century England was the biological-environmental element of epidemic disease, and that one disease, plague, was of particular importance. What made plague so crucial was its aetiology. It does not strike in isolated epidemic form, but rather in linked series of epidemics called pandemics. Pandemics last for hundreds of years; and within a pandemic, epidemics will strike in cycles of anywhere from three or four to twenty years. Thus, while plague is one of the most virulent of all infectious diseases, it is the frequency of plague cycles and not the virulence of any single epidemic which makes the disease so deadly. Between 1430 and 1480, the dates covered within, it was reported in England in twenty-seven of the fifty years. Through this frequency of appearance, plague was capable of preventing population from recouping its losses.

Population is a complex subject, and in a brief introduction such as this, it is not possible to discuss even the most basic principles of pre-industrial demography in any detail.[9] But since this study will emphasize the importance of demographic factors in fully understanding fifteenth century England, and since it purports to lay some sort of empirical framework, it will be useful to provide a short overview of some of the issues of pre-industrial demography.

Intensive research has not only allowed demographers to make some generalizations about the complicated issue of population, but also put to rest many misconceptions which modern observers had held about pre-industrial populations. Contrary to general opinion, conjugal family size was generally small. This was the result of a variety of fertility limitation measures, the most common and effective of which was late age of first marriage. Women, except perhaps those from the "gentler" classes, did not marry immediately upon reaching puberty at fifteen and sixteen. Average age of first marriage for both sexes was probably after age twenty-five from at least the late fourteenth century on. In terms of fertility, late age of marriage meant that from one-third to one-half of a woman's potentially fecund years might occur outside of wedlock.

Numbers of children per conjugal family surviving to adulthood averaged between two and three, but the number of children born who failed to survive the rigors of infancy or early childhood were much greater, perhaps three times as many. Pre-industrial birthrates were high, often measuring over 30/1000. But death rates were not far behind, due to high levels of infant mortality and periodic bursts of spectacular crisis mortality—precipitous rises due to plague, famine or other disasters. Hence, population was kept in overall balance and demographic growth before industrialization was slow and inconsistent.

Historians and demographers have generally followed one of two theoretical approaches in pre-industrial demography, the Malthusian and what may be loosely described as the biological positions. The Malthusian position is well-known, and requires little explanation. Briefly, Thomas Robert Malthus, a late eighteenth and early nineteenth century English parson and his followers argued that in agricultural societies, production, especially production from the land, was the key to levels of population. A population ceiling was set, established by agricultural productivity and the level of technological expertise; and above this ceiling, population could not be supported and thus could not expand. Further, due primarily to "the passion between the sexes," the ceiling was usually approached as quickly as possible, in the absence of checks, since population levels grew more rapidly than did food supplies. When population existed close to or just below the limits imposed by production, economic and social growth was retarded. This, according to the Malthusians, was the natural direction of pre-industrial populations.

There are checks in the Malthusian system which can keep population above the subsistence level. Malthus envisioned two types in particular, preventive checks and positive checks. Preventive checks lower fertility; these would include birth limitation and late age of first marriage, itself a means of birth control. Positive checks are those which increase mortality, such as disease and famine. Both types of constraint come into play at different times in various situations, but Malthus advocated the more humane preventive checks as the best means of limiting population growth. In essence, the Malthusian advocates see fertility as the demographic pacesetter.

The biological position, on the other hand, envisions mortality as the key pre-industrial demographic factor. Its proponents stress that fluctuating mortality need not necessarily nor even usually have been the result of a Malthusian availability of dearth in resources. Rather, they claim it was often the product of the random onslaughts of that most potent environmental factor, infectious disease. Originally propounded by a number of Scandinavian social scientists, the biological interpretation was first systematically applied to England by J. D. Chambers.[10] It stresses the independent nature of disease in containing population levels, diseases whose occurrence and frequency were dictated by biological phenomena such as rodent and insect life cycles, and by climatic changes. These phenomena can operate independently of general socio-economic conditions, and at times strike without apparent rhyme or reason, without distinction as to class, wealth or patterns of human settlement.

Both the Malthusian and the biological schools generally agree that demographic growth was very slow. Even during the great expansion of the eleventh, twelfth, and early thirteenth centuries, annual growth rates rarely approached 1 percent. And advocates of both schools agree that in contrast with slow growth came periodic onslaughts of extreme mortality which occasionally reached 30 to 40 percent of the population. If fertility rose slowly, disease and famine caused mortality to fluctuate violently. Because of high fertility and to a lesser extent high mortality, the age structure of pre-industrial populations was heavily skewed toward the younger brackets. The proportion of young people in pre-industrial societies was greater than that in industrial societies.

Both the Malthusian and biological positions have their proponents, and there is little doubt that at given historical moments each theory can be applied and found satisfactory. Fifteenth century England has already attracted two basic positions on plague and population, exemplified in the works of J. A. Saltmarsh and J. M. W. Bean.[11] Saltmarsh stressed the frequency of plague and what he perceived as its devastating social and economic effects. This was fitted into a more general interpretation of decline and decay caused by depopulation. Saltmarsh envisioned a tripartite division of English population from 1200 to 1500. The first period, extending through the thirteenth and into the early fourteenth century, was a period of population growth. The second stage was a period of decline, beginning with a slight demographic downturn from the 1320's and becoming precipitous from 1348, the initial appearance of the Black Death and the second plague pandemic. This decline ended in the 1450's at a demographic low point. Finally, there was a period of stagnation, from 1450 until 1480, followed by an era of steady demographic growth which continued until the late sixteenth century. Extending his argument into a broader socio-economic picture, Saltmarsh called the fourteenth and fifteenth centuries a period of declining prosperity, denying even a per capita rise in standards of living after 1348. Although he did not claim that plague initiated the depression, he did feel that it perpetuated it, with population decline being the key element in the more general economic decline, and plague in turn being the cause of falling population.

Bean did not deny the presence of plague in the later Middle Ages, nor did he completely discount its overall effects on population. But he did feel that Saltmarsh overestimated its significance. First, Bean claimed that by the fifteenth century, the more lethal septicemic and pneumonic strains of plague had given way almost entirely to the less lethal bubonic strain. Second, he felt that certain supposed epidemics of plague were indeed not plague, but rather other, presumably less deadly diseases. In all, Bean claimed there were but twelve national epidemics of plague from 1348 to 1480. Finally, he alleged that in the fifteenth century, plague was an urban phenomenon, predominantly local, and that people were able to flee from it.

Bean therefore reduced the role of plague in molding the course of later medieval England. He claimed that a considerable portion of the adult population survived any given epidemic, and that after particular epidemics, people married sooner due to greater economic opportunity, that nutrition was better, and that birth rates rose, allowing population quickly to regain its former levels. Thus, Bean concluded that fifteenth century England was not markedly effected by plague, while Saltmarsh claimed that it was. One of the goals of this study will be to test the biological and the Malthusian models on the fifteenth century, and to provide further information in the Saltmarsh-Bean debate.

Unfortunately, the sources which are available for this task are poor and often frustrating. There are few censuses or mortality lists, thus eliminating direct demographic evidence. There are not even records of vital registration, such as parish registers, which those working in the early modern period may use. The demographer of medieval England must work with sources which were not made to give population information, and which therefore must be squeezed and exploited with great care to provide serviceable data. Some medieval records do exist which can be used for demographic studies. Perhaps the best are tax rolls, such as the famous English Poll Taxes of 1377, 1379 and 1381. But even these direct taxes, head or hearth, present serious problems for those who attempt to adapt them for demographic purposes. They are often incomplete, and, more important, usually list just adults, or only numbers of "heads and hearths." Rarely is the entire population listed. This means that a common denominator for household size must be calculated, which is itself the subject of great controversy.

There are other governmental and ecclesiastical documents which can be used for demographic purposes. Among them are manorial court rolls, and surveys and extents. For England there are a number of royal surveys, the most famous and one of the most useful being the Domesday Book of William the Conqueror. More common and more helpful for local population studies are the numerous manorial surveys taken by landlords to assess their estate holdings. But all surveys, royal or local, present the student with a record taken entirely from the lords' point of view. At best, they represent only property holders or tenants, generally adult males of importance to the lord. And of course, surveys are not demographic records *per se*: a considerable amount of extrapolation is necessary just to make them serviceable.

There is also a wide variety of peripheral demographic evidence. Much of it is indirect, such as secular trends in prices and wages, or patterns of land settlement, such as the levels of assarting. Rising prices and an expanding arable are usually signs of growing population. Stagnant prices and a shrinking arable, as occurred in fifteenth century England, generally point to a stagnant or falling population. Other peripheral sources include eye-witness estimates and physical evidence, such as numbers and geographic size of towns, expansion of town walls, numbers of buildings, and deserted settlements. There are archeological sources which are often of use, such as cemetery and tombstone evidence, and even skeletal remains. And occasionally, special series of records exist and afford a unique opportunity to investigate a wide swathe of medieval society. One of these special sources survives from fifteenth century England. These are tens of thousands of probated wills, and they form the heart of this study.

No medieval source, not even probated wills or those few existing censuses, can provide complete demographic data. It is clear that barring new and unforeseen documentary discoveries, the medieval demographic picture must remain in part incomplete. Rarely can direct demographic information on such things as fertility and infant mortality be obtained. Incomplete survival of records makes it imperative to work at a local or regional level. This is not a bad thing; in order to understand the demographic process completely, it is imperative to study local intricacies. Still, it would be helpful to have larger national or even European overviews, but the data do not permit this. Yet even with these reservations, much can be done within the limits of existing medieval data. Caution is the first prerequisite of anyone attempting to apply the methods of the social sciences to historical evidence. But the documents survive and wait to be exploited. Probated wills provide the opportunity to place fifteenth century English demographic movements in a larger pre-industrial and medieval context, and to test the models and theories proposed by others. Perhaps they will also help historians in their attempts to reconstruct a better picture of this difficult and still misunderstood period in English history.

## Notes

1. J. R. Lander, *Conflict and Stability in Fifteenth Century England* (London: Hutchinson and Co., 1969), p. 11.

2. It is not possible to list all 19th century studies of 15th century England. The interested reader is advised to see the bibliography in E. F. Jacob, *The Fifteenth Century* (Oxford: Univ. Press, 1961). Two books worth noting are W. Denton, *England in the Fifteenth Century* (London: George Bell and Sons, 1888); and J. R. Green, *A Short History of the English People* (London: Macmillan, 1874).

3. For a discussion of Shakespeare's histories and their relationship to the 15th century, see C. L. Kingsford, *Prejudice and Promise in Fifteenth Century England* (Oxford: Clarendon Press, 1925). For an introduction to Tudor historiography and 15th century England, see P. M. Kendall, *Richard III: The Great Debate* (New York: W. W. Norton, 1965).

4. As with the other references in the introduction, detailed notes cannot be given. Perhaps the most influential exponent of 15th century economic decline is M. M. Postan, "The Fifteenth Century," *Economic History Review (Ec.H.R.)*, IX, 1939, and "Some Agrarian Evidence of Declining Population in the Later Middle Ages," *Ec.H.R.*, 2nd series, II, 1950. Many articles in the *Economic History Review* address this problem.

5. G. R. Elton, *England, 1200–1640* (Ithaca, N.Y.: Cornell University Press, 1969).

6. For a discussion of the documentary weakness of the 15th century, see E. M. Carus-Wilson, "The First Half-Century of the Borough of Stratford-upon-Avon," *Ec.H.R.* 2nd Series, XVIII, 1965.

7. Among others, see S. B. Chrimes, *Lancastrians, Yorkists, and Henry VII* (London: Macmillan, 1966); F. R. H. DuBoulay, *An Age of Ambition* (New York: Viking Press, 1970); Lander, *op. cit.;* and R. L. Storey, *The End of the House of Lancaster* (New York: Stein and Day, 1967).

8. See, among others, A. R. Bridbury, *Economic Growth: England in the Later Middle Ages* (London: George Allen and Unwin, 1962).

9. For a more detailed discussion, see E. A. Wrigley, *Population and History* (New York: McGraw-Hill, 1969).

10. J. D. Chambers, *Population, Economy and Society in Pre-Industrial England* (Oxford: Oxford Univ. Press, 1972).

11. J. A. Saltmarsh, "Plague and Economic Decline in England in the Later Middle Ages," *Cambridge Historical Journal,* 7, 1941; J. M. W. Bean, "Plague, Population, and Economic Decline in England in the Later Middle Ages," *Ec.H.R.,* 2nd series, XV, 1962–1963.

# CHAPTER I

# *Methodology*

## 1.1 The Will

It has been over fifty years since C. L. Kingsford first urged historians to turn to new, relatively unused sources, sources without the ulterior motives of narrative records, in order that they might at last come face to face with the common people, and "discover the truth and discern the promise of the fifteenth century in England."[1] Among the new sources Kingsford suggested were wills. Although their importance as an historical source needs no stressing, and although several historians have made excellent use of them,[2] there has been a general reluctance to analyze large numbers of wills in an orderly, quantitative manner. It is my intention to use about 20,000 probated, registered wills, loose probates, letters of administration, and items on intestacy lists in an attempt to assess the effects of epidemic disease in Norfolk, Suffolk, the archdeaconry of St. Albans in Hertfordshire, and those parts of Cambridgeshire which fell under the jurisdiction of the bishop of Norwich.[3] These areas have been chosen because of the large-scale survival of registered wills from the various ecclesiastical courts, and because of the large numbers of wills from poor and middling testators surviving alongside those of their wealthier counterparts. This is especially true for Norfolk and Suffolk, where wills from the prerogative, consistory and archdeaconry courts,[4] as well as those from a peculiar court, exist in great number. In terms of sheer numbers and comprehension of registration of testamentary evidence, Norfolk and Suffolk are unique in fifteenth century England; and, with the possible exception of Kent, a survey of this sort could not be done for any other county. Throughout the text, the term "East Anglia" will be used in a limited sense to delineate those parishes contained exclusively within the jurisdiction of the consistory court of Norwich, and not to any parishes in Essex, or those parishes in the fenlands and Cambridgeshire which were not within the authority of the bishopric.

The period 1430–1480 was chosen for particular reasons. Before the 1430's, wills from the archdeaconry court jurisdictions in East Anglia and the peculiar court of Bury St. Edmunds survive only in bits and pieces. Although probated wills from the two Norfolk archdeaconry courts exist only for a few years even within the period 1430–1480, those from the Suffolk archdeaconry courts and Bury St. Edmonds begin to appear in considerable numbers from the late 1430's onward. The selection of the date 1480 as the terminating point was made on both historical and practical grounds. First, there were limited numbers of wills that could be read and a limited number of files that could be placed on a computer tape and used readily in the computer time available.[5] But there was also more historical reasoning which went into the selection of 1480. The most virulent epidemic of the fifteenth century was the plague of 1479–1480, and it was essential to include this date within the survey. More important, for at least a generation after 1480, plague epidemics occurred less frequently than they had in the period 1430–1480, and in fact less frequently than they had since 1348. This is extremely important, since the most crucial aspect of plague in the fifteenth century was not the virulence of any particular epidemic, but rather the frequency with which these epidemics came, one after another, rarely at intervals greater than four or five years. A cursory examination of the period 1480–1510[6] shows that minor plague epidemics occurred in 1486, 1491 and 1493, but that the next major epidemic after 1479–1480 did not strike until 1499–1500, and the next after that not until 1510. While this hardly marks an era of total respite from plague or infectious disease in general, it does indicate a considerable slackening from the pace of the preceding fifty years, and possibly an aetiological change in the character of plague itself. Plague came to England less frequently after 1480, and this must be accounted as a major demographic landmark. There is some justification for extending the study to 1485, to include the sweating sickness of that year, and the author hopes to do this in the near future.

Of the approximately 20,000 testamentary documents used, about 15,000 were wills. All of these were registered and proved, and only the wills were computerized. A statistical breakdown of the data by county, decade and some occupations is provided in Chapter 6.

This initial chapter explains the methodology used. The second and third chapters set the chronology of epidemic diseases in the period 1430–1480, and attempt to assess their individual aetiological identity and survey the contemporary medical response. Literary and narrative sources, rather than wills, are used in Chapters 2 and 3. Chapters 4 through 7 analyze the wills quantitatively. Chapters 4 and 5 discuss the virulence of the individual epidemics of the period under study and their seasonal frequency, propose a model of the mortality pattern of bubonic plague, chart the path and distribution of individual epidemics, and investigate those areas which were most severely afflicted, and where infectious diseases may have been endemic, as well as epidemic. Chapters 6 and 7 look at the demographic characteristics of the sample. Chapter 6 discusses the age, wealth and nuptial patterns of the testators themselves; while Chapter 7 analyzes the testators' children and tries to project the long-term trends of population between 1430 and 1480. Chapter 8 discusses the implications of these results, and tries to apply them in general terms to fifteenth century England. Because of the lack of basic population data for England in the period 1430–1480, and the lack even of parish registers, it becomes vital to take the greatest care in explaining the methodology, starting with the will itself, the main source used.

By the middle of the thirteenth century, the form of the will as it was to prevail until the Reformation became approximately fixed in character.[7] It was usually a deathbed statement dictated in the first person. This was called the original will. The individual or group of persons named in the will as executor or executors then took the original will to the appropriate court, where it was proved. A probate copy was made and then placed in a bound register—hence the name "registered copy will"—with the executor presumably keeping the original. All this was done for a fee, without payment of which the will might not be registered. Theoretically, the amount of the fee seems to have varied. In the fourteenth century, Edward III had fixed it at between 2s, 5d and 5s, but in the early fifteenth century, Commons complained that the fees were far too high, often ranging between 40s and 60s.[8] Lyndwood, in his compilation of ecclesiastical laws, wrote that the scribe who copied down the will got 6d for his efforts.[9] If the estate were worth less than 30s, there was in theory to be no fee. If the estate ranged between 30s and 100s, the fee was to be 12d; if the estate was valued between 100s and £20, the fee was to be 3s, and so on up the scale. In practice much larger fees were undoubtedly charged or extorted, and many executors or families of the deceased either refused or were unable to pay the registration fee, and a registered copy may not have been made. Several registers have what appear to be original wills inserted in them, and some record offices have bundles of original wills alone.[10]

In the event of intestacy, the deceased's next of kin were supposed to go to the appropriate court and apply for a letter of administration. The court would then appoint an executor, entitled to dispose of the estate less the necessary fee. A number of registers have long lists of intestate deaths, letters of administration, or simply just probated wills, undoubtedly via these circumstances.[11] It is possible that in the event of intestacy and perhaps even of testate death, the local parish cleric may have come to the dwelling of the deceased, and himself taken the document or news of intestate death to the appropriate court.[12]

Occasionally, *testamenta* accompany the wills in the bound registers. The distinction between *testamenta* and last wills had become blurred by the later Middle Ages. Originally, the *testamenta* were devoted to movables, and the *ultima voluntas* to land.[13] Also, the *testamenta* were made earlier than the *ultima voluntas*, as the last will was a deathbed document. By the fifteenth century, the *testamenta* had become rare, and are to be found mostly from the wealthier testators and primarily in the Prerogative Court of Canterbury (P.C.C.). They were almost always accompanied by the last wills, which were nearer to the date of probate.[14]

Fifteenth century wills followed a common form. Generally, they were written in Latin, although occasionally and more frequently from 1460 onward, they were in English. A few P.C.C. wills from before 1450 were in French. Initially, the testator began by stating his name and any aliases, the date and the place of domicile. Townsmen who were citizens would state that fact, and both urban and rural testators might list an occupation. Almost always, it is stated that the testator was sound of mind and memory, though sick of body. The testator then bequeathed his soul to God, the Blessed Mary and all saints, and stated the name of the place at which he wished to be buried. Usually, this was the place of immediate residence, but there were exceptions. At times, if the testator had migrated from the place of his birth, he would say so, and request burial in the parish of his origin. Many rectors living away from their benefices, for example, asked to be buried there.

Often the specific church of burial within a particular village or town was listed. This was necessary if the testator lived in a settlement with more than one parish church, such as Forncett in Norfolk, or if he lived in a large town, such as Norwich. It was also necessary for the many testators who lived in villages with similar or identical place names, such as Aldeburgh, or the many Thorpes and Stokes scattered about East Anglia. Finally in the introductory section, the testator might ask to be buried within the parish church itself, rather than in the graveyard, or perhaps in a neighboring monastery or deanery. At times, a special spot, such as behind the high altar, would be particularly delineated and carefully provided for. Deceased spouses are sometimes mentioned here, and this is of great importance in deducing such things as marriage ratios.

The first bequests listed were pious[15] or charitable. Most germane to this study was the bequest to the high altar of the parish of burial "for tithes forgotten." This is encountered almost without exception. Occasionally the bequest was made in kind, especially grains, but generally it was made in cash. Next came the bequest to the fabrics of the church of burial, another donation almost universally encountered. This was followed by a wide variety of further pious bequests, ranging from lights in the church to moonlight processions, to series of masses and special clerics to sing them. Occasionally, provisions of a few pence were provided for anyone who attended the funeral of the deceased. As with the bequests to the high altar, other pious donations were usually in cash, with those bequests in kind generally being bushels or quarters of wheat, barley or malt. Parish guilds were another favorite recipient, but although the guilds were almost always incorporated under the aegis of a favorite saint, it is sometimes difficult to decipher their precise nature and function. Hospitals, private chantries, lazar houses, prisoners in gaols and religious houses were other favorite recipients of pious bequests.[16]

The initial explanatory phases and the pious bequests were the *pro forma* opening of most wills. Next, the testator's family was provided for. First came the spouse, then the sons, perhaps in direct order of birth, and then the daughters. When land was left in the will and there were no progeny of age, the spouse, if the testator were married, would be given most or all of it.[17] If one or more of the children, most particularly a son, were of age, he or she would get the bulk of the land. But a female spouse was generally left with something all to her own, such as a toft, a messuage or a chamber in the main house, and may have been provided for in advance of the will. Some or all of the children also may have been provided for in advance of composition, although, especially in the case of the male children, this would not preclude their presence in the last will.[18]

Sons took preference in inheriting land. Generally the eldest, if of age, would get the bulk, or if not of age at the making of the will, would inherit it from his mother when she died or when he came to his majority. Although younger sons would occasionally be "paid off" in movables, they were frequently given nonintegral pieces of land, such as a *pratum* or even an extra *tenementum,* and a lump sum of cash, depending on the wealth of the individual testator. Movables generally went to the spouse and daughters; when they were given to male progeny, they often took the form of farm tools, equipment or livestock. When included, daughters were most likely to get household possessions or cash. Occasionally, they too were left bits and pieces of land.

The disposal of land by will was freer in fact than theory. Legally, fifteenth century Englishmen were forbidden by Crown and Church, if not custom, from leaving what was not theirs. As Maitland wrote about an earlier period, it was believed that "only God, not man, could make an heir."[19] In practice, land was regularly passed on, increasingly so by the 1450's, and generally by the 1460's without even the formality of enfeoffment. Land was virtually always left within the nuclear family, if possible. If no immediate heirs survived, relatives, especially brothers and nephews, were the favorite recipients. Mortmain was not common in the wills, but did occur despite legal sanctions against its unlicensed practice. The land left varied from very large to very small. In the P.C.C. and consistory courts there were instances of entire manors being bequeathed, and in the consistory and archdeaconry courts cases of mere tofts and crofts. In towns, whole shops and businesses were left. Though not land, one "immovable" bequest encountered was from a rector, who saw fit to leave his benefice to his nonclerical brother.

Other relatives were often included among beneficiaries in the wills, though less frequently when these were direct male heirs, especially if those heirs were of age. Brothers and sisters of the deceased and their children were favored. If the parents of the testator were still alive, they too were usually mentioned, and were often asked to act as executors. If a daughter were married, her husband may have been included, and acted as an executor if there were no male heirs of age. Servants of a variety of types and friends made up the last group who often received bequests, almost always in movables, but not in cash.

Debts were paid when necessary, and any other desire, such as the wish for someone (always amply paid) to go on a pilgrimage, be it to Walsingham or Jerusalem, were indulged. Usually, the latter sections of the will were in quite rambling, almost free form. Finally, the testator named his executor or executors, generally the spouse, a son of age, a parent, friend or cleric. Probate form was standardized, mentioning the probate clerk, the place where the will was proved and whether all the executors were present. It was quite rapid, usually taking less than a month.[20]

## 1.2 The Wills and the Ecclesiastical Courts

The wills used in this study have been taken from four levels of ecclesiastical courts:[21] the prerogative court, the consistory court, archdeaconry courts, and a sacrist's peculiar court. Additionally, about twenty wills from the city court of Norwich have been used for completeness' sake. The Prerogative Court of Canterbury has been searched for all probated wills from Norfolk, Suffolk, Essex, Kent, Hertfordshire, the city of London, and Southwark falling between 1430 and 1480. The wills proved in the *Register of Henry Chichele* falling within the above guidelines have also been read. To register in the Prerogative Court of Canterbury a testator was supposed to have held land in two or more bishoprics totaling £5 or more in value. Almost without exception, the testators encountered in the P.C.C. were very wealthy; if the three major types of ecclesiastical courts can be said to fall into a hierarchy, then the P.C.C. was at the top. The P.C.C. group as a whole, including the testators from London, Southwark and the other urban centers, were in general large property owners. Those from London, and most of those from Southwark were citizens of the city of London, and mostly members of the great livery companies, especially the mercers, grocers, drapers and fishermongers. A great many of these big city testators held land in adjoining areas, especially within the bishopric of Rochester.

The testators from Kent, Essex, Hertfordshire, Suffolk and Norfolk whose wills have been registered in the P.C.C. fell into distinct social and geographic groups.[22] A great many of them were armigerous, mostly gentry, and are hereafter called the rural élite. The second group consisted of provincial townsmen, primarily being citizens from Norwich, King's Lynn, St. Albans and Canterbury itself. There were a disproportionate number of wills from testators living in Canterbury and Kent, who may be said to form the third group of non-Londoners registered in the P.C.C. They seem to have been somewhat less well off than the others in the P.C.C., and many of them did not possess land worth more than £5 in two or more bishoprics. It may be surmised that these testators were permitted to register their wills in the P.C.C. because of convenience or proximity to the archbishop's court, or because they elected to pay the necessary fees for personal or status reasons. The fourth group of non-Londoners using the P.C.C. were clerics of all varieties, with the majority being rectors.

The consistory court, as the name implies, was the court of the bishop. The only one used here was that of the bishop of Norwich, which provided the largest and most complete block of wills in the survey. In general, it appears to have been the next wealthiest ecclesiastical court, after the prerogative court. Officially, the £5 rule was to have held here, this time distinguishing the consistory court from the archdeaconry courts; legally, if the testator had land valued at £5 or more in at least two archdeaconries, he should have registered his will with the bishop's court. In fact, testators in the Norwich Consistory Court (N.C.C.) came from many wealth levels, with both extremes of the population represented, and by the latter half of the fifteenth century the £5 rule seems to have been stretched to include movables as well as land.

The existence of registration fees, or rather, the exemption from registration fees, made for a significant quirk in the demographic makeup of the testators in the consistory court. Clerics were exempted from paying them, and were supposed to register in bishop's court rather than archdeaconry courts.[23] Apparently, clergy (and gentry) who did not have lands valued at more than £5 were still entitled to register their wills in the N.C.C.[24] While there were practically no clerics in the archdeaconry courts, there were many in the peculiar court of Bury St. Edmuds. In the N.C.C., in certain seasons in the 1440's, clerics made up a disproportionate segment of the will-making population, and it has been necessary to program them out when taking family related statistics. It should be noted, however, that most clergy and gentry in the N.C.C. had lands and movables worth far more than £5.

The registration of wills in the N.C.C. was generally in chronological order of probate, in contrast to the random ordering in any of the archdeaconry courts. The decennial distribution of the N.C.C. testamentary data was more even than the distributions of the data found in the lower courts, also. Although there were more wills in terms of raw numbers from the modern county of Norfolk than from the modern county of Suffolk, with the exceptions of a few years in the 1450's due to preemption and a general decline of Suffolk wills in the late 1470's, there was a consistency in proportion and numbers between Norfolk and Suffolk records throughout the period under study. The N.C.C. has the most extensive lists of intestate deaths. These lists are generally encountered in the beginning of the registry volumes. With the exceptions noted in the graphs accompanying Chapter 4, they cover most of the period 1430–1480, and have been used as an independent check on the mortality exhibited by the wills. Although N.C.C. wills were generally proved in Norwich itself, at one time or another in the fifteenth century they were also proved at Aylsham, Butley, Charing, Eccles, Gaywood, Hoxne, Ipswich, Lynn, Sudbury, Terling, Thetford, Thornage, Thornham, Thorpe Episcope, Woodbridge and Yarmouth.

The archdeaconry courts were the lowest ecclesiastical courts available for probate of wills in East Anglia. An executor generally registered in the archdeaconry court physically closest to him, or the court under whose jurisdiction his deanery, parish or hamlet fell. Because it was lowest in the court hierarchy, the possibility of inhibition due to a visitation by the bishop was very real, and there are accompanying gaps in the Suffolk and Sudbury archdeaconry courts at the time of the increase in will registration in the N.C.C. in the late 1450's. The poorer families probably tried to prove their wills in the lowest, that is, the cheapest court possible, as shown by the following verse:

For who so will prove a testament
That is not all worth tenne pound
He shall pay for the parchment
The third of the money all round.[25]

However, per capita testator wealth in the archdeaconry courts was quite close to that shown by consistory court testators.[26]

The archdeaconry court wills are shorter, and less embellished than those from higher courts. Often, there are several wills to the page in the bound registered volumes. They are rarely in chronological order for more than short periods of time, although this may be due to delays in copying and binding. Many original wills are inserted in the bound volumes. Either executors resented paying the registration fees, did not have enough cash, or simply did not feel that registration of the original will was necessary. It is certain that many original wills have been lost, though a great number survive randomly for the archdeaconry of Suffolk. There are numerous intestate deaths reported in the registers of the archdeaconry of Suffolk, and a number of probate notices without corresponding wills in the archdeaconry courts of Sudbury and Norfolk. As with the list of intestates from the N.C.C., these have been used as an independent check on mortality as deduced from the wills themselves.

As stated earlier, the archdeaconry courts in Suffolk provide a fuller record than those in Norfolk, having extensive registrations from the late 1430's to the late 1470's. Less than one hundred wills remain between 1430 and 1480 from the archdeaconry court of Norwich. Some are from the year 1469, but most are from 1479 and 1480. The archdeaconry court of Norfolk has more survivals, which comprise an excellent, essentially chronological sample, but only from 1459 to 1477. The best collection of archdeaconry court wills used comes from the archdeaconry of St. Albans, in Hertfordshire. Over 1,300 St. Albans archdeaconry court wills exist from the period 1430–1480, in generally chronological order. The individual wills in the 1430's and early 1440's are extremely short and may not be demographically reliable until the mid-1440's.

It remains only to discuss the peculiar courts, especially that of Bury St. Edmunds, the jurisdiction of which was restricted almost without exception to the town of Bury itself. Demographically, the wills which have survived make up the most comprehensive sample for all the courts being covered. Many of the testators included listed their occupations, and a large number were simple laborers and shepherds, as well as grocers and drapers. Judging from fourteenth century tax returns, the will totals may be 70–80 percent complete for the adult male population during the period 1430–1480.[27] There are a large number of clerics in the sample, and they form the only group of testators who sometimes lived outside of the town itself. The wills are beautifully written, generally arranged chronologically according to date of probate, and are quite often long and detailed. The peculiar court of Bury St. Edmunds (B.S.E.) is different from the other courts discussed thus far in that the complete letter of administration, rather than the simple note of intestacy, was included in the registered copy volumes. As with other intestate and probate listings, the letters of administration have been used as corroborating evidence for the mortality exhibited by the wills.[28]

Other peculiar court and borough court jurisdictions within the geographical bounds of this study include the wills registered in the city courts of King's Lynn and Great Yarmouth, and the peculiar jurisdictions of Castle Rising and Great Cressingham, none of which have wills surviving from 1430 to 1480. About twenty wills survive from the city court of Norwich from 1430 to 1480, all among the records of enrolled deeds. They are generally from the citizen and aldermanic segments of society, and have been included in the sample.

## 1.3 The Will as a Demographic Source

The question of who left wills and the validity of the extent of their family composition is crucial to this study. Demographers aside for the moment, this question has been debated by historians and genealogists. Camp believed that many of the poorer peasants simply did not bother to make them.[29] Maitland, on the other hand, felt that practically all persons, regardless of wealth or legal status, made a will.[30] Legally, the distinction between the right of free and nonfree Englishmen to leave wills appears to have lost significance by the late Anglo-Saxon period, and to the great legal historian there was little question as to the total, all-pervasive nature of the will-making population.[31] Speaking about Kentish wills, Dulley felt that only the richer inhabitants had enough goods to justify will making, and that perhaps one-third or even one-half of the adult population did not leave them.[32]

It is the author's belief that virtually all adults, including females, had the opportunity to make an original will in East Anglia, from the 1450's onward. The most crucial factor appears not to have been will making, but rather the motivation and subsequent incidence of will registration. It was the registration, not the making of a will, which drew a significant fee, and the church preached strongly against intestacy.[33] It is clear, however, that most East Anglia female wills were not registered, while those of adult males, by the 1460's, excluding the poorest 25–30 percent of the population, were.[34] Most important, about 20,000 testamentary documents have been used in this study of a fifty-year period, and the sheer magnitude of numbers makes for a viable demographic sample.

A statistical assessment of wealth levels of the individual testators has been conducted. The results can be seen and are discussed in detail in Chapter 6.[35] These wealth data show the inclusive nature of the will-making population. Of the five categories of wealth, the modal figure was always in the next to the last, or second poorest, category. With a bequest of only 5d being required for admission into this category, membership in the club of will makers can hardly have been too exclusive. At the same time, the lowest wealth category, requiring a bequest of only 1d, constituted a very small proportion of the will-making population, indicating perhaps that the 25–30 percent of the total adult male population who did not have wills registered may have been the most destitute segment.

About 14 percent of the will-registering population was female, and only certain distinct female groups appear to have gone to the trouble to ensure the registrations of their wills. The most predominant and perhaps most obvious of the female groups to leave wills were widows. They made up about 38 percent of the female population. Another group were unmarried, seemingly never-married women. A few of these testators actually called themselves "single-woman," but the majority of them simply did not mention children or a living or deceased spouse. It is possible that some of these women were at one time married, but experience has shown that dead or married children and especially dead spouses were rarely forgotten. The final group of female testators had husbands alive at the time of the will. They were distinguished from the bulk of married females who did not leave wills by the fact that most of them had dowries or goods settled upon them at the time of their marriage or earlier, the income of which they shared with their husbands in life, but which they still had the power to bequeath at the time of their death. Sometimes this would go to a daughter or female relative, thus perpetuating one segment of the group of female testators.[36]

The will-making population was "adult." The definition of being "of age" at least in part meant "of age to make a will." An attempt to assess the ages of the will-registering population as a whole has been made, and is discussed at length in Chapter 6.[37] Less than 2 percent of the sample were clearly unmarried with parents alive at the time the will was made, and are estimated to be from sixteen to twenty-five years of age. The rest of the will population was in their late twenties and older.

Demographically, the historian is on surest ground when using wills to discuss mortality. When graphed, the wills can provide a yearly, seasonal, and even monthly barometer of mortality over extended periods of time.

The greatest problem is in determining the exact date of death of the testator. Is the date of the will's composition the date of death, or is it the date of the will's probate? In fact, precision cannot be achieved by using the wills alone, except for the intestate listings, and a special technique had to be devised to ascertain the date of death.

In a compromise between historical certainty and statistical precision, season of death, as opposed to month or year of death, was chosen. The seasons of the year were divided as follows: December through February, winter; March through May, spring; June through August, summer; and September through November, autumn. The "year" for purposes of this study, runs from 1 December to 30 November. The year 1468, for example, will run from 1 December, 1467, through 30 November, 1468. The year 1469 will run from 1 December, 1468 through 30 November, 1469. This was thought to be the most accurate seasonal division "climate-wise."[38]

Generally, the season of death was taken as the mean between the date the will was made and the date of probate. If, for example, a will was made on 1 September and proved on 1 November, the date of death was considered to be on 1 October, and the season of death, autumn. If the will was dated 10 August and the probate was 10 September, the date of death was considered to be 25 August and the season of death, summer. There are, necessarily, modifications to this system. If the will antedated probate by more than six months, the date of probate was taken as the date and season of death, unless the probate death were one of the first five days of the new season. Thus, a will made on 1 April, 1468, and proved on 6 December, 1468, would be considered as a winter death; a will made on 1 April, 1468, and proved on 4 December, 1468, was considered to have been an autumn death. Only wills that have been proved have been included in the sample; wills without probates cannot be used as there is no positive evidence when the testator died. Any will proved after the first twenty-five days of a new season was considered part of that new season, regardless of the date of will composition. Thus, a will made on 6 July, 1468, and proved on 26 September, 1468, was considered to have been an autumn death; but a will made on 6 July and proved on 24 September of the same year was considered as a summer death.

Obviously, many of these distinctions are quite artificial, but no other proposed system seemed as comprehensive. The difference of one day may seem too arbitrary to cast two wills into different seasons of death, but no other option was available. In actual practice, none of the more Byzantine methods had to be employed too regularly. The will-making and will-probate dates were usually fairly close together, seldom being more than three weeks to a month apart, especially in the lower courts.

Likewise, the frequency of probate was overwhelming; in the arch-deaconry court of Suffolk in the 1430's and early 1440's there were sizeable numbers of wills without probates, but many of these wills were crossed out. Wills from the archdeaconry court of Sudbury and the peculiar court of B.S.E. were not used for the early and mid-1430's because too many of them lacked probate. Only in the P.C.C. were long gaps between the date of the will and date of probate frequently encoun-tered, and it was in the P.C.C. that many of the above described measures had to be used. Even here, many of the long gaps were bridged by series of *testamenta* which got closer and closer to the date of probate. It can be said in general that while there exists great danger of inaccuracy in attempting to divide will mortality into monthly intervals, there is a great degree of certainty in dividing them into seasonal divisions. There are no such problems in graphing the intestate deaths listed in the will registers, or by definition, the single probates and letters of administration. They tell the precise date of death, or give but a single date to work with. The same seasonal scheme was used here as was outlined above.

The wills may mention illness, and often provide indirect clues to the cause of death. In times when the chronicles report epidemics or crisis periods, the date of will making and the date of probate invariably draw closer together than they do in times of "normal" mortality. The gap between the numbers of probates and intestate deaths shrinks—or the increase in intestate deaths becomes so large that there can be little doubt that a period of crisis mortality was in progress. Moreover, during a crisis period, the wills are entered in closer chronological order in regard to both date of composition and date of probate. More wills are crossed out, perhaps indicating a greater desire to ensure registration of the will, as does the oft-decreasing frequency in intestacy listings. Further, during crisis periods, more wills are usually crammed on to less folio page space than during normal times. Finally, daughters were more diligently re-corded when the likelihood was many times greater that one or all the male heirs would not survive.

Many factors relating to marriage, including crude numbers of hus-bands and wives, the frequency of first-time marriage and remarriage, numbers of widows and widowers, and approximate ages of first marriage can be gleaned from the wills. Dead spouses are commonly mentioned in the wills via prayer or pious bequest. A female testator will usually give her surnames from any previous marriage or marriages if she was or had been a widow, and may ask to be buried next to the predeceased partner or partners. There are a number of other ways in which a dead spouse can be included in the wills, such as a series of utensils or a dowry left by a dead female to her daughter, perhaps as reported in someone else's will. The role of the spouse, regardless of sex and especially as executor, was crucial, and it is probable that there was very little marital underenumeration in the wills, be the spouse dead or alive. Several different types of marital and remarital ratios have been used. In some instances, only living mates were taken; in others, all spouses directly mentioned in the wills; and in others still, all spouses, living or dead, implied or celebrated. The specifics of the marital replacement ratio methodologies and other particulars about marriage and the wills will be discussed in detail, below.[39]

Questions of fertility are more difficult to answer from the wills than are those of mortality and marriage. Do the wills present an accurate portrayal of the family, nuclear or otherwise? Before the late 1440's, the answer is almost certainly no. As the number of wills and the extent of the will-registering population rises from the 1440's onward, however, the portrayal of family size within each individual will also rises to give a fairer assessment of family numbers. But at no time in the period 1430–1480 do the wills give a totally accurate picture of the number of live births in fifteenth century families, with the possible exceptions of the P.C.C. testators from the late 1450's, and certain groups of N.C.C. testators in the 1470's. The principal reason for this is the chronic underenumeration of female progeny; they simply were not included in most non-P.C.C. fifteenth century wills in what surely were their actual numbers, even in the 1470's. Nevertheless, by using the replacement ratios, much useful data can be gleaned from the testamentary data about both family size and long-term population movements.

At least one son—one male heir—and probably all sons were mentioned in the wills. Unless the male progeny were very, very young, it does not seem reasonable to conclude that a person who had gone to the trouble to ensure the registration of his will would not mention at least a solitary male heir, even if the estate were very small and the heir were a cleric. Sons who were rectors or vicars were frequently appointed as executors, and got a cash bequest, if nothing else. Additionally, the probates and phraseology of the wills indicate that even those sons who had migrated elsewhere to seek their fortunes were included in the last testament. A key element in the inclusion of all male progeny in the will must have been the tenuous nature of life itself in the fifteenth century. The documents reflect the enormous pride of the testators in their possessions, and the strong desire to keep them, especially land, within the family. Bequests in mortmain were rare, especially when children survived. When there were no heirs in the conjugal family, the testator searched for other remembered relatives, especially brothers and nephews. The very large number of friends mentioned and bequeathed gifts in the wills makes it difficult to believe that these nonconjugal and nonextended family members would be given goods to the exclusion of children and relatives. Rather, they point to the lack of heirs or kin to whom the testator could bequeath his or her possessions.

This strong desire to ensure succession is nowhere better illustrated than in the detailed and exacting provisions made in the event of the death of one of the designated heirs. Will after will has long lists saying that if son number one should die, then son number two should take his place, and if son number two should die, then son number three should take his place, and if son number three should die, then daughter number one should take his place, and so on. Often, these formulas carry on through a half dozen places in the line of succession. Many wills makes a point of saying that a bequest is valid only if the designated heir reaches a certain age well before the official age of majority. The machinelike provisions for continued succession conform closely to the ideas expressed by Ariès in his discussion of childhood.[40] Additonally, the numbers of friends and relatives included in the wills can be seen to drop dramatically with the increasing number of progeny. But the most convincing evidence that most if not all sons were included in the wills from at latest 1450 onward, are the data themselves. As will be discussed, the numbers and distribution of surviving sons cast doubt on major underenumeration from the 1440's onward.[41]

It is far more difficult to measure numbers of daughters from the wills. Just as the data show "sufficient" numbers and distribution of sons, they show "insufficient" numbers and distribution of daughters. Assuming that there were no biological reasons for there to be up to 50 percent fewer female than male progeny, it is apparent that daughters simply were not listed in their full numbers, especially if there were brothers alive. Many females must have been dowered off or provided for in advance of the wills, and, in the less wealthy families, daughters would be most likely to be omitted should there be nothing of the estate left to divide. When they had no brothers, however, daughters came into their own. As was suggested above, they were usually mentioned more often during crisis periods than in normal times for fear of a male heir's failing to survive. Brotherless females were left land, and if they were of age, were sometimes named as executors. If daughters married and had sons, their male children would often be left considerable bequests. Therefore, there is some importance in measuring numbers of female progeny, and they have been included in the analysis in Chapter 7. The methodology used for taking female replacement ratios will be discussed as appropriate in the text.

Occasionally, the wills state that the testator has "pueros," but give neither the sex nor the precise number of progeny; at other times, testators will say only that they have "sons and daughters." In the case of "children," the minimal—and modal—figure, one son and one daugher, has been recorded. When the term "sons and daughters" is used, two sons and two daughters have been counted. Grandchildren have been recorded only when they are specifically said to have been the progeny of one of the particular children of the testator. The term *confilius* has not been interpreted as grandson. Those so designated have been included in the respective categories of male and female progeny, but their numbers proved negligible. *Nepos* and *neptis* and nece[42] were taken to mean nephew and niece, but the usual method for expressing such relations in the wills was to say son or daughter of a brother or sister. Statistically, nephews and nieces were lumped together.

It is necessary to be aware of the demographic limitations of the wills. Because of the flaws in recording of daughters, no true assessment of family size can be made, except in the case of the P.C.C. and special group wills. The age of first-marriage, a crucial factor as Hajnal has shown, can only be approximated.[43] As the wills give no clues as to births and only indirect clues as to the age of the progeny, any attempts to work with fertility factors must be severely limited. Factors of infant mortality cannot be approximated through use of the wills alone. Because there is no base population, and no accurate hypothesis of population looming on the historical horizon for fifteenth century East Anglia or England, no age-specific mortality rates or even crude mortality rates can be constructed. But what the wills do offer—accurate, long-term data when viewed proportionally—can be extremely useful in answering the questions about fifteenth century English population problems, and the demographic effects of epidemic disease.

## 1.4 The Demographic Record from the Wills

For purposes of this study, the wills were read for particular pieces of information. This information was then divided into eleven categories: testator's name, home, occupation, date of will, date of probate, season of death, spouse, male progeny, female progeny, other relatives, and bequest to high altar. For purposes of computer identification, a five-digit I.D. was affixed to each individual will.

Each of the original eleven categories was then further broken down, according to the nature of the wills themselves. Category 1, the testator's name, was broadened to include the testator's sex as well. Category 2 was divided into three basic subgroups. First, the name of the village, hamlet or town was recorded. Next came the name of the parish church. In most cases the will did not mention which parish church was dedicated. Usually, this is not a problem, since most of the villages, which constitute the bulk of places in the wills, had only a single church. When a village had two or more parish churches, such as Forncett in Norfolk, the name of the parish church was invariably listed, and there is no problem of confusion. When the testator lived in a town, such as St. Albans or Norwich, the parish church in which the testator desired burial is usually identified also. In some cases, as with the wills proved in the peculiar court of B.S.E., the parish of burial is quite frequently omitted, and only the name of the town can be recorded. But with few exceptions, there is little difficulty in identifying particular villages.

Occasionally, different villages are named by the testator as his place of residence, and his place of burial or place of birth. In this case, all villages or towns were recorded; but, for demographic purposes, the village in which the testator claimed to be living was used as the "home" residence. The final distinguishing subcategory used in category 2 was for county. For the sample under a consideration, N was used for Norfolk, S for Suffolk and H for Hertfordshire. The wills from the P.C.C. were broken down by county also, with L standing for the city of London and Southwark, and E and K for those P.C.C. wills from Essex and Kent used for comparative purposes.

Occupational data, category 3, have been divided into two main groups: those testators who listed occupations and called themselves citizens of a particular town or city, and those testators who simply listed occupations. The citizen occupations are three digital, with the first number being odd, e.g., 1--, or 3--, etc. The noncitizen occupations are also three digital, with the first number being even, as with 0--, or 2--. Clerics, for example, are 001, armigerous testators 002, and blacksmiths 052. Citizen drapers are 118, and citizen mercers 135. Nothing has been entered for the bulk of testators who listed no occupations, and it is not assumed that they were "peasants." One of the first things that becomes obvious from reading a vast number of wills is that while the testator will readily and with great pride list his occupation, nothing in the fifteenth century was "absolute." The various crafts and occupations often mixed with small scale husbandry, and many husbandmen appear to have practiced a craft, such as weaving. Surnames were seldom occupationally accurate by 1430, and John Baker may as readily have been a carpenter or smith as a baker.

Categories 4 and 5 are the date the will was made and the date of probate. Dates have been recorded in both the fifteenth and twentieth century manners. Thus, the medieval dates from 1 January to 24 March have been updated in the following notation:

dd/mm/y1/y2

For example, the date 12 February, 1468, from the will has been written:

12/02/68/69

When only *testamenta* are encountered, the date closest to probate was selected.

Category 6 is season of death. For the reasons described above it is rarely possible to determine the exact date of death or even month of death of the testator. Consequently, the elaborate system of determining season of death has been devised.

Category 7 is spouse. This has been divided into two subcategories: number of spouses, and whether or not any of these spouses were dead at the time the will was made. Categories 8 and 9 concern male and female progeny respectively. Each was then further subdivided into three more categories: total number of progeny, children of age or married, and grandchildren. Grandchildren were included in the total number of progeny, both male and female. In general, they were a rather infrequent phenomenon; and for practical purposes, the raw data for the progeny may be considered as reflecting only the testators' children. The incidence of grandchildren is important, however, because they give a clue as to the testators' ages.[44]

Category 10 is a potpourri of subcategories. Their unity is in their common reason for being—the hope that they too can help in the estimate of the testators' ages. Subcategory 1 is the ascendant generation. This includes parents of the testator alive at the time of the will, and any aunts or uncles. Subcategory 2 consists of any relation of the same generation as the testator. This would include brothers and sisters, and anyone called *consanguineus, cognatus,* 'cosyins,' or described as being the son or daughter of an aunt or uncle. As the precise meaning of all but the last of the terms listed above will always be in some question, this subcategory's accuracy is open to some doubt. Further, it is probable that cousins were the kin group most frequently omitted from the wills, especially from the will of a testator with several children

Subcategory 3 of category 10 is for descendant generation. This includes primarily nieces and nephews. Unfortunately, this subcategory was least helpful in assessing the age of the testator, as a niece or nephew could be had at virtually any age. Subcategory 5 is a further attempt at determining the testators' age. It lists all the godchildren of the testators who themselves had children. This too is a somewhat nebulous method, but it is probably fair to assume that a man or woman was not asked to stand as a godparent before adulthood.

Subcategory 4 of category 10 is an assessment of wealth, and more logically should have been included in category 11. A lack of foresight during the research stages of this study was responsible for this; however, for computer purposes it has been lumped with category 11. It lists any testator who has in his or her employ a serving person or farm laborer, as revealed by the will. Persons listed as *serviens, ancilla* or *famulus* are included in this subgroup.

The final grouping, category 11, lists the bequest to the high altar of the parish of the testator's burial. It is an attempt to discover the deceased's approximate wealth. Category 11 is especially useful because almost all testators, regardless of content in the wills, left something for this purpose. Whenever there has been an obvious discrepancy between this bequest and the rest of the will maker's wealth as indicated by the testament, the bequest has been recorded, but not used statistically. When the bequest was made in kind, it was recorded but used only when it was in grain, the price of which could be obtained, preferably from the testamentary data. Fortunately, both of these problems, and those few instances where no bequest at all was made to the high altar, accounted for under 10 percent of the totals. The bequest itself was recorded literally, in pounds, marks, shillings and pence, and then reclassified for computer purposes.

## Notes

1. C. L. Kingsford, *Promise and Prejudice in Fifteenth Century England (Oxford: Clarendon Press, 1925),* p. 21.

2. For two examples, see W. K. Jordon (1959), *Philanthropy in England, 1480– 1660* (London: George Allen and Unwin 1959); and S. L. Thrupp, *The Merchant Class of Medieval London* (Chicago: University of Chicago Press, 1948).

3. See Map 1.

4. Not all the archdeaconry courts existed for all or even most of the fifty-year period discussed. For the chronological extent of the archdeaconry court wills, see the graphs accompanying Chapter 4.

5. For a discussion of the computer methodology and the programs used, see Appendix D.

6. "A Cursory" in this instance means relying on the not always reliable Charles Creighton's, *History of Epidemics in Britain,* 3d. ed. (London: Frank Cass, 1965).

7. For a discussion of the development of the English will from the early Middle Ages, see Michael Sheehan, *The Will in Medieval England* (Toronto: Pontifical Institute of Medieval Studies, 1963).

8. *Rotuli parliamentorum ut et Petiones et Placita (Rot. Parl.)* (London, 1761–1783), IV, p. 84.

9. William Lyndwood, *Provinciale seu Constitutiones Anglie. . .* (Oxford, 1679), p. 181.

10. This is particularly the case with the archdeaconry of Suffolk wills.

11. This is especially so for the registers of the consistory court of Norwich. For the extent of the intestacy lists, see the graphs accompanying Chapter 4.

12. These observations are based on the author's own work with the wills. For additional interpretations, see A. J. Camp, *Wills and Their Whereabouts* (Canterbury: Phillimore, 1963); and E. F. Jacob, ed., *The Register of Henry Chichele,* II (Oxford: Oxford Univ. Press, 1937).

13. Jacob, *op. cit.,* pp. xix–xxi.

14. It is possible that the *testamenta* were made at some previous time of sickness from which the will makers had recovered.

15. By custom, one-third of the estate went to the church in the form of pious bequests, one-third to the spouse and one-third to the progeny. See Sheehan, *op cit.*

16. For a discussion of pious bequests as viewed from printed 15th century wills, see J. T. Rosenthal, *Purchase of Paradise* (London: Routledge and Kegan Paul, 1972).

17. The topic of landholding and inheritance patterns is extremely complex. The author's intention is simply to describe some of the more obvious aspects, as noted in the wills. For detailed information, see Michael Sheehan, "The Influence of Canon Law on the Property Rights of Married Women in England," *Medieval Studies,* XXV, 1963); Andrew Jones, "Land and People at Leighton Buzzard," *Ec. H.R.,* XXV, 1972; and J. A. Raftis, *Tenure and Mobility* (Toronto: Pontifical Institute of Medieval Studies, 1964).

18. Gwyn A. Williams, in *Medieval London: From Commune to Capital* (London: Athlone Press, 1963), takes issue with this. This will be discussed in detail, pp. 124–125.

19. F. Pollack and F. W. Maitland, *History of English Law,* 6th ed. (Cambridge: Cambridge Univ. Press, 1968), II, p. 315.

20. Jacob, *op cit.,* p. xxv.

21. For a discussion of wills in manorial courts, see A. E. Levett, *Studies in Manorial History* (Oxford: Clarendon Press, 1936), pp. 208–223. She claims that by the 1430's even unfree peasants had the right of making and leaving wills. Large groups of manorial wills survive from the archdeaconry of St. Albans, but the numbers fall off by the 1430's. The author knows of no large groupings in East Anglia for the mid- and late fifteenth century.

22. For further classification, see Jacob, *op. cit.,* pp. v-xix. No distinction has been made in the tables between peers and gentry; they are lumped together as "rural elite."

23. Camp, *op. cit.,* p. xii.

24. *Ibid.,* p. x.

25. Thomas Wright, ed., *Political Poems and Songs Relating to English History* (London: Longmans, 1859), I, p. 325.

26. See below, pp. 162–175.

27. This estimate is based on the 1377 Poll Tax returns of the Public Record Office, London (P.R.O. E. 359). A total of 2,445 taxpayers are listed for Bury; ostensibly, they were all persons of both sexes over the age of fourteen. From 1460 through 1480, there were approximately 325 males who died both testate and

intestate from Bury; all but four were clearly over twenty-five. J.C. Russell, in his *British Medieval Population* (Albuquerque: Univ. of New Mexico Press, 1948), pp. 132 and 142, projects a population of 3,668 for the town. If a decrease of 20% from 1377 to 1460 is assumed, a death rate of 40/1000, and the adult male segment of the population is calculated to be about 21%, the will population constitutes about 66% of existing adult males. When Bury testators from the archdeaconry, consistory and prerogative courts are added to the peculiar court total, it rises to about 77%. Needless to say, if the Russell figures are incorrect, if the population of Bury decreased by more or less than the projected 20%, or if the death rate is lower than 40/1000 and the segment of the adult male population was higher than 12%, the final figures would be different. This method is meant to provide only a rough estimate.

28. For a discussion of some aspects of life in Bury St. Edmunds in the later Middle Ages, see M. D. Lobel, *The Borough of Bury St. Edmunds* (Oxford: Clarendon Press, 1935).

29. Camp, *op. cit.,* p. ix.

30. Pollack and Maitland, *op. cit.,* II, p. 360.

31. *Ibid.*

32. A. J. F. Dulley, "Four Kentish Towns at the End of the Middle Ages," *Archeologica Cantiana,* LXXXI (1966), pp. 95–96.

33. For details, see Pollack and Maitland, *op. cit.,* II, pp. 356–363.

34. This estimate is based on the 1377 Poll Tax returns (P.R.O. E. 359). Norfolk had 97,817 taxpayers, and Suffolk 62,562. The will survey yielded 5,714 Norfolk testators and 6,744 Suffolk testators, about 86% male and over 98% 25 years and older. The intestacy lists add about 28% to the Norfolk totals and 24% to the Suffolk figures. If the proportions of Norfolk to Suffolk testators were the same in the fifteenth century as they had been in 1377 (and the 1524–25 tax returns cast some doubt on this), then the Norfolk totals which are minus all of the Yarmouth and Lynn peculiar court wills, virtually all of the city court of Norwich and archdeaconry court of Norwich wills, and most of the archdeaconry court of Norfolk wills, would rise to at least 10,500. Taking just the Suffolk wills and intestacy listings, the male testamentary population over twenty-five is approximately 7,141, about 4,013 of whom were recorded between 1460 and 1470. Using the same methods and figures employed in footnote 27, and adding about 25% to the Suffolk testamentary total to make up for the losses of the Suffolk will registers in the 1470's, the figures come to about 70% of Russell's 1377 figures. Again, the totals vary depending upon the mortality rates and proportion of the adult male segment of the population used, and the projected percentage decline from 1377 to 1460. And once again, it is stressed that this is just an estimate, provided for comparative purposes.

35. See below, pp. 162–175.

36. Sheehan, "Influence of Canon Law," gives extensive information on the subject of dowries and wills.

37. See below, pp. 159–164.

38. This method of classification is not as arbitrary as it may initially seem. Fifteenth century Englishmen dated their new year from 25 March, not 1 January,

and many economic historians date their years from Michaelmas. There is even a debate about precisely when the Michaelmas year should begin. See J. Z. Titow, *English Rural Society* (London: George Allen and Unwin, 1969), pp. 27–30.

39. See below, pp. 175–183.

40. Philippe Aries, *Centuries of Childhood* (New York: Vintage, 1965).

41. About 10% would be the maximum amount of underenumeration, although there is no reason nor evidence to support this view. See below, pp. 187–196.

42. These terms can designate grandchildren, and because of this possible source of confusion, little was done with *nepos, neptis,* and nece.

43. J. Hajnal, "European Marriage Patterns in Perspective," *Population in History,* edited by D. V. Glass and, D. E. C. Eversley (London: Edward Arnold, 1965), pp. 101–143.

44. See below, p. 161.

# CHAPTER II

# *The Chronology of Epidemic Disease,*
# *1430–1480*

## 2.1 Epidemic Disease from the Literary
## and Narrative Sources

It has been said that the fifteenth century was characterized by a dearth of literary and narrative sources;[1] and certainly, this was the case with the recording and discussion of epidemic disease. A search through fifteenth century chronicles, various governmental calendars, parliamentary rolls, church visitation records, bishops' registers, private correspondence, documents of state and calendars thereof, exchequer records, and even the calendars of two non-English archives has produced little more than the mere mention of the presence of epidemic disease. When an epidemic was mentioned, it was generally referred to by the almost generic names of "epidemiae pestem,"[2] "a gret pestelens,"[3] "a grete dysease,"[4] "pestilence,"[5] "morbi pestiferi"[6]—or, on occasion, merely "a gret dethe of peple."[7] Surely, the first five expressions refer to epidemic disease, and probably the last one does as well, but the nature of the diseases in question remains something of a mystery. Rarely does the investigation find something as graphic as "pestilencie plagum,"[8] and missing indeed are the touching yet revealing descriptions of fourteenth century epidemics left by Boccaccio and Galfrid Le Baker.[9]

It is possible that fifteenth century narrative writers do not describe epidemic disease as fully as do their fourteenth century predecessors because fifteenth century infectious diseases, especially plague, were not always epidemic, but also endemic. Perhaps plague was no longer the dreaded, unknown scourge of the Black Death, but rather a persistent, nagging sore, another of the recurring hazards of medieval life which annually or every two or three years cropped a small but significant segment of the population, and only in certain years in particular areas actually reached epidemic proportions. Only then would infectious diseases draw the attention of at least some of the chroniclers and poets, and hence compel them to record its presence in the community. Another factor which curtailed the actual recording of epidemic diseases was the limited space that many of the fifteenth century urban chroniclers—and it is the urban chronicles in this century which are the richest and most useful for the social and economic historian—seem to have had in their calendarlike, mayoral year format. Political events captured the imagination more than bacilli and viruses did, and the Battle of St. Albans, or even the exposure of more strumpets in the streets of London usually took precedence in their limited space over yet another epidemic.

The decade before the commencement point of this study, the 1420's, was a period of frequent epidemics, especially plague and influenza. There are reports of disease in 1420, 1423, 1426, 1427, 1428 and 1429.[10] *The Calendar of Papal Registers* is filled with complaints from parishes scattered throughout England claiming that rents had been drastically reduced, or had fallen far behind, because of epidemics and other natural disasters.[11] One letter, dated 9 April, Kal. 1430, is especially vociferous in its outcries—outcries which appear to be applicable to the entire decade before the date of the letter.[12] It is likely then, as we enter the period 1430–1480, that the English populace had been besieged in the previous decade by epidemic disease.

The decade of the 1430's offered little respite, at least in terms of epidemic frequency, if not epidemic virulence. The first reference comes from John Amundesham, the current St. Albans chronicler. Although Amundesham, perhaps prior of the Benedictine monks at Gloucester Hall, Oxford, is alleged to have written several years after the events he described took place—an allegation which may apply to many fifteenth century chroniclers[13]—his descriptions seem to speak of first-hand knowledge. In 1431, he reported pestilence in Hertfordshire:

*Pestilentia apud Codycote, et diversis locis hujis dominii, hoc anno.*[14]

An independent entry in the *Papal Registers,* admittedly the least reliable of the narrative sources in regard to chronology, corroborates the presence of pestilence, probably plague, in 1431. Dated 10 October Kal. 1431, and directed to the Bishop of Rochester, it claims that a recent petition of the master, chaplains, clerks, and choristers of the church of St. Michael Royal, London, stated that while there was a cemetery on the east side of the church, nevertheless, in 1431, due to the smell and infections of the dead bodies, the master could not sleep in the church.[15] The incidence of pestilence in Kent in 1431 is further substantiated by the obituary list of the Canterbury Cathedral Priory (C.C.P.).[16]

Between 1433 and 1440, England was beset by natural disasters, extreme weather conditions, at least two major epidemics of a national character, and two further epidemics of more local natures. Further, the mid and late 1430's are unique in the demographic history of mid-fifteenth century England for yet another reason: in the entire fifty-year period 1430–1480, it is only during the years 1434–1435, 1437, and 1438–1440 that there were food shortages on a national level which led to famine conditions. The disasters began in 1433, when a "gelu magnum et pestilentia magna" are said to have occurred.[17] The Rolls of Parliament speak of an adjournment of Commons, due to the presence of an epidemic in London:

> ... *Dominus Cancellarius ... ulterius declaravit ... quod in Civitate London' et Suburbiis ejusdem, gravis pestilentia ceperat jam oriri ...*[18]

It is difficult to generalize on such meager evidence, but it is obvious that the London area and its immediate environs, at least, were suffering from some sort of epidemic. England as a whole was suffering from other natural disasters. The years from 1433 to 1436 were a period of exceptionally cold weather. There are no less than fifteen different references to particularly inclement and freezing weather in these years. The *Chronicle of London (C.L.)* tells of a "gret frost" which began of "Seynt Kathereyns deye" (25 November), and lasted more than eleven weeks, until "Seynt Scholastyce dey" (10 February[19]), an event which is corroborated *inter alia* by William Gregory's *Chronicle*[20] and the *Great Chronicle of London (G.C.L.)*,[21] in similar but not identical words. Unusually cold weather appears to have persisted more or less until 1440, with the winters of 1434–1435 and 1435–1436 being the most severe.

With the cold came disease. *The Brut: Chronicles of England,* while mentioning the frosts, says also of 1433–1434:

> And in this same yere was a grete pestilence in London, bothe of men and women and children, and namely of worthy men, as aldermen and other worthy communiers; and also thurgh England the peple deyed sore, bothe pore and riche, which was grete hevynesse to all peple...[22]

Here then, early in 1434, is the first distinct suggestion in the period 1430–1480 of something more than a local or regional epidemic. The presence of the epidemic in the city of London is aptly echoed by the 1434 ordinances of the Privy Council of Henry VI, which mention a "pestilencie mortal '. . . in Civitate . . . London' jam existen' . . ."[23]

While the frost of the winter of 1434–1435 abated with the coming of spring and summer and then began anew in the autumn and winter of 1435–1436, the narrative sources hint at the continued presence of infectious disease throughout the entire two-year period. The *Chronicles of the Grey Friars* reported that in the year of the Duke of Bedford's death, there was a "gret pestelens, and a gret frost."[24] But the duration of the pestilence nonwithstanding, by all accounts the years 1434 to 1436 seem to have been a time of great hardship and high mortality. *Great Chronicle of London (G.C.L.)*, perhaps the best continual narrative for the period covered, sums up the situation best:

> . . . and in this yere [1434–1435] was a passing grete wynter and a colde frost. . . . It was so strong that no ship myght saile. And that yere [1436] was a passyng grete froste. And oon of the strengest that hath be seyen. For brede was frore so harde to gyder that but men wold thawe yt by the fire. . .[25]

It is not possible to state in absolute terms precisely what the epidemic or epidemics of 1434 to 1436 were, although Creighton has attempted to do so.[26] Bean seems to think the epidemic was one of plague,[27] and the testamentary mortality patterns, to be presented in Chapters 4 and 5, support this view.[28] The connection with the extremely cold weather may indicate that if the epidemic or epidemics were plague, then the pneumonic strain could have been present. Typhus is another possibility, as is smallpox. In France, in 1434:

> *mais très gran mortalitié estoit en celui temps, especialment sur petit enfants de boce ou de verole platte.*[29]

Influenza, or just plain pneumonia, brought on or aggravated by the protracted cold weather are further possibilities.

London was visited by epidemic disease once more in 1437. The reference to this outbreak comes from the St. Albans chronicler Amundesham, and the author hints at the continuing connection between cold weather and epidemic disease:

> . . . *propter epidemiae pestem, quae pro tunc regnabat in Civitate Londonarium.*[30]

Also:

> . . . *subito et ex insperato supervenit tanta sterilitas frugum, in tantunque invaluit fames ubique locorum per universum regnum* . . .[31]

But the worst was still to come. In 1438–1439, there was an epidemic of pestilence, and for one of the rare occasions in the period 1430–1480, severe and widespread famine. For one of the few times in this period— perhaps the only time—the possiblity of death brought on by famine, directly or indirectly, existed for a large proportion of the population. Vicars and rectors bemoaned their dwindling revenues.[32] William Gregory, the skinner and one-time mayor of London, stated in his chronicle that in the sixteenth year of the reign of Henry VI there:

> was great dyrthe of corne, for a buschelle of whete was worth 2/6. And that yere was grete pestylaunce, and namely in the northe contraye.[33]

The Rolls of Parliament attest to the fact that the south of England suffered as well as the north:

> . . . in this present Parlement for the Comuns of this youre noble Roialme assembled: howe that a sekeness called the Pestilence universally through this youre Roialme more comunely reyneth than hath bien usuell bifore this tyme, the whiche is an infirmite most infectis . . .[34]

And *The Brut: Chronicles of England* sums it up best, once again:

> And moche worthy people dyed in thes yere [1438] of pestilence, and other commune pepl . . . And thys yere and the year of grace . . . [1438–39] . . . on St. Clementes day [23 November] betwene iij and iiij after None ther fell such wedring of wynde and reyne . . . And in thys yere all greynes of corne were at an high price: for whete was at xxxijd, barly at xvjd, and rye at iis . . .[35]

The hardship of this period should not be underestimated. The *Chronicle of London* (C.L.) speaks of great dearth extending throughout England for 1439 also, and William Gregory tells us that the dearth lasted throughout the country into 1440.[36] Letters from the *Papal Registers* from 1438 through 1442 speak of local parishes and monasteries all across England being impoverished by famine and pestilence.[37] The decade 1431–1440 must have been a very harsh one indeed for the English people.

By comparison, and only comparatively, the next two decades and the early years of the 1460's were relatively "disease-free." There are references in the narrative sources to at least sixteen epidemics in the next twenty-two years, but all save two seem to have been relatively localized in their presence. In 1442, 1445 and 1446 the *Papal Registers* and the *Register of Edmund Lacy, Bishop of Exeter (Lacy)*, once again discuss the predicament of the parishes and monasteries devastated by pestilence, though they still may have been referring to the awful years of the 1430's.[38] More concrete in regard to 1442 are references in the Exchequer records and Chancery proceedings. The former speak of pestilence in London in 1442 and the early part of 1443, and tell of people fleeing from the city:

> . . . *par cause de pestilence qi fuist en loundres qar ils demoyent en pays.* [39]

The Chancery proceedings corroborate this story of flight, at least among those who could afford to do so, with the tale of a draper who departed with all his household "frome the said citie for this dethe."[40]

The *Paston Letters* also refer to an epidemic in 1443. On 28 September, 1443, Margaret Paston wrote from Oxnead in Norfolk to her husband John, in London, inquiring anxiously about his health, "desyring hertly to her of your welfare, thanckying God of your amendying of the grete dysesse."[41] There is no evidence that the "dysesse" from which John Paston was recovering was an epidemic disease, nor, if it were, that it extended beyond London. But in 1444, the Rolls of Parliament mention, *quod in Civitate London' et Suburbiis ejusdem, gravis pestilentia ceperat jam oriri.*[42] Certainly, London must have been an unhealthy place in which to live in the early 1440's.

The Canterbury Cathedral Priority Obituary List (C.C.P.) names several monks who died from *pesta epidemia* in 1447, and in 1448 there is a report of plague in Oxford.[43] In 1449 the Rolls of Parliament again mention an epidemic in the city of London and its immediate environs:

> . . . *Aeres corruptas et infectas evitantes et fugientes. Quaproper dictus Dominus Rex, de Aeris corruptione ac pestilentia, ad tunc in diversis Locis infra Civitatem suam London', ac etiam in Villa. Westm . . .*[44]

If this reference confirms the presence of yet another epidemic in London, perhaps bubonic plague, a notation from the same source for the following year is more mysterious. The Rolls state that Parliament once again fled from Westminster, this time to Leicester, because of *necnon insalubritatem aeris in Villa. Westm. et Locis adjacentibus.*[45] Although it cannot be stated, as Creighton has, that foul air meant plague, one cannot rule it out, as Bean has done, especially in the light of the previous year's conditions, as described by the same source.[46] There are two additional references to the presence of pestilence in 1450, in July and November. Both are from the diocese of Exeter, in southwestern England, and one claims that parishioners refused to bury the dead because of the virulence of the pestilence.[47]

The period 1449–1452 must have been a bad one in the city of London. In 1452, Parliament again found it necessary to flee from the city because of "infectious air," this time adjourning in November to meet in Reading.

Perhaps infectious air or pestilence was present throughout England on a national scale, for in February, 1453, Parliament adjourned from Reading itself: *de magna mortalite in dicta villa Redyng jam regnante.*[48] As we shall see in Chapters 4 and 5, the testamentary evidence shows a heavy, protracted period of mortality throughout East Anglia and Hertfordshire, indicative perhaps of the only national epidemic of infectious disease from 1439 to 1458.[49]

Flight from urban areas into the country during the fifteenth century was a common, if not necessarily sound, medical practice.[50] On 6 September, 1454, John Paston advised fleeing from London to more hospitable, rural climes:

> I tolde hym her is pestelens and sayd i fard the better he was in good hele, for it was noysyd that he was ded . . . Her [London] is gret pestelens. I purpose to flee in to the contre.[51]

There is one final record of epidemic disease in the 1450's. Toward the end of the decade, John Herryson, chancellor of Cambridge University, wrote about a severe pestilence, probably plague, although he did not mention the geographical distribution of the epidemic. The following are the only entries in his chronicle for the years 1458 and 1459:

> *Hoc Anno pestilencia quasi universalis per quem plures regiones.*

And,

> *Pestilencia magna et sevis.*[52]

Probably, the pestilence extended to Ely. The Infirmary Rolls from the Benedictine monastery in the town survive from the years 1458 to 1459, and indicate a high incidence of pestilence mortality.[53] More will be said about the extent of this pestilence in Chapter 4.[54]

There are no other references in the narrative sources to epidemic disease from 1454 to 1462. In the third year of the 1460's, however, the grim combination of cold, inclement weather and epidemics reappeared, indicative perhaps of pneumonic plague, which with its accompanying high levels of mortality would jolt the chroniclers used to the milder effects of endemic bubonic plague and draw their attention away from the Wars of the Roses. In November, 1462,* there is an isolated report of

---

*There is some doubt as to this date. Writing many years later, Fabyan seems to have been referring to 1462, but Creighton dates it as 1463, and that is when Edward IV was on campaign. The year 1462 will be used in the text, but there must be some question as to the veracity of Fabyan's chronology.

Edward IV coming down with a case of "the sykeness of pockys," while on expedition against the Scots and Lancastrians.[55] Nothing more is said about the "pox," nor are there any other references to its presence in any part of England. As we shall see in Chapters 4 and 5, however, mortality as measured by the testamentary evidence was very severe.[56]

In 1463, John Warkworth wrote in his chronicle of a freezing cold winter, and subsequent conditions ominously similar to those of the 1430's:

> . . . the thyrde yere of the reynge of Kynge Edwarde . . . [1463] . . . ther was ane fervent froste thrugh Englonde, and snowe, that menne myght goo overe the yise, and a fervant colde . . .[57]

This was followed in 1464 by what appears to have been a national epidemic of plague. According to the anonymous author of *A Short English Chronicle*, there was first a great drought which "dured from mydness of Marche tyll the morn after Mydsomer day that never reyned."[58] This was followed, later in the year by "a grete pestilence through the realme."[59] Confirmation is supplied by a document from the Sforza archives in Milan. Writing on 5 October, 1464, from Bruges, a Venetian merchant who had to leave London on 26 September reported plague in the city at a rate which he assessed at 200 deaths *per diem*, no doubt something of an exaggeration.[60]

This combination of bad weather and epidemic disease continued into 1465. *A Short English Chronicle* speaks of another "grete frost and grete snow" for the fourth year of the reign of Edward IV, of a winter so cold that "where thorowe mych catell and bestis and shepe for fawte of mete were destroyed."[61] The epidemic may have lingered on through the late summer. Another Paston *Letter*, dated 18 August, 1465, reads as follows:

> Item my cosyn Elisabeth Clere ys at Ormesby and your moder purposyth to be at her place at Caster thys wyke, for the pestylens ys so fervent in Norwych that thay ther [dare] no longer abyde there.[62]

In 1467 another epidemic swept through parts of England, and was possibly national in its scope. If the Rolls of Parliament are to be believed, it was unquestionably an epidemic of plague:

> *Dominus Cancellarius . . . declaravit . . . necton pestilentie plagum regnare incipientum, qualiter quosdem de Domo Communitatis plaga ille infectos . . .*[63]

In the same year, Herryson reported that *hoc anno venit magna pestilencia in Anglia*,[64] and *Ingulph's Chronicle of the Abbey of Croyland* mentioned an infection covering the whole of England, making the familiar connection between cold weather and epidemic disease.[65] And correspondence dated 5 Kal. November, 1468, from the *Papal Registers,* possibly looking back on the previous year, makes the perpetual complaint of further impoverishment due to decimation by pestilence.[66]

There is an interesting passage in one of the chronicles for the year 1462, which in a way prophesies the forbidding years to come. According to the chronicle, in that year, a boy, while walking in a lane near Clare College, Cambridge, met an old man *cum prolixa barba,* who warned:

> *Vade jam et dic cuicumque quod infra istos duos annos erit tanta pestilencia et famis ac interfectio hominum quanta nullus vivens videt perantea.*[67]

Worse was indeed yet to come. Like the 1430's, the 1470's were a disease-ridden decade. There were at least three virulent epidemics on a national scale, two probably of plague, and the other almost certainly of dysentery. Judging from the testamentary data, mortality from each of these epidemics was greater than at any time since 1439. Further, there is literary and testamentary evidence indicating the possibility of two further national epidemics in the decade, and if Tickell's *The History of the Town and County of Kingston-upon-Hull* is to be believed, there may have been but a single epidemic-free year in the entire decennial period 1471–1480.[68]

The reintroduction of epidemic disease into England on a massive scale in the 1470's was summed up nicely, if not necessarily chronologically, by *The Brut.* The author has just finished describing Edward IV's expedition into France in 1475:

> And in that Iorney our Kynge lost many a man that fylle to the lust of women and wer brent by them: and there membrys rottyd away and they dyed. And after that ther fylle a gret dissese in Engelond callyd the "styche" and moche peeple dyede sodeynly therof. And also another dissese reyned aftyr that called the "fflyx" that neuer was seen in Engelond before; and peple deyde hogely therof iij yer togedyr in on place or other. And aftyr that ther bred a Raven on Charyng Crosse at Londen; and neuer was seen noone brede there before. And aftyr that cam a gret dethe of Pestilence that lastyed iij yer; and peple dyed myhtely in euery place, man, woman, and chylde on whois soulys God haue mercy! Amen![69]

The French Pox, as the disease caused by the "lust of women" is called in the marginal headings of *The Brut,* can probably be dated at 1475.[70] Its epidemic nature, if the French Pox were truly epidemic at all, seems to have been highly restricted, and the testamentary evidence, even for the Prerogative Court of Canterbury (P.C.C.), does not indicate a great upsurge in mortality.[71] It does not appear from the other narrative sources or the testamentary data that either a stitch or a flux appeared between 1475 and 1480. Possibly *The Brut* chronicler was merely listing in sum the epidemics of the disease-ridden 1470's. The flux can almost certainly be redated with the aid of other sources to 1473.[72] *The Brut* is probably correct in saying that the flux was not familiar to the people of the 1470's. With the exception of one solitary reference to *fluxu dissentirico* in 1475, the last recorded outbreak was that reported by Thomas Walsingham in 1411, and also revolved around an expedition to France.[73] By the seventh decade of the fifteenth century, only a few very old men or women would have remembered that far back. The stitch was probably the epidemic of 1471, though evidence to be presented below indicates that this epidemic was one of plague. Another possible explanation of stitch is pleurisy, with the stitch referring to the associated severe pains in the side. As for the pestilence, this is almost certainly the great epidemic of plague of 1479.

The epidemics of the 1470's are more carefully dated in other narrative sources. As mentioned above, what appears to be an outbreak of epidemic disease on a national scale flared up first in 1471. At Southwell Minster, a college for secular clerics in Nottinghamshire, the church visitation records tell of the priests fleeing the college for a period of one month because of a *morbi pestiferi*.[74] More ominous is another of the Paston letters:

> Item I praye yow sende me worde iff any off owr frendys or welwyllers be dede, for I fear that ther is grete dethe in Norwyche, and in other Borowgh townese in Norfolk, ffor I ensur you it is the most unyversall dethe that evyr I wist in Ingelonde: for by my trowthe I kan not her by the pylgrymes that passe the contre nor noon other man that rydethe or goethe in any contre that any Borow town in Ingelonde is ffree ffrom that sykeness . . .[75]

In 1473 there was another epidemic of national proportions. Bean was quite certain that this was dysentery, which does seem to be the case, judging from Warkworth's vivid description:

> . . . ther was a gret hote somere bothe for manne and beste; by whiche ther was a gret dethe of menne and women, that in feld in harvist tyme men fylle downe sodanly and unyversalle feveres, axes [probably agues], and the blody flyx, in dyverse place of Englonde.[76]

As we shall see, Forestier's contemporary medical treatise defines the "blody flyx," or flux, as intestinal dysentery.[77] The *Paston Letters* also discuss the epidemic of 1473. In 1472, there were many references to crop failures, and in 1473 there are references appropriately enough not to pestilence, but to "dysese."[78] Further, the independent testamentary evidence bears out the incidence of excessive mortality.[79]

In 1474, there is a reference to plague in Bangor diocese;[80] and in 1475, *The Brut* mentions the French Pox, and Worcestre mentions the flux. Leaving aside Tickell's generally uncorroborated views,[81] and testamentary evidence indicating heavy mortality in 1477,[82] the next major epidemic according to the narrative sources came in 1479. This was the fifteenth century's most severe outbreak of epidemic disease. It was almost certainly plague, and not even the stately *G.C.L.*, which failed to name another incidence of epidemic disease in the entire period 1430 to 1480, omits a reference to it.

Most of the accounts of the 1479 pestilence are depressingly similar, and speak well enough for themselves:

> And this yere was grete deth of people: wherefore the kynges courts were not kepte at Westm' frome Easter to Midsomer, nor in the Guyldhall from Easter to Midsomer.[83]

> Thys yere [mayoral year] the ducke of Clarans was put to dethe. And the term defferd from Ester to Myhylmus be cause of the grete pestelens.[84]

> In Thys mayers [Richard Gardyner] tyme was an huge mortalyte and deth of people, The which aloonly contynuyd not wy'n the Cyte, But alsoo In many other partyes of this Realm, To the grete mynsysshyng of the people of all maner and agys.[85]

> Thys yere was a gret mortalytie and dethe in London and many other partyes of this realme, the whiche beganne in the latter ende of Senii (September) in the presedynge yere [mayoral year] and contynued in this yere tylle the begynnynge of Novembre, in whiche the passetyme dyed innumerable people in sayd citie and many places ellys where.[86]

At Southwell Minster, the priests were again granted a leave of absence, this time not for a single month, but for the entire summer:

> . . . *quod dira pestilentialis strages in villa Suthwell verismiliter continuare estimature: quod que ipse venerabiles viri cum eorum familiaribus infectionem dictae pestiferae stragis timent gravissime incurrere, justo metu ipsuis futuri morbi dispensaverunt et eorum alter dispensavit . . .*[87]

The epidemic of 1479 seemed to have been quite familiar to the clerics of Southwell Minster. The *Paston Letters* contain several references to the disease also. A letter dated 21 August, from Edmund (II) to John(II) tells of the death in Norwich from disease of three members of the Paston clan.[88] On 29 August, when the pestilence must have been at its most virulent, John (II) wrote to Margaret a letter containing one of the most interesting comments in regard to epidemic disease to be found in the entire period 1430–1480:

Please it yow to weet, that I have been heer at London a iiii nyght whereoff the ffyrst 4 dayes I was in suche feer off the syknesse and also ffownde my chambr and stuffe nott so clene as I demyd, which troblyed me soor . . .[89]

One important, independent mortality record does exist for at least parts of the fifteenth century. This is the obituary list of the monks of the Canterbury Cathedral Priory.[90] It cannot be used as a definitive record of mortality, as Creighton tried to do.[91] The cause of death of the monks is not always given, and the dating is not always clear. Some monks, said to have died in one part of the record, are listed in another part as alive or as having died at another time, often several year later.[92] The years of death are sometimes not given even when the cause of death is, but rather referred to only obliquely as the "same as above." Further, for the period 1430–1480, the obituary list is useful only from 1430 to 1447.

Nevertheless, with all these reservations considered, the C.C.P. obituary list is a useful, independent source, and conceivably one for which an age specific mortality record could be constructed for a wealthy, relatively closed society. For purposes of this study, it provides another record of the presence of epidemic disease within the community. Three monks are said to have died in the late summer 1431 as the result of *pestilentia*. One of these monks, a certain John Bernard, was buried quickly, so that the spread of pestilence might be averted.[93] Two other monks in 1435 and one other monk in 1437 died from *epidemia*. Nothing further is said in the obituary list about the nature of the mysterious *epidemia*, although once again the monks were buried hastily to help prevent the spread of the disease.[94] Additionally, two more monks may have died from the *epidemia* in 1435, as their names follow hard upon the other *epidemia* stricken monks. On the basis of such scanty evidence, it is not possible to state specifically what *epidemia* was, but Bean's assertion that it could not possibly have been plague because plague was referred to in the C.C.P. list only as *pestilentia* is equally unacceptable. To the contrary, in his medical treatise, the physician John La Barba uses the terms pestilentia and epidemia—in this case, as in so many others, almost certainly plague—interchangeably.[95] The final reference to epidemic disease in the Canterbury Cathedral Priory Obituary list comes in 1447, when one John Cranbrooke is said to have perished as the result of *peste epidemia*, probably plague.[96]

## 2.2 A Table of Chronology*

The occurrence of epidemic disease, and the more sensational climatic events which may have affected the frequency of epidemic disease in the period 1430–1480, may be tabulated as follows:

1420's background—1420, 1423, 1426, 1427, 1428, 1429.

| | | | |
|---|---|---|---|
| 1431 | pestilence | Hertfordshire | Amundesham |
| | pestilence | Kent | *Papal Letters* |
| | pestilence | Canterbury | C.C.P. |
| 1433 | pestilence | national | 3 15 |
| | pestilence | London | *Rot. Parl.* |
| | pestilence | London | *The Brut* |
| | pestilence | London | Arnold |
| 1434 | pestilence | national? | *The Brut* |
| | pestilence | national? | Herryson |
| | pestilence | London | *Privy Proc.* |
| | weather (cold) | | *Ingulph's* |
| | weather (cold) | | *C.L.* |
| | weather (cold) | | *The Brut* |
| | weather (cold) | | Gregory |
| | weather (cold) | | 3 15 |
| | weather (cold) | | *G.C.L.* |
| 1435 | pestilence | national | *The Brut* |
| | epidemia | Canterbury | C. C. P. |
| | weather (cold) | | *The Brut* |
| | weather (cold) | | *C.L.* |
| | weather (cold) | | *G.C.L.* |
| | weather (cold) | | 3 15 |
| | weather (cold) | | Gregory |
| | weather (cold) | | Fabyan |
| 1436 | weather (cold) | | *The Brut* |
| | weather (cold) | | *G.C.L.* |
| 1437 | pestilence | London | Amundesham |
| | epidemia | Canterbury | C.C.P. |
| | weather (cold) | | *The Brut* |

| | | | |
|---|---|---|---|
| 1438 | pestilence | national | *The Brut* |
| | pestilence | national | Gregory |
| | pestilence | national | *Papal Registers* |
| | weather (cold, rain) | | *The Brut* |
| | weather (cold, rain) | | Gregory |
| 1439 | pestilence | national | *The Brut* |
| | pestilence | national | *Rot. Parl.* |
| | pestilence | Devon | *Lacy* |
| | weather (wet) | | *Ingulph's* |
| | weather (wet) | | *C.L.* |
| | weather (wet) | | *The Brut* |
| | weather (wet) | | Gregory |
| 1440 | weather (wet | | *The Brut* |
| | weather (wet) | | *C.L.* |
| 1442 | pestilence | London | P.R.O. Exchequer |
| | pestilence | London | P.R.O. Chancery |
| | pestilence | Lancashire | *Papal Registers* |
| 1443 | disease | Norfolk | *Paston Letters* |
| | pestilence | London | Exchequer |
| | pestilence | London | Chancery |
| 1444 | pestilence | London | *Rot. Parl.* |
| 1445 | pestilence | Wales | *Papal Registers* |
| 1446 | pestilence | Devon | *Lacy* |
| 1447 | pestilence | Canterbury | C.C.P. |
| | weather (floods) | | 3  15 |
| 1448 | pestilence | Oxford | Wood[97] |
| | weather (wet) | | *The Brut* |
| | weather (wet) | | *C.L.* |
| 1449 | pestilence | London | *Rot. Parl.* |
| 1450 | pestilence | Devon | *Lacy* |
| | unhealthy air | London | *Rot. Parl.* |
| 1452 | great death | London, Reading | *Rot. Parl.*[98] |
| 1454 | pestilence | London | *Paston Letters* |

| 1458 | pestilence | Ely | Herryson |
|---|---|---|---|
| 1459 | pestilence | Ely | Herryson |
| 1462 | pox | north country | Fabyan† |
| 1463 | pestilence | national | 3  15 |
|  | weather (cold) |  | 3  15 |
|  | weather (cold) |  | Warkworth |
| 1464 | pestilence | national | 3  15 |
|  | pestilence | London | *Calendar . . . Milan* |
|  | weather (cold) |  | 3  15 |
| 1465 | pestilence | Norfolk | *Paston Letters* |
| 1466 | infection | London | *Rot. Parl.*[99] |
| 1467 | pestilence | national | *Ingulph's* |
|  | pestilence | national | Herryson |
|  | pestilence | London | *Rot. Parl.* |
|  | weather (wet) |  | *Ingulph's* |
| 1468 | pestilence | Coventry | *Papal Registers* |
| 1471 | pestilence | Southwell | *Visitations* |
|  | great death | national | *Paston Letters* |
|  | stitch | national | *The Brut* |
| 1473 | flux, axes | national | Warkworth |
|  | flux | national | *The Brut* |
|  | sickness | national | *Paston Letters* |
|  | weather (heat) |  | Warkworth |
| 1474 | pestilence | Bangor | *Papal Registers* |
| 1475 | French Pox | soldiers | *The Brut* |
|  | dysentery (flux) | London | William of Worcestre |
| 1479-1480 |  |  |  |
|  | pestilence | national | *Visitations* |
|  | pestilence | national | *Grey Friars* |
|  | pestilence | national | Arnold |
|  | pestilence | national | *The Brut* |
|  | pestilence | Norwich | William of Worcestre |
|  | pestilence | national? | medical remidies[100] |

| | | |
|---|---|---|
| great mortality | national | G.C.L. |
| great mortality | national | Fabyan |
| great death | national | *C.L.* |
| great death | national | Kingsford[101] |
| sickness | London | *Paston Letters* |

*Elements in the table appear in the following order: type of epidemic or nature of climatic abberation; location of event; source in which it was reported.

†Possibly autumn, 1463

We may conclude that there were at least seven, probably ten, and perhaps even eleven outbreaks of epidemic disease on a national scale in the fifty-year period 1430–1480. The seven "certain" national epidemics occurred in 1433–1435, 1438–1439, 1463–1464 or perhaps 1465, 1467, 1471, 1473, and 1479–1480. The "probable" national epidemics were the pestilences of 1452–1453 and 1458–1459 and the pox of 1462, and the "perhaps" was the French Pox of 1475. It has been argued elsewhere that the epidemic of 1473, called the "bloody flyx" by Warkworth and others, was intestinal dysentery, and that is how it was identified by Forestier in his medical treatise of the late fifteenth century.[102] It is not possible to identify definitively what the other six certain national epidemics were, but it is most likely, based on the descriptions of the narrative sources and testamentary evidence to be presented in Chapters 4 and 5,[103] that they were plague. The epidemics of 1463–1465 and 1467 were almost certainly bubonic plague. Initiating and terminal dates are given in the chronicles and letters for the epidemic of 1463–1465 which restrict the periods of extreme virulence to the late summer and early autumn, and the epidemic of 1467 is actually called a pestilence of plague.[104] Further, the mortality patterns established from the testamentary data follow the plague pattern.[105]

Despite the reference to the name "styche," used by *The Brut*, the epidemic of 1471 was also probably bubonic plague. The dates given in the visitation records of the Southwell Minster restrict the epidemic to the summer and autumn, and the testamentary mortality patterns are of the plague type.[106] The great epidemic of 1479–1480, the most virulent of the fifteenth century, also seems to have been plague, but perhaps pneumonic plague in some regions, as well as bubonic. In London, it was said to have persisted only from September through October, but other narrative sources say it began in the spring, and the testamentary evidence indicates that in East Anglia, at least, it may have persisted through the winter, into 1480.[107] Further, William of Worcestre's stepson died in January, 1480, apparently only two days after contracting the pestilence, a characteristic sign of pneumonic plague.[108] The wills for the winter 1479–1480 show that mortality was much higher than usual, and there is little evidence of severe conditions or famine being the cause of the heavy death toll.

It is probable that the national epidemics of 1433–1435 and 1439 were of plague, bott bubonic and pneumonic. Both persisted through at least one winter; and if the ambiguous *The Brut* is to be believed, the epidemic of 1433–1435 lasted through no less than three winters. Despite the deficiencies of will registration in all ecclesiastical courts, save perhaps the P.C.C., for the decade 1430–1440, there is still considerable testamentary evidence for high "plague-type" mortality—that is, late summer, early autumn for bubonic plague, and winter for pneumonic plague.[109] Although the role of famine must be stressed for the 1430's, the fact that there is such overwhelming literary evidence of the unusually cold winters in this decade tends to support the idea that pneumonic plague was present within the community. The 1458–1459 pestilence epidemic was also probably bubonic plague, although there is some doubt as to whether pneumonic strains were present.

It is more difficult to determine the nature and scope of the epidemics of 1452–1453 and 1462. For 1452, the Rolls of Parliament speak only of a great death, and apparently are the only source to yield even that. However, this "great" mortality was said to have taken its toll in both London and Reading, and the testamentary evidence in East Anglia, especially from the archdeaconry courts, shows protracted and extensive mortality in the fall and winter, 1452–1453. The case of the pox of 1462 is almost identical to that of the epidemic of 1452–1453. There is but a single, fleeting reference to its presence in the narrative sources, a reference even more nebulous than that for the 1452–1453 epidemic. But the mortality evidence from the testamentary data shows a dramatic and pronounced rise in deaths in the spring, 1462, a pattern which is almost certainly the result of a nonplague epidemic. Both of these epidemics, and a significant rise in testamentary mortality in 1477–1478, uncorroborated by any of the narrative sources, will also be discussed in Chapters 4 and 5.[110]

As is the case with the poorly documented "national" epidemics of 1452–1453 and 1462, the thirteen or so local epidemics in the period 1430–1480 are more difficult to deal with than the seven major national epidemics. One, that of 1475, is specifically referred to as the French Pox, and must have been a cutaneous manifesting disease, such as yaws or smallpox, if not syphilis or gonorrhea. *The Brut's* reference to lust with women and the particular affliction of the privy "member" would seem to favor one of the last two diseases. The only other reference to a pox in the period is the already mentioned contraction of the "pockys" by Edward IV in 1462. Edward has received a well-deserved reputation as a womanizer, and was certainly a prime candidate for any venereally contracted disease.[111] Unfortunately, the reference from Fabyan is too vague to be of any more aid in deciphering the nature of Edward's ailment.

At least five of the remaining thirteen epidemics, those of 1437, 1442, 1444, 1449–1450 and 1454, seem to have been restricted mostly or entirely to the city of London and its immediate environs, although there are independent references to pestilence in Lancashire in 1442, and Devon in 1450. One can guess from the descriptions, and do no more, that they were all epidemics of bubonic plague. The Norfolk pestilence of 1465 may actually have been part of the larger national epidemic of 1463–1464. The "local" epidemic of 1431 seems to have been quite widespread throughout Kent and Hertfordshire, but there are no surviving references to its presence in London. A period of extensive mortality from the testamentary evidence is not indicated for 1431 either, but this may be due to faulty will registration in East Anglia and Hertfordshire. The wills are not a reliable demographic source until the 1440's.[112]

The other local epidemics, those in Lancashire in 1442, Norfolk in 1443, 1445 in the west country and Wales, 1446 in Exeter, 1447 in Canterbury, 1448 in Oxford, 1468 in Coventry, and 1474 in Bangor diocese,[113] all seem to have been quite restricted in their scope. One thing that is apparent, however, is that epidemic disease was by no means limited solely to urban areas, as has so often been dogmatically stated;[114] and this is so despite the fact that it is the nature of many of the narrative sources, the best of which are the so-called urban chronicles,[115] to restrict mention of epidemics to their local areas. All urban areas in fifteenth century England were very small in any case, and the testamentary evidence indicates that epidemic diseases, especially plague, were as much a phenomenon of the countryside as they were of the country town. For a more detailed analysis of this we must turn to the contemporary medical reaction and response to epidemic diseases in the fifteenth century, and to a study of its geographical distribution.

# Notes

1. G. R. Elton, *England, 1200–1640* (Ithaca, N.Y.: Cornell University Press, 1969), pp. 16–17; C. L. Kingsford, *English Historical Literature in the Fifteenth Century* (Oxford: Clarendon Press, 1913), pp. 1–11.

2. John Amundesham, *Annales Monasterii S. Albani*, edited by H. T. Riley, 2 vols. (London: Longmans, 1870–1871), p. 27.

3. *Chronicles of the Grey Friars of London,* edited by J. G. Nichols (London: Longmans, 1827), p. 16.

4. *Paston Letters,* edited by James Gairdner, vols. I–III (London: Chatto and Windus, 1904), I, p. 48.

5. *Proceedings and Ordinances of the Privy Council of England (Privy Proc.),* edited by N. Harris Nicholas (London: Eyre and Spottiswoode, 1835), IV, pp. 282–283.

6. *Visitations and Memorials of Southwell Minster,* edited by A. F. Leach (Westminster: Camden Society, 1891), n.s. XLVIII, p. 11.

7. *Chronicle of London, 1089–1483,* edited by N. H. Nicolas (London: Longmans, 1827), p. 146.

8. *Rot. Parl.,* V, pp. 618–19.

9. Giovanni Boccaccio, *The Decameron,* trans. by Frances Winwar (New York: Modern Library, 1955); E. M. Thompson, ed., *Chronicon Galfridi Le Baker de Swynebroke* (Oxford: Clarendon Press, 1889).

10. References to and discussions of the epidemics of the 1420's can be found in *Calendar of Papal Registers,* edited by J. A. Tremlow (London: H. M. Stationery Office, 1906–1955), III, pp. 458, 522, 525; *Privy Proc.,* III, pp. 261–263; Charles Creighton, *History of Epidemics in Britain* (London: Frank Cass, 1965), I, 3rd ed.; and J. M. W. Bean, "Plague, Population and Economic Decline in England in the Later Middle Ages," *Ec.H.R.* 2nd series, XV, 1962–1963.

11. *Papal Registers,* as cited above, footnote 10.

12. *Ibid.,* VIII, pp. 158–159.

13. Amundesham, *op. cit.,* II, p. ix.

14. *Ibid.,* I, p. 62. "Pestilence toward Codicote, and diverse places of this territory, in this year."

15. *Papal Registers,* VIII, p. 341.

16. *Canterbury Cathedral Priority Obituary List,* Ms.d 12F., f. 23.

17. *Three Fifteenth Century Chronicles,* edited by James Gairdner (Westminster: Camden Society, 1880), n.s. XXVIII, p. 149. See also John Herryson, *Abbreviata Chronica ab Anno 1377 Usque ad Annum 1469,* Caius College, Cambridge, Ms., edited by J. J. Smith (Cambridge Antiquarian Society: Publications, 1840); Richard Arnold, *Customs of the City of London* (London: F. C. and J. Rivington, 1811). Herryson refers to a "magnum gelu et pestilencia" in his calendar format for 1433, and Arnold mentions a "grete pestilence" and a great frost in the mayoral year of John Brokle (1433–1434).

18. *Rot. Parl.,* IV, p. 420. "The Lord Chancellor . . . further declared . . . that in the city of London and in the suburbs of the same, a grievous pestilence already had begun to arrive."

19. *Chronicle of London,* p. 120.

20. William Gregory, *Chronicle,* in *Historical Collections of a Citizen of London in the Fifteenth Century,* edited by James Gairdner (London: Camden Society, 1876), n.s. XVII, p. 178.

21. *Great Chronicle of London,* edited by A. H. Thomas (London: G. W. Jones, 1938), p. 171.

22. *The Brut: Chronicles of England,* edited by F.W.D. Brie (London: Oxford Univ. Press, 1960), II, p. 467.

23. *Privy Proc.*, IV, pp. 282–283.

24. *Grey Friars*, p. 16.

25. *Great Chronicle of London*, p. 173.

26. Creighton, *op. cit.*, I, pp. 227–238.

27. Bean, *op. cit.*, pp. 428–429.

28. See below, p. 96, and 146–148.

29. *Journal D' Un Bourgeois De Paris sous Charles VI et Charles VII*, edited by André Mary (Paris: Henri Jonquières, 1929), p. 265, ". . . but very many people were dying, especially small children, from the plague or smallpox."

30. Amundesham, *op. cit.*, II, p. 127, ". . . on account of the pestilence of an epidemic which then was reigning in the city of London."

31. *Ibid.*, p. 157, ". . . suddenly and unexpectedly there came over a great barrenness; and in as great a measure, hunger prevailed all over the whole realm."

32. *Register of Edmund Lacy, Bishop of Exeter, 1420–55*, 5 vols., edited by G. R. Dunstan (Torquay: Canterbury and York Society and Devon and Cornwall Society Publications, 1967), III, p. 316.

33. Gregory, *op. cit.*, p. 181.

34. *Rot. Parl.*, V, p. 31b.

35. *The Brut*, II, pp. 473–474.

36. Gregory, *op. cit.*, p. 124.

37. *Papal Registers*, VIII, pp. 242, 633; IX, p. 268.

38. *Ibid.*, IX, pp. 268, 486; Lacy, *op. cit.*, p. 259.

39. P.R.O.E. 101/128/31, as cited by S. L. Thrupp, *The Merchant Class of Medieval London* (Univ. of Chicago Press, 1948), pp. 226–272.

40. *Ibid.* Also see S. L. Thrupp, "Aliens in and Around London in the Fifteenth Century," in A. E. J. Hollaender, ed., *Studies in London History* (London: Hodder and Stoughton, 1969), p. 259.

41. *Paston Letters*, I, p. 48.

42. *Rot. Parl.*, V., p. 67b.

43. *Canterbury Cathedral Priority*, f. 25; Creighton, *op. cit.*, I, p. 228. Creighton took the latter reference from Anthony Wood, although he did not specify which particular work.

44. *Rot. Parl.*, V, p. 143b, ". . . avoiding and fleeing the corrupted and infected air. On account of which the said Lord King [was called?] from the corruption of the air and the pestilence at that time in different places within his own city of London and even in the town of Westminster."

45. *Ibid.*, p. 172b.

46. Creighton, *op. cit.*, I, pp. 229–230; Bean, *op. cit.*, p. 427.

47. *Lacy, op. cit.*, III, p. 273; III, p. 9.

48. Creighton, *op. cit.*, I, pp. 229–230. This epidemic is not discussed by Bean, *op. cit.*, and the author did not find the reference in the *Rotuli parliamentorum*. It reads, "from . . . the great mortality already reigning in the town called Reading."

49. See below, pp. 97–98, and 126–138.

50. See below, pp. 138–142.

51. *Paston Letters*, I, pp. 302–303.

52. *Abbreviata Chronica*. The entry reads, "In this year was a virtually universal

pestilence throughout a great many regions," and "Great and serious pestilence." The original chronicle is in Caius College, Cambridge. The printed edition, edited by J. J. Smith, was not available to the author. Therefore, years rather than page numbers will be cited, when appropriate.

53. John Herryson, "Appendix X: Infirmarer's Roll," in T. D. Atkinson, *An Architectural History of the Benedictine Monastery of St. Etheldreda at Ely* (Cambridge: Cambridge Univ. Press, 1933).

54. See below, p. 98.

55. Robert Fabyan, *New Chronicles of England and France,* edited by H. Ellis (London: F.C. and J. Rivington, 1811), p. 653. The chronologically questionable quotation reads as follows: "When the kynge was aware of the queens [Margaret, wife of the deposed Henry VI] thus avodynge he entered to haue folowed, and to have made warre upon the Scottys, but he was then vysited with the sykenesse of pockys, that he was forced to leve that iournaye."

56. See below pp. 99–100, and 148–149.

57. John Warkworth, *A Chronicle of the First Thirteen Years of the Reign of King Edward the Fourth,* edited by J. O. Halliwell (London: Camden Society, 1839), X, p. 3.

58. *Three Fifteenth Century Chronicles,* p. 80.

59. *Ibid.*

60. *Calendar of State Papers Relating to Milan,* edited by A. B. Hinds (London: H.M. Stationery Office, 1912), I, p. 113; *Calendar of State Papers and Manuscripts Relating to English Affairs: Venice,* edited by Rawdon Brown (London: H. M. Stationery Office, 1864), I, p. 114.

61. *Three Fifteenth Century Chronicles,* p. 80.

62. *Paston Letters,* II, p. 226.

63. *Rot. Parl.,* V, pp. 618–619, "The Lord Chancellor declared that death was reigning from a pestilence of incipient plagues, just as the same men of the House of Commons had been infected by that plague."

64. *Abbreviata Chronica,* the year 1467.

65. *Ingulph's Chronicle of the Abbey of Croyland,* edited by H.T. Riley (London: H.G. Bohn, 1854), p. 443.

66. *Papal Registers,* XII, p. 644.

67. *Three Fifteenth Century Chronicles,* p. 163, "Go now and tell anyone the fact that within those two years there will be such pestilence and famine and killing of men, as no one living has been before."

68. J. Tickell, *The History of the Town and County of Kingston-upon-Hull* (Hull: 1798), p. 132. See the excellent discussion of the validity of Tickell's work in Bean, *op. cit.,* pp. 436–37.

69. *The Brut,* II, p. 604.

70. For the chronology of Edward's expedition to France, see E. F. Jacob, *The Fifteenth Century* (Oxford: Oxford University Press, 1961), pp. 572–579.

71. For the evidence of the wills from the Prerogative Court of Canterbury (P.C.C.), see below, pp. 108–110. For a discussion of soldiers enrolling their wills in the P.C.C. before an overseas campaign, see E. F. Jacob, ed., *The Register of Henry Chichele* (Oxford: Oxford University Press, 1937), II, p. xviii.

72. Warkworth, *op. cit.,* p. 23.

73. There is one reference, on page 255, in William of Worcestre, *Itinerum,* edited by John Harvey (Oxford: Clarendon Press, 1969). The other reference is Thomas Walsingham, *Chronica Monasterii S. Albani,* edited by H. T. Riley (London: Longmans, 1867–1869), II, p. 285.

74. *Visitations,* p. 11. The passage reads as follows: ". . . residentianes certas causas legitimas et necessarias, gracia speciali voluerunt quod quilibert Canonicus Residentiarius per unam mensem . . ." (". . . the residents with respect to certain legitimate and necessary causes, that is, on account of the fear of the pestilence-bearing disease, each and every resident canon was willed by special grace and sent away for one month.")

75. *Paston Letters,* III. pp. 14–15.

76. Warkworth, *op. cit.,* p. 23.

77. Thomas Forestier, *Tractus contra pestilentiam, thenasmonem et dissenterium* (Rouen: 1490), chapter 8. For a discussion of the treatise, see below, pp. 68–69.

78. *Paston Letters,* III, pp. 48–49; III, pp. 99–101.

79. See below, pp. 101–102.

80. *Papal Registers,* XIII, p. 279.

81. See above, footnote 68.

82. See below, pp. 102–103.

83. *Chronicle of London,* p. 146.

84. *Grey Friars,* p. 22. See below, pp. 95–96, for a discussion of the dates of this reference, and that of Richard Arnold *(op. cit.).*

85. *Great Chronicle of London,* p. 226. The marginal notes refer to a "pestis."

86. Fabyan, *op. cit.,* p. 666.

87. *Visitations,* p. 40. ". . . because the dire pestilential slaughter in the town of Southwell which was thought likely to continue and because the venerable men themselves with their relatives fear grievously to incur the infection of the so-called pest-bearing slaughter, by the justified fear for themselves of the future disease, they have collectively made arrangements for each of them to privately leave."

88. *Paston Letters,* III, pp. 251–252.

89. *Ibid.,* p. 254.

90. *Canterbury Obituary List,* f. 15 seq.

91. Creighton, *op. cit.,* I, p. 226.

92. *Canterbury Obituary List,* f. 15 seq. Particular attention should be given to the case of J. Cranbrooke, monk, listed as having died in 1437, and again in 1447.

93. *Ibid.*

94. *Ibid.*

95. Bean, *op. cit.,* p. 433n; John La Barba, British Museum Sloane Ms. 3449, f. 5b. Also, see below, pp. 63–65.

96. *Canterbury Obituary List,* f. 25.

97. See above, footnote 43.

98. See above, footnote 48.

99. Creighton, *op. cit.,* I, p. 230. As Bean *(op. cit.,* p. 427) has commented, there is no record of this in Creighton's alleged source, the *Rotuli parliamentorum.*

100. See below, p. 74.

101. Kingsford *op. cit.*

102. Forestier, *op. cit.*, Chap. 9.

103. See below, pp. 104–105.

104. *Paston*, II, p. 226; *Rot. Parl.*, V, pp. 618–619. In regard to the latter, the expression "pestilencie plagum" is used.

105. See below, pp. 118–121.

106. *Visitations*, p. 11.

107. Fabyan, p. 666. For the chronology from the narrative sources, see above, pp. 45–46; for a discussion, see below, pp. 95–96.

108. Worcestre, p. 255.

109. See below, pp. 96–97.

110. See below, pp. 97–98; 98–99; 102–103; 148–149.

111. Still the best biography of Edward IV, including discussion of his personal life, is Cora Scofield, *The Life and Reign of Edward the Fourth*, 2 vols. (London: Longmans, 1923).

112. See above, pp. 22–23.

113. *Papal Letters*, IX, p. 486; XIII, p. 279.

114. Among modern historians who have restricted plague in fifteenth century England to urban centers are Creighton, *History of Epidemics*, I; Bean, "Population and Economic Decline"; J. F. D. Shrewsbury, *A History of the Bubonic Plague in the British Isles* (Cambridge: Cambridge University Press, 1971); and J. R. Landers, *Conflict and Stability in Fifteenth Century England* (London: Hillary House, 1969). For a full discussion of plague and its fifteenth century distribution, see below, pp. 142–150.

115. Kingsfold, *English Historical Literature*, provides a detailed analysis of this.

# CHAPTER III

# The Medical Response to Epidemic Disease

## 3.1 The Aetiology of Plague

Plague was the epidemic disease which was not frequent and which posed the greatest threat to fifteenth century Englishmen.[1] Probably because it is no longer of major danger to Western man, plague is also one of the diseases about which modern epidemiologists write least. Consequently, historians have eagerly leaped into the medical gap, and have written so much about the aetiology of plague in recent years that is no longer seems necessary to "write for the benefit of the uninitiated," as one historian recently phrased it.[2] For convenience's sake, however, it will be useful to summarize the basic medical characteristics of at least plague, if not the other epidemic diseases of fifteenth century England.

Pestilence was a generic name for epidemic disease in fifteenth century narrative sources, as shown in Chapter 2, although it probably was used for plague more often than for any other epidemic disease. Correctly speaking, plague is the disease caused by the bacillus *pastuerella pestis,* which presents itself in three forms: bubonic, pneumonic and septicemic plague.[3] It is possible that a fourth form, enteric, or abdominal plague, also exists.[4]

There have been at least three pandemics of plague in recorded Western history. A plague pandemic is generally rather slow in spreading—compared, for example, with influenza—taking about ten years to make its way around the world.[5] When plague does arrive, however, it comes to stay. The first pandemic began sometime in the early or mid-sixth century in Europe, and lingered on for at least two hundred years.[6] The second, the one with which we are concerned in fifteenth century England, erupted in Western Europe late in 1347, and persisted in the West until the early eighteenth century. The most recent pandemic began in the Far East in the last decade of the nineteenth century, and has had little effect on Western Europe.[7]

There is considerable medical evidence to indicate that plague is endemic to certain regions of the world for protracted periods of time.[8] It has been argued from the medical evidence that late medieval Europe was one of the historical regions of endemic, as well as epidemic, plague, a point relevant for fifteenth century England.[9] A very mild form of bubonic plague—or at times simply enlarged glands without even a fever—called *pestis ambulans* or *pestis minor* is known in the endemic regions.[10] Areas in which plague is or has been endemic in the twentieth century include Central Asia, Siberia, Mongolia, the Yunan region of China, and parts of Iran, Libya, the Arabian peninsula and East Africa.[11] Endemic plague can be very localized, and restricted to extremely small geographical areas. In Arabia, Clemow claimed that in the southwestern part of the peninsula, plague was confined (around 1900) to a narrow, twenty-mile-wide mountainous strip.[12] Biraben localizes endemic plague to even smaller areas, saying that at times only particular villages in a small area will be afflicted, depending upon rodent epizoötic conditions.[13]

As mentioned above, the causative agent in plague is a bacillus called *pastuerella pestis*. It is long and rectangular in shape, and easily visible through a microscope. *P. pestis* grows in chains and is spore-producing.[14] It lives in the bloodstreams of warmblooded animals, or in the digestive tract of the flea, especially the flea *Xenopsylla cheopis*. Plague generally appears first as an epizoötic or glandular infection among the rodents which *x. cheopis* inhabits; it is important to realize that *p. pestis* is first and foremost a parasite of rodents and rats in particular, and not of the fleas who carry it, nor of man. When *p. pestis* is endemic to a rodent population, it is called silvatic plague. In those regions of the world where plague is endemic, a similar condition of silvatic plague is usually to be found among the rodent population.[15]

*P. pestis* then is transmitted from host to host through the medium of the flea *x.cheopis*. Since *x.cheopis* prefers rodent hosts, especially the black rat, *rattus rattus*, and the brown rat, *rattus norvegius*, it is only when the primary host of the flea dies that the flea will search for a new host, sometimes man. The flea most common to man, *pulex irritans* does not seem to carry *p.pestis* except during the rare outbreaks of septicemic plague, when the human bloodstream is loaded with the bacilli.[16] *X.cheopis* is itself not susceptible to the plague, but may starve to death if the bacilli multiply in the flea's stomach in sufficient numbers to block the disgestive tract. When this happens, the blocked flea, as it is called, when feeding will regurgitate *p.pestis* into the bloodstream of its victim, and hence pass on the plague. It is crucial that the skin of the victim be broken by the flea, as it has been demonstrated by Hirst that *p.pestis* cannot survive on the surface of the skin.[17] *P.pestis* may also be transmitted by the defecation of the flea, which is generally loaded with the bacilli; if the victim scratches the irritation caused by the flea's presence, and breaks the skin, then infection can occur.[18]

Most observers believe that *x.cheopis* is the only type of flea which an transmit the plague.[19] According to MacArthur, this is due to the four-stage life cycle of most fleas.[20] The first three flea stages are not parasitic, but are dependent on the adult fourth-stage flea for nourishment. A nest is needed for this purpose, and hence, according to MacArthur, most fleas would not inhabit a completely mobile animal such as a deer (nor presumably a very stray dog, although this dog would undoubtedly have lice).[21] The adult flea feeds its young by defecating almost pure blood of its victims. *X.cheopis*, however, is an exception to this four-stage cycle of development. It's young are not dependent on excreted blood or on a nest, and hence *x.cheopis* is more mobile than other types of flea, and is therefore able to infect a wider range of hosts.[22]

Just as *p.pestis* seems to thrive in the stomach of *x.cheopis*, *x.cheopis* thrives on the black house rat, *rattus rattus*.[23] Because the black rat lives close to man, it is most dangerous to him. Being an excellent climber, the thatched roofs of a medieval peasant dwelling, or the high roof beam or dark corners of a medieval urban house must have been an ideal home for it. It is only when the rat or other rodent host dies that *x.cheopis* will adopt a new host. In addition to man, Liston has claimed that *x.cheopis* will readily inhabit pigs, cats, dogs, cattle, hens and other animals,[24] though Biraben believes that this flea is repelled by the odor of certain animals, including horses, sheep and goats.[25] Thus man, far from being a preferred host, is the victim of a rat epizoötic. A few medieval observers, including painters,[26] did seem to note the presence of large numbers of dead rodents during plague epidemics, but the connection between the rodent epizoötic and the human epidemic was only vaguely made.[27]

The incubation period from the time of infection to the first symptoms is between two and ten days. *P.pestis* then manifests itself in one of three or even four ways—bubonic, pneumonic, septicemic and possibly enteric plague—dependent perhaps upon the initial area of infection and probably on a variety of environmental conditions.[28] Bubonic plague was far and away the most common form in fifteenth century England, and at least one historical epidemiologist has argued that it was the only form of plague present.[29] With bubonic plague, *p.pestis* attacks the lymphatic gland system, once it is in the bloodstream. Depending upon the point of penetration, a large, discolored swelling will appear in either the groin, the armpits or, less commonly, in the neck. The tell-tale buboes and dark blotches will appear with the swelling, caused by subcutaneous hemorrhaging. Intoxication of the nervous system may also occur, and this in part may explain some of the macabre dance rituals which the literary sources tell us so often preceded death during an epidemic of plague.[30] Bubonic plague is strictly insect-borne; it is transmitted only by fleas.[31] Hirst reports that even in incidents of cannibalism among rats, plague is not transmitted if blocked fleas are not present.[32] Bubonic plague runs its course in four to seven days, and is usually fatal in 50–80 percent of the cases.

Pneumonic plague is far deadlier than bubonic plague, but also far less frequent. The precise reason as to why pneumonic plague develops in some epidemics and not others is not yet fully understood, but it may be connected with a pneumonial infection, and is most common during the winter months.[33] It seems to cause a consolidation in the lungs, resulting in rapid cyanosis and the expectoration of bloody sputum. Because of this, pneumonic plague is air-borne as well as insect-borne, and is directly contagious from one human to another. It is the only form of plague which is directly contagious, and is said to be second only to smallpox in the ease in which it is contracted.[34] Hirst has associated the presence of pneumonic plague with territory experiencing its first epidemic, and with burrowing rodents.[35] Pneumonic plague runs its course in about three days, and sometimes the buboes do not have time to form. It is almost 100 percent fatal to those who contract it.[36]

Septicemic plague, like bubonic plague, is insect-borne. Like pneumonic plague, it is not yet fully understood. For reasons as yet unkown, *p.pestis* sometimes enters the bloodstream in enormous quantities, causing septicemic plague.[37] A rash forms, and the victim can be killed within a matter of hours, well before the buboes have time to form. It appears to be literally 100 percent fatal, but is even rarer than pneumonic plague. Because *p.pestis* is present in the bloodstream in such enormous quantities during septicemic plague, there exists the possibility that the human flea, *pulex irritans,* as well as *x.cheopis,* can transmit it.[38]

There are certain conditions necessary for the presence of plague, most of them contingent upon its animal hosts. In regard to the primary rodent host, usually *rattus rattus,* sufficient numbers of rodents must live close enough to man so that when the rodent dies, *x.cheopis* may next infect man himself. Since bubonic plague, by far the most common strain, is insect-borne, and the fleas stick close to the rodent primary host, it is necessary, if man is to contract plague, that an epidemic rather than silvatic conditions prevail.[39] Rodent migrations may also be a key factor, especially with wild rodents and the course of the pandemics. But *x.cheopis* is not totally dependent on the primary rodent host for transport, and can be moved about by men or human transport, as in bales of hay or merchandise. The hearty flea can survive for long periods without any host whatsoever, and there have been cases of *x.cheopis* known to survive for up to fifty days without food, and for far longer in piles of dung, which must have been common in medieval barnyards and stables.[40]

A more effective control of the blocked flea harboring *p.pestis* is temperature. *X.cheopis* seems to flourish between 68–78°F, and the occurrence of bubonic plague in England is almost always in late summer and early fall.[41] During the winter, the flea generally becomes more sluggish and hibernates, though a relatively well-heated house, especially a kitchen, could produce an artificially warm climate, even during the winter. At 55°F the flea's eggs do not hatch, and at 45°F the eggs die.[42] Perhaps the warm winters account for the infrequency of pneumonic plague in fifteenth century England.

Several other epidemic diseases were present in fifteenth century England. Dysentery—the flux, or "bloody flyx"—was the cause of at least two epidemics in the century, one in 1411 and another in 1473.[43] From 1485, there was the English Sweat, or sweating sickness, perhaps a form of influenza.[44] Toward the end of the fifteenth century there was the French Pox, first reported by *The Brut* in 1475, perhaps part of the great syphilis epidemic of the late fifteenth and early sixteenth century, or perhaps yaws or gonorrhea, but an infectious skin disease in any case.[45] Further, there is little doubt that England also felt the ravages of typhus, smallpox and influenza in the fifteenth century, to name but a few.[46] Typhus, a winter disease which seems to have become very frequent in late Tudor England,[47] may have been equally prevalent in the fifteenth century.[48] All of the above-mentioned diseases, with the exception of the English Sweat, which lies beyond the chronological limits of this work, are also scourges of the modern world, and as such have been well studied and well documented by modern medical authorities. There is no need for the historian to discuss their aetiological characteristics.

One final factor must be discussed in regard to the aetiology of fifteenth century English epidemic diseases. When a disease is mentioned in the narrative sources or even in a contemporary medical treatise, it is usually called by the generic name "pestilence," and identified by its symptoms. Therefore, historically speaking, typhus, caused by a series of microorganisms called *Rickettsia* and transmitted by the body louse, is often confused with enteric fevers such as typhoid fever and, appropriately enough in the medieval sense, food poisoning, which are caused by various bacteria and sometimes transmitted through water. Since both types of disease exhibit toxaemia, high temperature and a rash, they were often lumped together by medieval chroniclers.[49] The same can be said about measles and whooping cough; and smallpox, syphilis, yaws and leprosy.

## 3.2 The Fifteenth Century: The Medical Response

As we have seen, for the half-century 1430 to 1480, there were probably eleven outbreaks and eighteen years of national epidemics. There were at least twenty other outbreaks and fifteen other years of epidemics on a local scale, giving parts of England, such as London, up to twenty-seven years at the very minimum in a fifty-year period during which there were outbreaks of epidemic diseases.[50]

The written medical response to epidemic disease was spare indeed, and, in many respects, a contradiction in terms to the aetiological patterns of the century. While continental Europeans immersed themselves in medical studies and went back to the writings of classical antiquity to seek solutions, English scholars did practically no original writing or even thinking, if we are to judge from the surviving source material, on the topic of infectious disease. The most interesting, influential and apparently most popular treatises circulating in England during this period came from two Frenchmen, a Norman and a Swede.[51]

Two of the most popular medical treatises of the period came from fourteenth century France. They are the tractates of John La Barba, or John of Burgundy, as he is alternatively called, and John of Bordeaux. Both treatises deal with what the authors refer to as "pestilentia," in this case almost certainly plague. Both were recopied many times throughout the fifteenth century, with the British Museum (B.M.) being one of many institutions having several copies from the period studied by this thesis.[52] Both writers, while wrong if quite imaginative in regard to the causes of pestilence, were strong in their chapters on sanitation and the prevention of infectious diseases. Some of the copies which circulated throughout England were written in Latin, but most were composed or copied in English.[53]

John La Barba calls himself a physician and professor of medicine in Liège.[54] He divides his treatise into eight well-organized chapters, and takes an especially strong, preventive, public health attitude about epidemics. Bathing, the taking of medicine, and strenuous labor are considered dangerous during epidemic periods—measures which may to some degree have accounted for the treatise's overwhelming popularity.[55] The reason for the prohibition of bathing, which was considered to be the most dangerous single factor, was fairly logical, if not necessarily medically sound. John believed the pestilence entered the body through opened pores, a process facilitated by hot-water bathing.

The observational powers of John La Barba were striking. He divided the body into three principal members—the brain, the heart and the liver.[56] When pestilence attacked the body, bearded John wrote, the three principal members "put out things," and these things, the symptoms of the disease, were revealed by a swelling in the neck, the armpits or the groin, depending upon where the disease entered the body.[57] In fact, these observations are medically correct for plague, with the buboes appearing in the neck, the armpits or the groin, depending upon the location of the fleabite. Even John's principal cure for pestilence, phlebotomy, was rooted in sound, observatory diagnosis. He believed that bloodletting would drain the buboes brought on by the plague.[58]

Unfortunately, in diagnosing the causes of pestilence, John La Barba's medical insight leaves him. In common with his mid-fourteenth century predecessors, and his successors for another two hundred years and more, John saw the causes as being astral and cosmological, and subject to the conjunctions of the planets, or in terms of the miasma-contagion theory of Galen and classical antiquity.[59]

John's greatest contribution, however, at least in the historical sense, lies neither in his policies of public health nor in his medical observations; rather, it is his diagnosis of the endemic nature of the "pestilentia," the predominant form of most epidemic diseases which remains after and between the more virulent but much rarer epidemics. His statement needs quotation in full:

> Not that the aire was corupte in his substance, for hit is a symple thing or an unmedled body, but hit corupteth by encheson of the evyl vapours medled togyders. Wherfor epidemia or pestilentia in many costes folowith, and yit in many places his traces and steppes apparen as hit shewth wele. For many mane is infecte and namely suche as has been replete and stuffed with humors than ben mystempled with evyl quantite. but yit coruptyng of the aire is not alone cause of moreyne but also haboundance of humors corupt in them that dien. As Galen saith in his boke of fevers[60] the body suffreth no corupcion but if the matier of the body be prompt or redy ther to and in a maner subiect or obiedient to the coruptible cause ffor right as the fyre may not brene but in mater that is combustible or able to brene right so nouther pestilence ne pestilencial aire noyeth not but if it finde mater ready and obeying to corupcion.[61]

John La Barba seems to have been aware, if for all the wrong reasons, of the continuing presence of the bacilli within the community in an endemic or silvatic form, probably flaring up into epidemic proportions when a new, virulent strain of bacilli was introduced into the area. In light of this statement, the corrupt and insalubrious air which forced Parliament to flee from London in 1450 may have been, as Creighton suggested, an epidemic of plague.[62] Once again, one must be impressed with the powers of observation of John La Barba.

The tractate of John of Bordeaux, written originally about twenty years later than that of John La Barba (1360's to 1380's), is quite similar to its predecessor.[63] John of Bordeaux's work also is strong on diagnosis, observation and prevention, and appallingly weak on causation. Like John La Barba's treatise, many of the copies of John of Bordeaux's work survive in both English and Latin.[64] The Bordeaux manuscript is shorter than La Barba's, being divided into four chapters: diet; "hou the pestilence coumthe and infects"; "trewe medicine to withstande the pestilence"; and a further chapter on diet and medicine.

In addition to condemning baths and hard work, as did John La Barba, John of Bordeaux tells his readers that honey and especially fruit are to be avoided; a light diet and, as Aristotle advises, a generally temperate lifestyle are the best ways to avoid pestilence.[65] In fact, one senses in this treatise an increasing feeling of helplessness in attempting to understand the true nature of epidemic disease, brought on no doubt by the recurring epidemics of the later Middle Ages. Attempts to explain the causation of epidemics are particularly feeble, relying heavily on astrology and cosmology.[66] Little is known about John of Bordeaux's personal background or training, but he refers to physicians throughout the treatise as "leches." This seems to have been an expression of general usage throughout the fourteenth and fifteenth centuries.[67]

Despite the apparent popularity of numerous editions of the works of both John La Barba and John of Bordeaux, the most popular treatise of all in fifteenth century England seems to have been that of the Swedish bishop of Vatoras, Bengt Knuttson, or Kanuti. This treatise, of which there are several surviving copies, was first written in 1460, after a serious outbreak of plague in Sweden.[68] It was one of the earlier books printed in England, with the first editions dating about 1485.[69] Knuttson claims to have studied and practiced medicine at Montpellier, and says that he wished to write what he had learned from the greatest and most learned physicians of the day, so that he might help others in times of "pessulaunce."[70] In the best medieval tradition, the treatise itself was largely taken from yet another of those fourteenth century French works, that of John of Jacobus, himself a physician and one-time chancellor of the medical school in Montpellier.[71]

The treatise was divided by Knuttson into four parts: tokens of the infirmity, the causes, remedies, and comfort of the patient. Almost as an afterthought, he adds a fifth part on "when it schall be season to lett blode." This division is maintained in the first printed editions, and all the various treatises and early printed editions are essentially the same, despite slight differences in vocabulary and syntax. As with the previous works discussed, the bishop is excellent on disinfection and prevention, and weak on causation, relying mostly on astrology and cosmology to explain the existence of epidemic disease.[72]

In his alternatively titled *Passing Gode lityll boke necessayre and behouveful agenst the Pestilence*, or *A Litell Boke the which traytied and reherced many gode things necessarie . . . for the Pestilence*, or in Latin, *Regimen contra pestilentium . . .*, Bengt is aware of the need for proper hygiene in combating epidemic disease, and even recognizes the harm of vermin in general, if not rats, fleas and lice—to name a few—in particular.[73] Both stagnant water and "stynkyng dede caryon" are to be avoided, and sweet odors to be sought.[74] The bishop also mentions the significance of house structure, though, once again, there is no specific reference to thatched roofs being an ideal home for black rats. The essence of avoiding disease, according to Bengt, is to keep "infect aire" and "putrification" away from the places "where most folkes sleepe."[75] One must keep his home clean at all costs, and keep it clear of the fire of flaming wood.[76] Herbs, especially the "levys of baye trees," are to be sought.[77] This remark is of particular interest because during the years of the great frosts and epidemics of the 1430's, the chroniclers continually lamented the "bay trees, rosemary, sauge, tyme and many other herbes which deyed."[78] The leaves of the bay tree were thought to be an effective remedy against pestilence.

Knuttson offers further remedies. Frequent washing of the mouth and face and "evyn the handes" in a solution of rosewater and vinegar is highly recommended, as is the drinking of vinegar and treacle.[79] The eating of cheese and meat, and the drinking of "clene" wine is advised, if each of the items is taken in moderation; if they are consumed in excess, they will "putrify" the body's humors, and lead to pestilence.[80] Hot things like peppers and garlic are to be avoided because they too will upset the delicate balance of the humors.[81] This is so despite the fact that ordinarily both pepper and garlic were considered to be valuable apothecarial aids, since it was believed that pepper "purgeyth the Brayne," and garlic, even though it could make one's body too hot, was effective against evil humors.[82] Knuttson agrees with John of Bordeaux in advising his readers to avoid fruit, but if the patient must indulge, cherries, pomegranates and a bit of apple were thought to be least harmful.[83]

Unlike most of his contemporary treatise writers, Knuttson was fairly well-disposed toward the medical profession of his day, due perhaps to his own training at Montpellier. It is essential, he felt, that every patient have a good physician.[84] Application of any of the recommended cures by a layman could lead to upsetting the humors or to a too great opening of the pores.

One of the most interesting aspects of the treatise is Bengt's continual cautions about the transmission of the pestilence orally. He was convinced that the pestilence to which he was referring could be transmitted from person to person:

> . . . the people as moche as is possible is to be eschewed lest of infecte brethys som may be infecte [by others] . . .[85]

And,

> . . . the pestilence sores be contagious because of the enfecte humours . . . and because of corupte aire it is good to flee from those persons as be infecte.[86]

Further, physicians are cautioned from getting too close to infected patients. When treating the very ill, the physician is advised to stand very far away, holding his face toward an open door or window, and especially toward the north.[87] One wonders if Bengt had not correctly deduced the nature of the transmission of pneumonic plague.

It is hard to imagine a fifteenth century bishop being as clinical as Knuttson, and not moralizing just a little bit; and indeed, he does just that. The first thing one ought to do, he says, is stay home all day, probably the worst thing one could have done for bubonic plague or typhus, given the state of the average medieval dwelling, but not bad advice for sweating sickness, influenza or smallpox.[88] He paraphrases Scripture (Jeremiah), saying the "heist [best] remedye in time of pestilence is penaunce and confession to be p'ferred over all other medicynes"; after "penaunce," the best thing to do is avoid all possible "putrification and stynkyng," the most dangerous of which is "fleschly lust with wymmen," followed closely by "the gret repleccacions" [meals].[89] Also to be avoided are the south and the southern winds, not surprising in view of his land of birth, which are "naturally infectyf."[90] Possibly this statement may indicate that bubonic plague and dysentery, diseases which occur in the summer and fall, were more feared in the fifteenth century than cold weather diseases such as pneumonic plague, influenza and typhus. Finally, common baths are to be avoided, although Knuttson does not specify if this is for medical or moral reasons.[91]

Despite the rantings about the dangers of women, food and warm weather, there is much good advice from Bengt Knuttson. It is interesting to note that in 1892, Charles Creighton, whose famous book of historical epidemiology has recently been reissued and called the most authoritative book of its kind, believed as did the fifteenth century bishop that plague came from "stinking and corrupt heaps."[92]

As was the case with Knuttson's work, another of the more influential fifteenth century treatises on epidemic disease, Thomas Forestier's *Tractus Contra Pestilentium, Thenasmonium, et Dissinterium,* was printed a few years after my period, probably in 1490.[93] The earliest manuscript copies are dated around 1485. Forestier's work is especially important because it discusses not only pestilence, which in this treatise as in so many others is almost certainly plague, and the sweating sickness, but also the flux, which he identifies as intestinal dysentery. The treatise was ostensibly written in response to the sweat of 1485, but both the manuscript and printed editions seem more concerned with pestilence, "sekeness," and the flux.[94] The work was dedicated to Henry VII, and Forestier, a Norman who styled himself a "medicine doctore," may have come from Rouen with Henry's triumphal army to Bosworth Market.[95] More is known about Forestier's departure from England. According to the *Calendar of Patent Rolls,* he is said to have been living and practicing medicine in Westminster until 1487, when he was forced to flee the country.[96]

Forestier's treatise is similar to Knuttson's, though longer, and it too was probably based on John of Jacobus's orginal.[97] The text of the printed edition is very well organized into twelve chapters, the last two of which are devoted toward advising the poor on how to avoid ignorant and corrupt physicians.[98] He is especially bitter at those "leches" who pretend to understand things when in reality they do not. The state of the medical profession in the fifteenth century seems to have genuinely troubled him, and he felt, probably rightly so, that most leches did more harm to their patients than good.[99] The manuscript editions of the treatise are shorter than the printed one, but in content are quite similar to it.

The treatise is similar to the other works discussed thus far in that it invokes celestial causation for pestilence on one hand, while pronouncing thoughtful, clinical observations and advocating sound conceptions about public sanitation on the other. The remedies that Forestier proposes are quite like those of Bengt Knuttson, but in this treatise—probably more so than in any of the others—there is a commendable detachment and lack of sensational outburst in discussing the symptoms of pestilence.[100] Forestier even admits at certain times to having something less than total knowledge of his subject, rather than feigning information.[101] His also differs from the other treatises of the period in not advocating phlebotomy,[102] and this may account for his sarcastically consistent usage of the derogatory expression "lech," meaning physician. However, Forestier stands almost alone among the treatise writers in advocating original sin as one of the causes of pestilence;[103] for every step forward, there is the inevitable step back.

Forestier was well read in the classics and works of his medieval predecessors. He constantly evokes the wisdom of Aristotle and Galen, as well as the Arab polymath Avicenna, from whom he takes his major reason for the causation of pestilence.[104] Further, to the standard dogma about astrological causation, he adds much new information about humidity and corruption of the air.[105] But perhaps Forestier's greatest contribution, at least to the historian, is in definitively identifying the "bloody flyx," or flux, mentioned by John Warkworth and others, as *dissinteria intestinale.*[106] In a long and detailed chapter of the printed edition of the work, he identifies and discusses dysentery in no uncertain terms, and has helped posterity in being able to identify at least one of the epidemics of the fifteenth century with some degree of surety.

Another important work is an anonymous treatise written in English, probably late in the fifteenth century, which takes the form of a general textbook on a variety of ailments.[107] Like most of the other treatises, the "textbook" stresses moderation, is weak on causation, and comparatively strong on prevention. This treatise is interesting in that it offers cures for almost all sicknesses current in fifteenth century England. The first three or four pages in depth, and the first fifteen pages in general refer to pestilence, which in this case once again seems to be plague. The manuscript in which the treatise itself is bound contains a potpourri of other treatises on a host of "biological" topics, including falconry, hunting the hart and a cookbook, which is comprehensive and precisely detailed. About midway through the manuscript, a "Treatise of Sikenesses" begins, and deals with remedies for such things as "amoletk, or a stone in the shuld," "ryngbone," "a strayte hove and lose hove," and "for to make a hors fitter," all of which give it more of a veterinary than a medical tone.[108] The format of the treatise can only be described as "chatty." It is in English, is very rambling and, in the custom of the day, calls physicians leches.[109]

As with Forestier's treatise, this anonymous work ultimately attributes the cause of pestilence to original sin and divine wrath.[110] Prayer and fasting, as advocated by the Swedish bishop Bengt Knuttson, are always the best checks on the ravages of disease.[111] Fasting aside, moderation is considered to be the best preventive measure.[112] The urge for moderation, which is perhaps the one overriding and common factor in all the treatises thus far discussed, stems from Aristotle, as well as from Galen's *Book of Fevers.*[113] Much is made of Galen in this treatise. His belief in discretion in life style and diet, and a moderate amount of daily exercise, is repeated in a series of eight steps. At times, the work seems to be more like a guide to good health than a treatise on preventive medicine.

Diet is a topic of considerable concern. The dangers of foul meat are emphasized, and the reader is told how to select good meats,[114] in steps similar to those used by Thomas Forestier when the latter advised his readers on how to select a good leech. Wines and ales in small quantities are recommended.[115] Bread in a cup with either wine or ale is also good.[116] Unlike the work of John La Barba, this treatise permits the consumption of fruits, especially apples, pears and plums; for La Barba, John of Bordeaux and, to a lesser extent, Bengt Knuttson, fruits were to be avoided at all costs.[117] The anonymous author warns against not only bad meat, but also oysters. "Beware of them," says the author, "eschewe to ete oysters,"[118] advice to be considered in light of the recent cholera epidemic in southern Italy. It is ironic that the cookbook which shares the manuscript with the pestilence treatise has several delectable recipes for oysters.[119]

If moderation, prayer and a sound diet do not succeed in warding away epidemics, the author has other solutions. He advocates phlebotomy, as do most of the other treatises, although he feels it must be done within twelve hours of the first sign of infection in order to be effective.[120] Finally, the author offers his last resort, "practical" remedies. Several prescriptions are given, among them:

3 finalie croppes or rewes
3 levys of yong tansay
3 levys off sauge and fayre washed to be chewed.[121]

This remedy is to be taken each day, promptly at noon.[122]

Throughout the treatise, the expressions "sikeness" and "pestilence" are used almost interchangeably. The author, obviously a man of learning and intelligence, writes as though all epidemics were essentially alike; and, in their ultimate result, they certainly were. With only a few exceptions, this is the habit of fifteenth century physicians and chroniclers alike; even though they might call a disease a pestilence or a flux or a stitch, all diseases were invariably considered to be caused by God, via corrupt heaps, foul air, original sin, or the conjunctions of the planets—and all remedies were in the long run just about the same.

To get a complete view of the scope of medical works on epidemic disease in fifteenth century England, one must briefly discuss two other early fifteenth century treatises. Both are quite short, anonymous, and in Latin. One, untitled, and following a short copy of John of Bordeaux's treatise[123] (falsely attributed in the manuscript to John La Barba), is distinguished mainly by its strong conviction that the fallen angel Lucifer is behind the whole business of epidemic disease. Rather than discussing cures or prevention of pestilence, the author concentrates on telling his public how to recognize the devil himself in disguise. The other treatise, entitled *De Signa Pestilentia,* concentrates on temperature as a major factor in the occurrence of epidemic disease, and there is some awareness of the seasonal frequency of various epidemic diseases.[124] It is otherwise quite similar to the treatise of Bengt Knuttson, or, more accurately, that of John of Jacobus.[125]

There were undoubtedly other medical treatises which were known and read in fifteenth century England. One of the manuscripts which contains a copy of the Knuttson treatise has a separate treatise on the flux within it, and a pestilence treatise by Benedict of Nursia, both of which may have been fifteenth century copies.[126] Judging from the numbers of surviving copies, however, the treatises which have been discussed above were the most popular and influential of the fifteenth century medical works.

In general, the medical sources in England from 1430 to 1480 were strong on clinical observations, reactions from and prevention of epidemic disease. There was a great deal of awareness of the necessity of proper sanitation, and hints that the surgeons and physicians had connected plague with the dirt and filth that attracts rats and fleas. On the other hand, there was an appalling lack of knowledge of the causes of epidemic disease, a weakness that persisted into the twentieth century.

## 3.3 The Fifteenth Century: The Popular Response

In all societies there is a gap between what the informed advocate and what the masses believe. In a basically illiterate society reliant on oral communication, such as fifteenth century England, this gap was likely to be especially large. The nonmedical world had its own remedies to combat epidemic disease.

Straddling the boundaries of the medical and nonmedical world is a splendid collection of popular and semimedical recipes or prescriptions, a fifteenth century leechbook.[127] Written in English, the leechbook was probably first compiled in the 1440's, after the plague-devastated 1430's.[128] The leechbook covers an enormous variety of maladies, ranging from gout and indigestion to what the compiler calls "palsy of the privy parts."[129] It is very pragmatic in its tone, designed it would seem for coping on a practical basis with everyday ailments. Most of the remedies it offers consist of herbs, which must have been both easy to obtain and cheap to purchase. Even the section on phlebotomy is sort of a "do-it-yourself" guide.

The disease covered most thoroughly and mentioned most frequently throughout the leechbook is flux. The author uses the expression flux in the broadest sense of the term, as a catch-all for stomach ailments. He tells his readers that there are four major types of flux: "collides"; "licentia, when ones mete passeth from him undigested"; diarrhea; and dysentery.[130] It is the "iiii maner of flux," dysentery, which will concern us here; as the author defines it, "that is when there cometh blode and shavings of gutties therewith togedir."[131] Two typical cures for dysentery are given as follows:

> For the bloody flux. Take yarrow and waybread and stamp them in a mortar and take juice of them and fair flour of wheat and temper them together and make a cake and bake it in ashes and make the sick to eat it as hot as he may suffer it. *Probatum est!*[132]

> Take a pennyweight of towncress and as much parsley seed and grind them in a pepper quern with a little pepper; then take small hedge sloes and seethe them in rain-water and ale, and then take a little of that water that the sloes were seethed in, as much as the sick may drink at once, and put therein three pennyweight of that powder aforesaid and let him drink it off and do so thrice. And if he shall live it is likely it shall stanch it.[133]

The final sentences in both prescriptions are worth noting. If the patient lives through the remedy, he shall certainly be able to survive the flux! Many remedies have the phrase *probatum est!* after them.

There are a great number and variety of other solutions for the flux. One stipulates that the patient's feet be washed in everfern—but not above the ankles.[134] Other recipes call for a variety of potions, salves and charms which include such elements as mint, plantation, mugwort, crab apples, beans, rye, wheat, honey, fresh swine's grease, peppers, oysters, a variety of roots and, of course, vinegar.[135] Most of the recipes seem a bit silly, but there is a sense of confidence, almost bravado, in these cures that is not present in the more professional treatises. It is as though the masses had turned from the advice of the "authorities"—if indeed they ever heeded them—and looked within their own ranks for solutions to their medical problems.

Poxes and skin diseases of all types from acne to leprosy are treated in the leechbook. Though the particulars of the pox are never discussed, pigeon dung was a favorite cure-all.[136] There are also favorite remedies for fevers of a "general nature." Peppers, kermes, ginger, raisons, mustard seed, ale and the omnipresent vinegar, the reader is told, can be used for virtually any fever.[137] For children, there are remedies which can be made into candy balls and liberally sweetened with honey.[138] The recipes are very rigid in the proportions of their contents, however, and in the time of day at which they are to be taken.

The recipes for pestilence, once again probably plague, are at the end of the leechbook, and the author is a bit more reserved when discussing their success.[139] Several of them end with expressions like "if they hold it, they shall have life."[140] One recipe has no less than thirty-nine separate ingredients in it,[141] and the cures for pestilence are in general far longer and more complicated than those for other ailments.[142]

Flowers are a unique, new ingredient in the pestilential cure-alls. Marigolds and dandelions are especially popular.[143] Other ingredients common to the pestilence remedies are rue, tansey, columbine, chives, eggs, treacle and ale.[144] One notable remedy for the pestilence is as follows:

> A medycine for the pestilence. Take 5 crops of rue if it be a man, and if it be a woman leave out the rue, for rue is restorative to a woman and wasting to a man [sic]; and take then thereto five crops of tansey and five little blades of columbine, and a great quantity of marigold flowers full of the small chives from the crops that are like saffron-chives. And if thou mayest not get the flowers, take the leaves, then must thou have more of marigold than all of the others. Then take an egg that is new laid, and make a hole in either end, and blow out all that is within. And lay it to the fire and let it roast till it may be ground to powder, but burn it not. Then take a quantity of good treacle, and bray all these herbs therein with good ale, but strain them not. And let the sick drink them three evenings and mornings. If they [the sick] hold it, they shall have life.[145]

In length, detail and generally pessimistic attitude, this recipe is fairly typical of the remedies used to combat pestilence. It is unusual in that it actually gives an alternative method for treating women. Generally, women were left out of the recipes at best, or, at worst, as in the treatise of Bengt Knuttson, were considered as out and out purveyors of epidemic disease.[146]

One last series of remedies in the leechbook have relevance in a study of epidemic disease and its demographic effects. These are the ones concerning conception, in one way or another. There is a special method listed for easing the delivery of a stillborn or dead child:

> Take leek blades and scale them, and bind them to the womb about the navel: and it shall cast out the dead child; and when she is delivered take away the blades or she shall cast out all that is in her.[147]

Stillborn births must have been a great problem. But in the underpopulated fifteenth century, impotence may have been considered even a greater problem. The leechbook proposes a solution:

> For the palsy in a man's pyntell (privy member). Seeth caster in wine and wash him therewith about the share [pubic region] and wet the cloth therein and upon the pyntell in a manner of a plaster.[148]

Either this was a time-proven and time-honored method, or the confidence which the author showed when dealing with the flux had returned, for this remedy is ended with a triumphal *probatum est!*"

More popular if less helpful were the various informal remedies to ward off *epidemia*. The best of these is the "Recipes for Edward IV's Plague Medicine." Written during one of the "reyning sekneys" of Edward IV's rule, it purports to tell the royal way for avoiding what is almost surely plague. First, one takes:

> a hanfull of rewe, a hanfull of marygoldis, halfe a hanfull of fetherfev, a hanfull of burnet, a hanfull of sorell, a quantite of dragenys—the crop or the route—then take a potell of ryngyng water. Fyrst wasche them clene and let then seethe easily tyl yt be a-moste cum from a potell to a quartre of lekker; then take a clene clothe, and strayne ytt and drynke yt; and yt be bitter, put ther-to a lytel suger of candy, and thys may be dronkyn ofttyme; and yf yt be dronkyn before eny purpel a-pere, by the grase of god ther schall be no perell of no dethe.[149]

Folk remedies are always popular in peasant societies, and they seem to have been especially so in the epidemic-ridden fifteenth century. The sources for such remedies are usually oral, and as such, are difficult to trace. They tend to come down to the historian in trickles, mostly through chronicles and private correspondence. The following were considered to be among the best remedies for pestilence: filed horse hooves, tin and mercury *(Crocus Joves)*, coral, crab's eyes and crab's claws, and a poultice of rue, flour, salt and pigeon's dung.[150] For the buboes caused by the pestilence, an ointment of honey, duck grease, turpentine, soot, treacle, egg yolks and scorpion oil was thought to be especially helpful.[151]

Remedies written for the "gentler" segments of society contain basically the same ingredients and the same strong dose of pragmatism that the remedies written for the masses do, but are geared for the activities of the upper classes. One of the most interesting recipes of this genre is "A Regiment Devicyed be Mastur John De Wymus, Doctor Servant of the Lady Margret of Borgon."[152] The regimen is of particular interest because it is dated early in 1480, "in tyme of the rayne of the haste sikeness called pestilence," or the plague epidemic of 1479–1480.[153]

In content, the regimen is similar to all the other contemporary pestilence recipes. But the noble lady is cautioned not to do certain things that less exalted figures may have considered a bit frivolous. She is not to walk at midday, especially when the weather is hot or cloudy.[154] And she must not walk at any time with a full stomach, nor sleep in the daytime.[155] Two new prohibitions are added to the food list: sweet milk and cheese.[156] Sudden temperature changes and the doing of anything at all at too fast a pace are also to be avoided.[157] If these recommendations are followed in full, Master De Wymus assures his noble readers that they have nothing to fear from the pestilence.

It remains to discuss the medical aspects of epidemic disease encountered in vernacular literature. With no Chaucer or Langland, this is more difficult for the fifteenth century than it is for the fourteenth century.[158] Lydgate and Hoccleve, probably the century's premier poets, seem to have been rather oblivious to epidemic disease. It is therefore necessary to turn to more obscure sources.

Indirectly, the problem of epidemic disease is covered in an old English stanza, "For helth of Body from Colde . . .," dating from the mid-part of the fifteenth century.[159] The remedies offered for the "colde" are almost identical to those offered for pestilence in other sources. The usual admonitions for moderation and against bad foods are voiced.[160] As was stressed by Bengt Knuttson in his treaties, lust with women is seen as a major cause of pestilence, and "women aged" are seen as the most dangerous females of all.[161] As with the anonymous textbook treatise of the late fifteenth century, general guidelines toward living a good and pure life, such as leaving one's neighbors in peace, eating slowly, avoiding liars and watching one's language are also felt to be extremely important.[162] In essence, it is a recipe for avoiding disease rather than one for curing a victim of it.

The last few stanzas of the poem are devoted exclusively to the "pestelens." In fact, however, only the names of the ailments are different; the remedies for cold and pestilence are almost identical, dwelling on lots of sleep and good food. Two new pieces of advice are added in the pestilence portion of the poem; the reader is cautioned against gossiping, and, significantly, a warning to change clothing frequently is given, although unless the body was likewise washed, the latter would be of little use.[163] Finally, the stanzas, like most of the other literary works discussed, are highly antiphysician, and do not recommend that the afflicted see a doctor.[164]

An excellent source on epidemic disease is a grammar book dating from the earliest years of the reign of Henry VII.[165] It is a fairly typical grammar in its structure, but its uniqueness lies in the fact that the author, probably John Stanbridge, assistant master at Magdalen College, Oxford, made a valiant attempt to make the subject matter of his grammar interesting to the boys who had to read it. He gave model sentences from the subjects of everyday life, and herein lies the importance of the book to the epidemiologist: he could not but help discussing some aspects of epidemic disease.[166]

One thing that is made apparent from the outset of the grammar is that even toward the very end of the fifteenth century, when the population had probably begun to grow again, there was no shortage of foodstuffs. The young scholars in the book are constantly dreaming about food, but this is because they are expected to abstain for disciplinary purposes rather than for lack of foodstuffs. Indeed, the central figure of the grammar is rather particular about what he eats, and generally disdains fish and despairs during Lent. He is especially fond of harvest time, when:

> It is a grete pleasure to be in the contrey for this hervist season in a goode husbondemanys house, for a man may fare well ther. for he shall lacke no Caponys, Chekyns, other pygens.[167]

There is an entire section devoted to the glories of crab meat, a dish fit for a king, but, at least in the fifteenth if not the twentieth century, one within the grasp of poor scholars.[168] At one point, the protagonist proclaims that food was so cheap that "no man alyve that can remembre."[169] Once again it is made clear that in the fifteenth century, with the possible exceptions of the 1430's and some years in the 1470's, death due directly or even indirectly to famine must have been rare indeed. The distinction during crisis mortality periods of death from epidemic disease and death from famine is not a major problem for the historian of the fifteenth century, as it is for historians of most other pre-industrial periods.[170]

The grammarian was aware that what he calls pestilence came in the autumn. Once again, it seems that the by now not so generic expression pestilence was used to refer to plague:

> I fere me lest the pleasyre of somer be overpast and the faire dais goo. For methynke the the colde wynter semyth to cum in, with his Company Rayne and Wynde. but this I could away withall and take it well at worth so that yf the storme of pestilence were seaside thrugh godys mercy, which that it may be sonner brought aboute I thincke we most praye . . .[171]

It was a common practice in the fifteenth century, to judge from the narrative sources, to flee to the countryside during epidemics. Men in the fifteenth century, as do many historians in the twentieth century, seemed to believe that the countryside was immune from the ravages of epidemic disease, especially plague. Flight from London and Norwich during times of pestilence within the cities is discussed in the *Paston Letters,* and in the Exchequer and Chancery proceedings.[172] But modern epidemiologists have shown that at least in regard to plague this is a misconception, [173] and our grammarian appears to have known so as well:

> I most ride within this ii or iij dais, yf I may gett me a hors into my Cuntrey for many errands that I have to done, but as they say they dye sore uponn the pestelence ther, wherfor I fere me hye to fast thyderwarde tyll I her other tydinges.[174]

Also:

> Feloue thoue art welcome home. thanke be to almygty gode thou were not vexede with no seknes sithen thou wentist into the contrey. . .[175]

There is of course some ambiguity in what the author meant by the terms "Cuntrey" and "contrey." But judging from the grammarian's own Latin translations and also from the content, it does seem that he meant the countryside—that is, rural areas.[176] Coupled with evidence from other literary sources, such as that from John La Barba about the endemic nature of epidemic disease, it would appear that not all fifteenth century figures believed that epidemic disease flourished in urban areas only. The question of the exclusive presence of epidemic disease in urban centers will be discussed in detail in Chapter 5, in light of the testamentary evidence.[177]

A connection is made between dirt and disease in the grammar book, like that made by John Paston.[178] Our grammarian was well aware that filth breeds pestilence:

> . . . but I passide over the teamys (Thames) ii tymes at lest, iiij tymes at most, for to go by londe it was to diseasful . . . and also durty.[179]

Finally, there are the usual references to physicians as leeches. The grammarian does use it as a generic expression, but seems rather well disposed toward the medical profession. Unlike so many of his contemporaries, he apparently felt that his fellow professionals were quite useful, and advised his friends and pupils to seek their advice in times of sickness.[180]

There is little that can be summed up without becoming redundant. Professional medical treatises and folk remedies alike were essentially pragmatic in the fifteenth century, with the aids and prescriptions for epidemic diseases consisting or being composed of everyday products. Physicians were scorned for their failure to halt the ravages of epidemics; and women were at best ignored, and at worst seen as purveyors of the epidemics themselves. Above all else, moderation was believed to be the key factor in preventing epidemic disease—moderation in eating, drinking, and generally in the way one conducted one's life.

# Notes

1. This appears to be a consensus opinion among most medical historians, although J. F. D. Shrewsbury, *A History of Bubonic Plague in England* (Cambridge: Cambridge Univ. Press, 1971), would diminish the historical role of plague. For a discussion of the Shrewsbury book, see below, p. 239. Among the better surveys which cover a wide range of epidemic diseases and their historical roles are: A. H. Gale, *Epidemic Diseases* (London: Penguin, 1959); and M. Burnet and D. O. White, *Natural History of Infectious Disease* (Cambridge: Cambridge Univ. Press, 1972). The author makes no pretenses toward first-hand medical knowledge of epidemic disease, even plague, and consequently has had to rely entirely on existing medical authorities. For this reason, a great number of sources were consulted and documented, as noted below, pp. 244–253.

2. Christopher Morris, "The Plague in Britain," *Historical Journal,* XIV, 1971, p. 206.

3. Among the books relied on most heavily by the author in regard to the aetiology of plague were L. F. Hirst, *Conquest of Plague* (Oxford: Oxford University Press, 1953); R. Pollitzer, *Plague* (Geneva: W.H.O., 1954); Burnet and White, *op. cit.;* and J-N. Biraben, *Les hommes et la peste* (The Hague: Mouton, 1975). At the time of writing, the Biraben book had not yet been published; Dr. R. S. Schofield was kind enough to let me see a copy in draft form. Therefore, only "Chap. 1," rather than page numbers, will be cited in the course of the notes.

4. F. G. Clemow, *Geography of Epidemic Disease* (Cambridge: Cambridge Univ. Press, 1903), p. 311. The Clemow book is old and no doubt outdated in many respects. Nevertheless, it purportedly deals with his first-hand experiences with the plague pandemic in the Far East in the 1890's, and is quite useful.

5. Burnet and White, *op. cit.*

6. For a discussion of the first pandemic of plague, see J. C. Russell, "That Earlier Plague," *Demography,* V, 1968.

7. See Hirst, *op cit.,* for a discussion of the late nineteenth century pandemic.

8. F. G. Clemow, "Endemic Centers of Plague," *Journal of Tropical Medicine,* II, 1900; Biraben, *op cit.*

9. Consensus opinion; see especially W. P. MacArthur, "Old-Time Plague in Britain," *Trans. of the Royal Society of Tropical Medicine and Hygiene,* XIX, 1926.

10. Clemow, *Geography of Epidemic Disease,* pp. 310–311.

11. *Ibid.,* p. 320.

12. *Ibid.,* p. 326.

13. Biraben, *op cit.*

14. Ronald Hare, *An Outline of Bacteriology and Immunity* (London: Longmans, 1956), chap. 17; Biraben, *op cit.*

15. For a good discussion of silvatic plague, see J. F. D. Shrewsbury, *Plague of the Philistines* (London: V. Gollancz, 1964), chap. 1; and Biraben, *op cit.* As will be discussed in Appendix C, one of the major shortcomings of the Shrewsbury books is his failure to discuss the transmission of plague by rodents other than rats; authorities now agree that a wide variety of animals are capable of carrying and

transmitting plague. It is possible that rabbits can be carriers, a factor which would have been of major importance in parts of fifteenth century East Anglia. For a discussion of late medieval rabbits, see Elspeth Veale, *The English Fur Trade in the Later Middle Ages* (Oxford: Oxford University Press, 1966), pp. 209–214.

16. MacArthur, *op cit.;* Hirst, *op cit.,* pp. 154–184. Biraben, *op cit.,* takes exception to this.

17. Hirst, *op cit.,* p. 154. Shrewsbury, *Bubonic Plague in England,* takes exception to this.

18. Shrewsbury, *Bubonic Plague in England,* p. 2; R. Sharpe France, "A History of Plague in Lancashire," *Trans. Historical Society of Lancs. and Ches.,* XC, 1938, p. 6.

19. Shrewsbury, *Bubonic Plague in England,* p. 2, adds another flea, *Nosopsyllus fasciatus,* although he feels that *x. cheopis* is by far more important.

20. MacArthur, *op cit.*

21. *Ibid.*

22. *Ibid.*

23. Hirst, *op cit.,* chaps. 5 and 6.

24. W. Glen Listen, "The Plague," *British Medical Journal,* 1, 1924.

25. Biraben, *op cit.*

26. For a discussion of plague and art, see Millard Meiss, *Painting in Florence and Siena After the Black Death* (Princeton: Princeton University Press, 1951); and Anna Campbell, *The Black Death and Men of Learning* (New York: Columbia University Press, 1931).

27. However, the Arab scholar Avicenna seems to have been aware of the connections between rats, men and plague, in *Liber Canons,* Book 4, Fin. 1, Tract 4.

28. Hirst, *op cit.,* chap. 9.

29. Shrewsbury, *Bubonic Plague in England.*

30. Giovanni Boccaccio, *The Decameron,* trans. by Frances Winwar (New York: Modern Library, 1955). Boccaccio has a graphic description of the more macabre aspects of the plague.

31. Hirst, *op cit.,* chap. 7.

32. *Ibid.*

33. *Ibid.,* chap. 9.

34. Gale, *op. cit.;* Burnet and White, *op cit.;* Shrewsbury, *Bubonic Plague in England.*

35. Hirst, *op. cit.,* pp. 33–35, 222.

36. Burnet and White, *op cit.,* p. 227; Morris, *op. cit.,* p. 206.

37. Hirst, *op cit.,* chap. 7.

38. *Ibid.;* Morris, *op. cit.,* p. 206.

39. Hirst, *op. cit.,* chap. 7.

40. *Ibid.,* pp. 322–338; Wu Lien Teh, J. W. H. Chun, R. Pollitzer and C. Y. Wu, *Plague* (Geneva: W.H.O., 1926), p. 269.

41. Hirst, *op. cit.,* p. 238.

42. *Ibid.,* chap. 10.

43. See below, pp. 101–102.

44. For a discussion of influenza, see F. L. Fisher, "Inflation and Influenza in Tudor England," *Ec.H.R.,* 2nd series, XVIII, 1965.

45. Gale, *op. cit.*, pp. 51–66.

46. See Shrewsbury, *Bubonic Plague in England;* and above, pp. 50–52.

47. A. B. Appleby, "Disease or Famine? Mortality in Cumberland and West-moreland, 1580–1640," *Ec.H.R.*, 2nd series, XXVI, 1973.

48. W. P. MacArthur, *op. cit.*, XX, 1926–1927.

49. For a good discussion, see Gale, *op. cit.*

50. Reference should be made to the table in Chapter 2.

51. This judgment was made on the basis of surviving treatise copies in England, and on cross-references among the treatise writers themselves. For a full discussion of this, and a more complete listing of surviving European treatises, see D.W. Singer, "Some Plague Tractates in the Fourteenth and Fifteenth Centuries," *Proc. Royal Society of Medicine*, 92, 1916. For a listing of the treatises used in chap. 3, see the bibliography.

52. *Ibid.*, p. 170.

53. *Ibid.*

54. John La Barba, British Museum, Sloane Ms. 3449, f. 5b, f. 7; also John of Bordeaux, British Museum, Sloane Ms. 965 (VIII), f. 132.

55. John La Barba, *op. cit.*, ff. 7–7b.

56. *Ibid.*, ff. 8b–9.

57. *Ibid.*

58. *Ibid.*, ff. 9b–10.

59. *Ibid.*, ff. 5b–6b.

60. R. R. Bolgar, *The Classical Heritage* (Cambridge: Cambridge Univ. Press, 1954) discusses the influence of Galen on late medieval thinkers.

61. John La Barba, *op. cit.*, f. 5b.

62. See above, p. 40.

63. John of Bordeau, *op. cit.*, f. 132. This manuscript is adorned with a frontispiece of a naked male, with astrological labels on various parts of the body.

64. Singer, *op. cit.*, p. 173.

65. John of Bordeaux, *op. cit.*, ff. 133–134b.

66. *Ibid.*, ff. 134b–137.

67. *Ibid.*, f. 137. Physicians are referred to throughout the John of Bordeaux treatise as "leches," and at one point, God is called the "head lech."

68. Bengt Knuttson, British Museum, Sloane Ms. 2276. One edition of the Knuttson treatise has been reprinted in the John Rylands Facsimiles collection as *A Litel Boke . . . for the . . . Pestilence*, edited by Guthrie Vine (Manchester: John Rylands Library, 1910). Also see Singer, *op. cit.*, pp. 183–184.

69. *A Litel Boke*, pp. xi–xii.

70. *Ibid.*, pp. xvi–xxxvi; Knuttson Ms. 2276, f. 191.

71. Singer, *op. cit.*, p. 179.

72. *A Litel Boke*, f. 1b.

73. *Ibid.*, ff. 6–6b. Knuttson was especially concerned with "fleys."

74. *Ibid.*, ff. 2–4b.

75. *Ibid.*, f. 3, ff. 4b–5.

76. *Ibid.*, f. 5.

77. *Ibid.*

78. See, for example, *The Brut: Chronicles of England,* edited by F.W.D. Brie (London: Oxford Univ. Press, 1960), II, p. 467.

79. *A Litel Boke,* ff. 5–5b.

80. *Ibid.,* f. 5–5b.

81. *Ibid.*

82. *Ibid.*

83. *Ibid.*

84. *Ibid.,* f. 3.

85. *Ibid.,* f. 6.

86. Knuttson, Ms. 2276, f. 191.

87. *A Litel Boke,* f. 3b.

88. *Ibid.,* ff. 4–5.

89. *Ibid.,* f. 4.

90. *Ibid.,* ff. 4–4b.

91. *Ibid.,* f. 6.

92. Charles Creighton, *A History of Epidemics in Britain* (London: Frank Cass, 1965), I, pp. 174–176.

93. British Museum, additional Ms., 27582, f. 70; printed volume, British Museum dated 1490, and said to have been printed then. Also, see Singer, *op. cit.*

94. British Museum, Ms. 27582, f. 70.

95. Singer, *op. cit.,* pp. 196–197.

96. *Calendar of Patent Rolls,* Henry VII, vol. I, p. 202. Forestier was pardoned for previous offenses.

97. Singer, *op. cit.,* p. 179.

98. Thomas Forestier, *Tractus contra pestilentiam thenasmonem et dissenterium* (Rouen: 1490). As there are no folio page numbers in the printed edition, it is not possible to list them when noting various statements. Therefore, only chapter numbers will be given, when possible. In this case, the chapters are Capitulum IX and Capitulum XII; they are entitled, respectively, "De Empericus ignaris et vetulis," and "De Apothecarius fidelibus quibus in firmi et pauperes . . ."

99. *Ibid.*

100. British Museum, Ms. 27582, ff. 76–77.

101. *Ibid.,* f. 72.

102. *Ibid.*

103. *Ibid.*

104. Forestier, *op. cit.,* Capitulum I.

105. *Ibid.;* also, British Museum, Ms. 27582, f. 70.

106. Forestier, *op. cit.,* Capitulum IX.

107. Cambridge University Library, Ms. LL1 18, *Medica,* f. 3.

108. *Ibid.,* ff. 3–14, 59–81, for pestilence and sickness; ff. 20–48 and 49–50 for "biological" treatises.

109. *Ibid.,* ff. 10–13.

110. *Ibid.,* ff. 3–3b.

111. *Ibid.,* ff. 3, 10–13.

112. *Ibid.,* ff. 10–13.

113. *Ibid.,* f. 12.

114. *Ibid.*, f. 9b.

115. *Ibid.*, ff. 3–4.

116. *Ibid.*, f. 3.

117. *Ibid.*, f. 3b.

118. *Ibid.*, f. 3.

119. *Ibid.*, f. 20.

120. *Ibid.*, f. 75b.

121. *Ibid.*, f. 3.

122. *Ibid.*

123. British Museum, Sloane Ms. 965 (IX), f. 143.

124. British Museum, Sloane Ms. 783B (XXIII), f. 206.

125. See above, pp. 63–65; for a discussion of the treatise of John of Jacobus, see Singer, *op. cit.*, p. 179.

126. British Museum, Sloane Ms. 404 (III) and 2276.

127. Medical Society of London, Ms. 136, ff. 1–95. It has been edited and printed as follows: W. R. Dawson, ed., *A Leechbook or Collection of Medical Recipes of the Fifteenth Century* (London: Macmillan, 1934).

128. Dawson, *Ibid.*, p. 3.

129. For a discussion of the text as a whole, see Dawson, *Ibid.*, pp. 1–17.

130. *Ibid.*, pp. 47–49, 126–127.

131. *Ibid.*, pp. 126–127.

132. *Ibid.*, pp. 46–47.

133. *Ibid.*, pp. 47–49.

134. *Ibid.*, pp. 148–149.

135. *Ibid.*, pp. 46–49, 126–129, 172–173, 194–195.

136. *Ibid.*, pp. 236–237.

137. *Ibid.*, pp. 135–143.

138. *Ibid.*, pp. 23–25.

139. *Ibid.*, pp. 318–319, 320–321, 326–327.

140. *Ibid.*, pp. 320–321.

141. *Ibid.*, pp. 326–327.

142. *Ibid.*

143. *Ibid.*

144. *Ibid.*

145. *Ibid.*

146. See above, p. 67, and p. 75.

147. Dawson, *op. cit.*, pp. 96–97.

148. *Ibid.*, pp. 234–235.

149. "Recipe for Edward IV's Plague Medicine," *Notes and Queries*, 1878, p. 343.

150. Most of these remedies come from Dawson, *op. cit.* Also, see France, *op.cit.*

151. France, *op. cit.*

152. Society of Antiquaries, Ms. 101, f. 1b.

153. See above, pp. 61–63.

154. Society of Antiquaries, Ms. 101, f. 1b.

155. *Ibid.*

156. *Ibid.*

157. *Ibid.*

158. Langland was especially interested in plague. See Langland, *Piers the Ploughman*, edited by J. F. Goodridge (Baltimore: Penguin, 1966), p. 26, for example.

159. Society of Antiquaries, Ms. 101, ff. 43–43b.

160. *Ibid.*

161. *Ibid.*

162. *Ibid.*

163. *Ibid.*, f. 43b.

164. *Ibid.*, ff. 43–43b.

165. John Stanbridge, British Museum, Arundel Ms. 249. Printed and edited as follows: William Nelson, ed., *A Fifteenth Century School Book* (Oxford: Clarendon Press, 1956).

166. Nelson, *Ibid.*, pp. 4–12.

167. British Museum, Arundel Ms. 249, f. 33. For other references to food, see ff. 32, 33, 44, among others.

168. *Ibid.*, f. 56.

169. *Ibid.*, f. 34.

170. See Peter Laslett, *The World We Have Lost* (New York: Scribners, 1965), and Pierre Goubert, *Beauvais et le Beauvaisis* (Paris: S.E.V.P.E.N., 1960), for the problem of distinguishing between deaths caused by disease, and those caused or abetted by food shortages and famine.

171. British Museum, Arundel Ms. 249, f. 45. See below, pp. 183–189 for a discussion of the seasonal frequency of plague.

172. See above, footnote 116.

173. Biraben, *op. cit.*, and Clemow, *Geography of Epidemic Disease*, discuss the frequency of plague among rural, "wild" rodents.

174. British Museum, Arundel Ms. 249, f. 19.

175. *Ibid.*, f. 29.

176. *Ibid.*, ff. 19 and 29. For the first quotation, for example, the phrase *solum natale* is used.

177. See below, pp. 118–121.

178. *Paston Letters*, III, p. 254.

179. British Museum, Arundel Ms. 249, f. 52.

180. *Ibid.*, f.12.

# CHAPTER IV

# *Patterns of Mortality, I*

## 4.1 The Graphed Testamentary Data: Testing the Accuracy of the Literary Sources

There is a striking correlation between mortality as indicated by the narrative sources' reports of epidemic disease, and mortality as indicated by the clustering of probated wills. Almost without exception, graphs made from the raw totals of probated wills and broken into the jurisdictions of their ecclesiastical courts and regions, peak during the periods of epidemic disease reported in the narrative sources, and then fall below normal levels almost immediately after the quarters of highest will mortality.

The most dramatic testamentary results occur in 1479, the year of the fifteenth century's most virulent epidemic. The Consistory Court of Norwich (N.C.C.) is especially complete for the 1470's. The graphed testamentary mortality (Graph 4.1.1,1.–4.1.1,3) for the five-year period preceding 1479 shows a typical fluctuating pattern of between 10 and 43 wills probated per quarter. This includes 1475, the year of the French Pox. The year 1479 itself began with a modest total of 21 N.C.C. deaths from December to February, 35 for March to May, and 28 for June to August. Between September and November, the number of probated wills shot up to 179, an increase of over fourfold from the highest level of any quarter year in the previous five years. Additionally, there were intestate recordings for the fall, 1479, the first such records in the N.C.C. in nine quarters, which add further to the death count. Mortality then dropped almost as rapidly as it had risen, falling to 86 for the winter quarter, 1479–1480, and then to 21 in the spring of 1420, a level approximately maintained for the rest of the year. As we shall see in section 4.3, this was probably the usual pattern of plague mortality in pre-industrial England.[1] It was particularly indicative of bubonic plague, with the relatively short duration of protracted, severe mortality in the fall quarter.[2] The comparative fall in numbers of deaths in the winter months of 1479–1480 may indicate that the pneumonial infections characteristic of pneumonic plague were not as important a factor in the epidemic as the narrative sources may lead the historian to believe.[3]

This pattern of high, autumnal 1479 mortality was repeated in the archdeaconry court of St. Albans (Graph 4.1.3, 3) and the sacrist peculiar court of Bury St. Edmunds (B.S.E.) (Graph 4.1.2, 3). In the Bury St. Edmunds court the numbers of probated wills were almost three times greater than the highest totals of previous five years, and rose by almost five times over the probates of the quarter June to August, 1479. As with the wills proved in the N.C.C., the number of probates in B.S.E. began to fall gradually in the winter quarter, 1479–1480, and dramatically in the ensuing spring quarter. Corroborating this pattern is a very large rise in the numbers of letters of administration filed independently in the court for the autumn, 1479. They increased in the fall quarter in far larger numbers than at any other time in the fifty-year period, 1430 to 1480.[4]

In the archdeaconry of St. Albans, the number of probated wills was nearly three times greater than at any other time in the preceding five-year period. Mortality, as in the N.C.C. and peculiar court of B.S.E., began to taper off in the winter quarter, and fall precipitously in the spring. However, the pattern in the archdeaconry court of St. Albans was different in certain respects. Numbers of deaths reached an apex in the autumn, 1479, but began to rise dramatically in the month of August. Further, deaths in the town of St. Albans itself, the seat and heart of the archdeaconry, as well as its largest urban center, not only began to rise in the summer quarter of 1479, but actually peaked in the month of August, and declined somewhat in the fall. Judging from this admittedly incomplete evidence, it may be that the epidemic of 1479 first struck in St. Albans, and then passed through Suffolk and into Norfolk.[5]

For a more thorough analysis of the path of the epidemic of 1479, a study of the patterns of mortality of the wills of the archdeaconry courts of the county of Suffolk is necessary. Unfortunately, in the archdeaconry courts of neither Suffolk nor Sudbury, the courts which would be most sensitive to the advances of the epidemic on the local level, do wills survive in complete form from 1477 to 1480. This is an intriguing problem, and will be discussed in some detail below.[6] Yet despite obvious deficiencies in registration or survival for both Suffolk archdeaconry courts for 1479,

*Graph 4.1.1, 1*

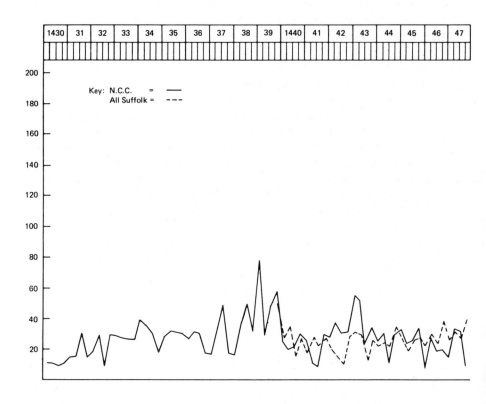

*Graph 4.1.1, 2*

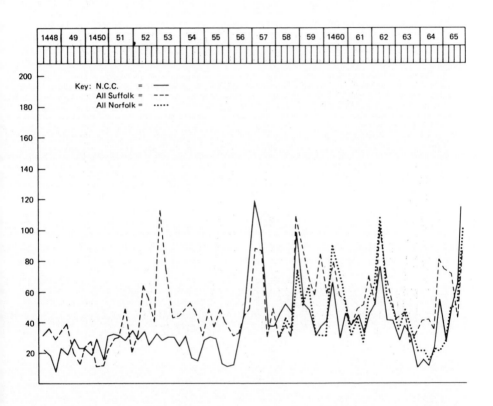

*Graph 4.1.1, 3*

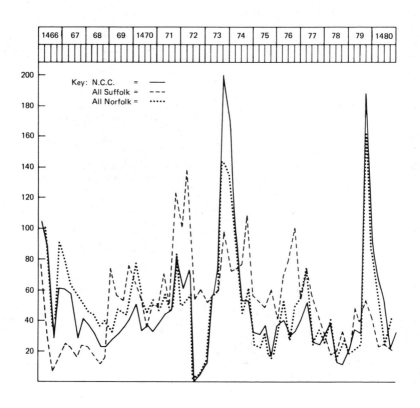

*Graph 4.1.2, 1*

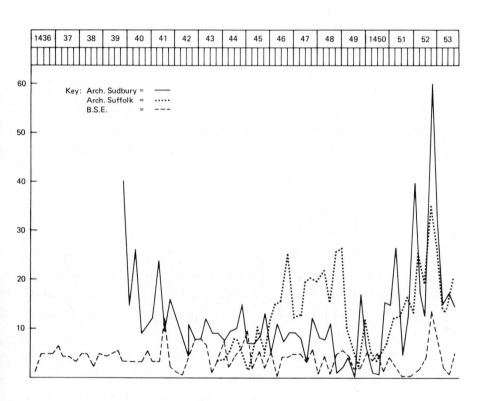

*Graph 4.1.2, 2*

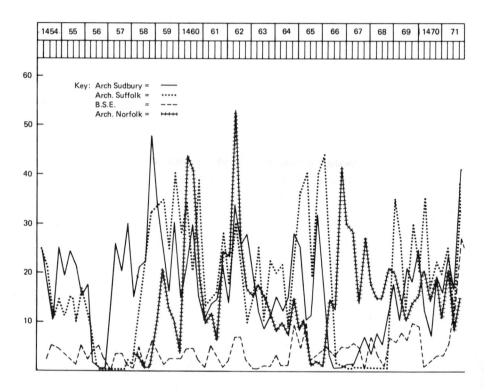

*Graph 4.1.2, 3*

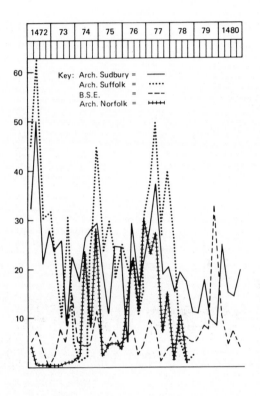

Key: Arch. Sudbury = ———
     Arch. Suffolk = ·······
     B.S.E.        = – – –
     Arch. Norfolk = ╟╫╫┤

*Graph 4.1.3, 1*

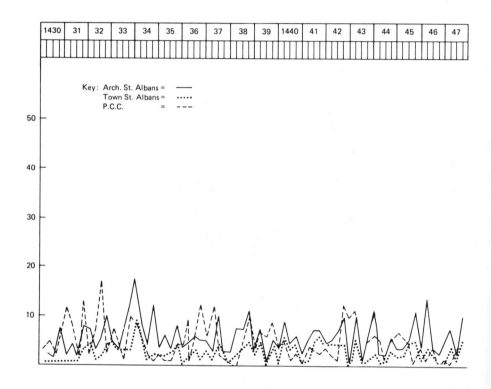

*Graph 4.1.3, 2*

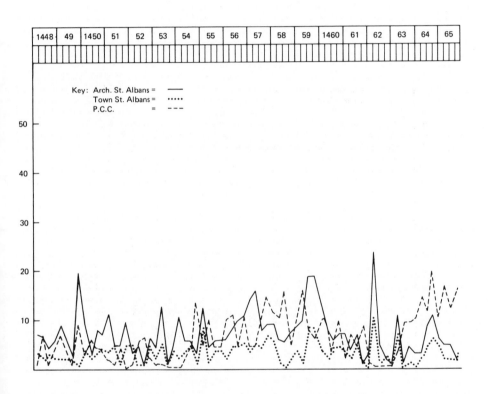

| 1448 | 49 | 1450 | 51 | 52 | 53 | 54 | 55 | 56 | 57 | 58 | 59 | 1460 | 61 | 62 | 63 | 64 | 65 |

Key:  Arch. St. Albans = ——
      Town St. Albans = •••••
      P.C.C.          = – – –

*Graph 4.1.3, 3*

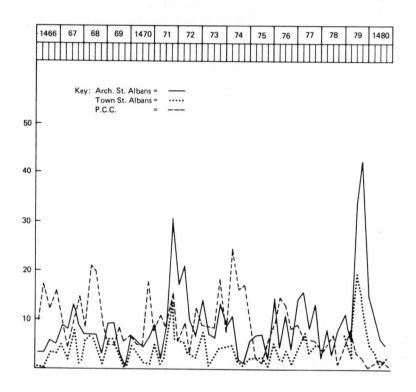

there is still evidence in them of increasing mortality. The rise in probated wills and letters of administration for B.S.E. has already been mentioned; but there was also a further rise in those few Bury wills which were registered in the archdeaconry courts. The total number of aggregate probated wills from all the courts having jurisdiction in Suffolk—that is, the N.C.C., B.S.E., and the two archdeaconry courts (Graph 4.1.1, 2)— also show a significant rise for the autumn, 1479, a rise of nearly fourfold from the totals of the previous quarter. Wills from the county of Suffolk, regardless of archdeaconry jurisdiction, appear in the N.C.C. in considerable numbers for the first time in over two years. For the archdeaconry court of Sudbury, where some wills do survive for 1478 and 1479, there was a noticeable mortality peak (Graph 4.1.2, 3) for late fall, early winter 1479–1480. Further, there is a separate listing of additional 1479–1480 wills from the Sudbury archdeaconry in a register which otherwise contains wills only from the sixteenth century. Finally, there was a considerable increase in the number of independently filed "probates only."

There is little question of the presence and virulence of the epidemic of 1479; it is reported by virtually all of the chroniclers writing at the time, and is apparent from the testamentary evidence. Its duration, however, is not as certain. According to two chronicles, it began in 1478, the year the "ducke of Clarans" was killed;[7] others say it began in the spring of 1479, and endured through the following winter;[8] and still others restrict it only to the fall, 1479.[9] The first claim can be safely dismissed. No original record other than the solitary recording in the *Chronicles of the Grey Friars* suggests that the epidemic began in 1478. Creighton's suppositions seem to be entirely unfounded,[10] as all of the testamentary and independent probate data indicate that 1478 was a year of unusually low mortality. For similar reasons, claims that the epidemic began in the spring, 1479, can also probably be discounted. That the epidemic may have begun in the summer of 1479 is a distinct possibility; wills from the town of St. Albans did show a mortality peak in the summer quarter. Also, we have substantial literary evidence from both the visitation records of Southwell Minster and the *Paston Letters* that the pestilence was in full swing by July and August. Further, Fabyan's restriction of the epidemic exclusively to the autumn, 1479, is made primarily for the city of London.[11]

It would seem for all the above reasons that the epidemic of 1479 had already broken out in some parts of eastern England by, at latest, August, 1479. The system used to determine the date of death from the wills is by its very nature bound to show at least a week or two lag in recording the testator's death. If this is so, and if the admonitions in the Southwell visitation records were not so much a report of things current as they were a rumor and a preventive measure for things to come, then the epidemic of 1479 began in early August, was at its most virulent in the early autumn, and persisted through at least the early months of the ensuing winter quarter.

The correlation between numbers of probated wills and their clustering patterns, and the chroniclers' observations, is strikingly close for almost all of the national epidemics which struck England during the period 1430–1480. The epidemics of the 1430's are not as well corroborated by the testamentary evidence as are those of the other four decades because of less complete will registration.[12] Nonetheless, the tell-tale zeniths and nadirs characteristic of epidemic periods and their aftermaths can still be seen from the graphed results. In Hertfordshire, probates rose in the autumn, 1433, and peaked in the winter, 1433–1434 (Graph 4.1.3, 1); in St. Albans town itself, the period of highest mortality was somewhat later, rising and peaking in the winter quarter, 1433–1434, and extending into the spring, 1434 (Graph 4.1.3, 1). For the N.C.C. (Graph 4.1.1, 1), total mortality as exhibited by the probates and intestate listings peaked during the winter, 1433–1434, and gradually fell to a nadir in the summer, 1434. It should be noted again, however, that the will data for much of the 1430's is incomplete even for the N.C.C.; for the archdeaconry courts of Suffolk and Sudbury and the peculiar court of B.S.E., there are no reliable probate data for most of this decade.

The national epidemic of 1438–1439 is a bit more fully documented than that of 1433–1435. Unlike the epidemic of 1479 and the epidemics of the 1470's in general, but like the epidemic of 1433–1435, mortality appears to have been protracted and drawn out, as the chronicles reported, and not short and sharp. The patterns of mortality set by the wills from the N.C.C. (Graph 4.1.1, 1) for the years 1438–1439 are especially interesting; this evidence is corroborated by the accompanying list of intestate deaths (Graph 4.1.1, 1), which in all cases paralleled the probate evidence. From a low point in 1437, mortality rose 4.5 times through the winter to a spring, 1438, peak. There was a drop in mortality in the summer, a rise to a twenty-year peak in the autumn of 1438, another drop for the next three quarters, and another rise in the autumn, 1439. This protracted period of epidemic disease was probably plague, but there were undoubtedly complications caused by the poor harvests mentioned by the chroniclers, and the prolonged period of bad winters that seem to have persisted, quite literally, for nearly a decade.[13] Ironically, it was not so much cold weather the chroniclers complained about in the period 1438 to 1440, but rather unusually wet weather. It is likely that the lack of severe cold during the course of the epidemic of 1438–1439 was responsible for the comparatively low winter death tolls; if plague were present, pneumonic plague probably was not a major factor. This is in contrast with the epidemic of 1433–1435, when mortality peaked during the winter months and when the meteorological complaints of the literary sources centered around unusually cold weather.[14] The two archdeaconry courts which have some probate data for this period also indicate a protracted time of high mortality. The record of wills from the archdeaconry court of Sudbury begins in the autumn, 1439, at a mortality peak it would not reach again for two decades (Graph 4.1.2, 1). In the archdeaconry court of St. Albans, where the data are admittedly very poor, will probates peaked during the autumn of 1438, the spring of 1439, and again in the fall of 1439 (Graph 4.1.3, 1).

The next series of major peaks in the testamentary mortality came in the early 1450's, at a time when the Rolls of Parliament say that Commons was constantly fleeing London because of pestilence, foul and unhealthy air, and high mortality.[15] Evidence from the wills indicates that the high mortality and perhaps epidemic disease were not confined to just the city of London and its suburbs. Suffolk in particular seems to have suffered during this period. In all four county Suffolk courts (Graph 4.1.1, 1; Graph 4.1.2, 1) there were prolonged and severe peaks in mortality. They are most evident in the archdeaconry of Sudbury, where, from a low point in summer, 1451, numbers of probated wills rose markedly and sharply to a peak in the winter quarter, 1451–1452. This peak was more than eight times higher than the summer, 1451, level. After a decline in probate numbers in the spring and summer, 1452, a new high in mortality was reached in the autumn, 1452, when the epidemic appears to have been at its most virulent; this peak was twelve times greater than the nadir of summer, 1451.

The dramatic patterns in Sudbury were repeated in the peculiar court of Bury St. Edmunds (Graph 4.1.2, 1). Here too mortality rose to an apex in the fall quarter, 1452. In the archdeaconry court of Suffolk (Graph 4.1.2, 1), the number of wills probated increased steadily from a low point in the winter, 1450–1451, again to a high in the autumn, 1452. The increase here was sevenfold, with another, slightly smaller peak in the spring, 1452. Taken together, and along with the county Suffolk wills from the N.C.C., the fall of 1452 was the period of highest numbers of wills probated in Suffolk from 1430 to 1470. And all the registers, though compiled independently of one another, show mortality peaks in the autumn, 1452, and the winter, 1452–1453.

London, if the literary sources are to be believed,[16] and Suffolk, if the testamentary sources are to be believed, suffered far more than Norfolk or Hertfordshire did in 1452–1453. Although there was a slight increase in testamentary mortality in Norfolk from 1451 to 1454 (Graph 4.1.1, 2), there were none of the dramatic peaks and troughs so evident in the Suffolk courts, and so characteristic of epidemic mortality. In Hertfordshire, the archdeaconry court of St. Albans (Graph 4.1.3,2) showed no rise which can be construed as characteristic of an epidemic period. This leaves an interesting problem: a period of limited, but more than local, epidemic. The repeated admonitions of the parliamentary rolls speak convincingly of an epidemic in the largest city in England, and the testamentary evidence does the same for the county of Suffolk. Yet the two other counties surveyed, Norfolk and Hertfordshire, and partial returns from two further counties, Kent and Yorkshire,[17] give no indication of high mortality nor of the presence of epidemic disease. Within the relatively small area covered, the epidemic of 1452–1453 appears to have been limited in scope, with no apparent geographical patterns to its distribution.[18]

Herryson's chronicle and the Infirmarer's Rolls from St. Etheldreda Abbey in Ely speak of pestilence in Cambridgeshire and Ely in 1458 and 1459.[19] The graphed data show widespread crisis mortality throughout all of East Anglia, not from 1458–1459, but from 1457 to 1459. Probate numbers were highest in the autumn quarters of 1458 and 1459 for all courts within the consistory court of Norwich jurisdiction, and particularly for the city of Norwich. In 1457, however, mortality was highest not in the fall, but in the winter. For the consistory court of Norwich itself, much of the "mortality" peak was due to the preemption and subsequent inclusion of the archdeaconry court wills in the bishop's court, but some of the rise was due to an actual increase in mortality. This is in accordance with the testamentary patterns in the archdeaconry of St. Albans, where there was also a late winter, early spring mortality apex in 1457. Taken as a whole, mortality levels in the winter, 1457, and autumn, 1458, the peak crisis mortality quarters, were approximate to those reached in 1452, 1462 and 1465. Although the numbers of N.C.C. wills were artificially swollen, there can be little doubt as to the extreme virulence of the epidemic or series of epidemics of the late 1450's, probably bubonic and perhaps pneumonic plague.

The narrative sources tell us that the next extended period of epidemic disease occurred in the 1460's. The earliest peak in mortality in the decade came in Hertfordshire. After a period of fluctuating but not atypical pre-industrial mortality,[20] there was a sudden and precipitous rise in will probates for the spring quarter, 1462 (Graph 4.1.3,2). This pattern of high spring mortality was repeated, somewhat less dramatically, for 1463, a reputed period of bad weather. In 1464, the plague pattern reappeared throughout the archdeaconry.[21] But, at least in Hertfordshire, the virulence of the plague epidemics of the 1430's was not repeated, and mortality soon dropped back to normal levels.

Mortality throughout Suffolk in the early 1460's was significantly greater. As in Hertfordshire, probate numbers for the three exclusively Suffolk courts (Graph 4.1.2,2) peaked in the spring, 1462. Interestingly enough, no plague or pestilence was reported in the narrative sources in this year, and the only epidemic which was recorded was called a "pockys."[22] Whatever the correct aetiological identity of the pox, it had a spring apex, and a decidedly nonplague pattern of death. The mortality patterns were especially severe in the parishes of the archdeaconry of Sudbury, where the peak in probates in spring, 1462, was merely the culmination of an extended rise in mortality dating back to the winter quarter, 1461, and in the archdeaconry of Norfolk. Further, in the archdeaconry courts of both Suffolk and Sudbury, there were additional peaks in the numbers of wills probated in the autumn, 1461.

The data from the N.C.C. (Graph 4.1.1,2) indicate that the "pockys" of 1462 was certainly regional and probably national in its scope. As was the case with the other courts, there was a peak in numbers of probates in the spring, 1462. Further, in Norwich, this was matched almost precisely by the accompanying record of intestate deaths (Graph 4.1.1,2). Thus, despite the lack of supporting references from the literary sources, the pox was an epidemic of major proportions. It infected large areas of eastern England, and was almost certainly not an epidemic of plague.

The chronicles report an epidemic in 1464–1465, and the testamentary sources indicate that it was plague. Like the wills of the archdeaconry court of St. Albans, those from the ecclesiastical courts of East Anglia peak in this period (Graph 4.1.1,2; Graph 4.1.2,2). A reference from a Venetian merchant tells us that a pestilence raged from the autumn, 1464, and a Paston letter speaks of "pestylens" in the following year.[23] In the archdeaconry of Sudbury, wills clustered in the characteristic autumnal patterns for 1464 and 1465; and in the archdeaconry of Suffolk, there were autumn and winter mortality peaks for both years. In B.S.E., mortality began to rise in the fall, 1464, but did not peak until the spring quarter of the following year. The wills proved in the N.C.C., the center of which was farther from London, where the Venetian observer felt the pestilence was at its strongest in the autumn, 1464, also peaked in both 1464 and 1465, and are corroborated by the accompanying intestate data. Curiously, in the wills proved in the N.C.C. from the city of Norwich itself, mortality reached a high point in the autumn, 1464. This period is reported by the chroniclers as being one of protracted cold, and not only plague but influenza, typhus, or pneumonial complications may have been responsible for the high mortality. Whatever the aetiology of the epidemic or epidemics of 1464–1465, it or they produced a long and extensive period of abnormally high mortality.

The narrative sources also reported a national epidemic of pestilence in 1467.[24] But unlike 1462 and 1464–1465, the testamentary evidence for 1467 shows few of the signs of high mortality caused by epidemic disease. Probates for all the courts surveyed ran at around normal levels, although the absence of large clusterings of wills may be due to the extensive periods of prolonged, severe mortality of the early 1460's. In Hertford-shire in general and St. Albans in particular there were slight mortality peaks in the summer of 1467 (Graph 4.1.3,2). In the N.C.C. there were winter, 1466–1467, and slight autumn, 1467, peaks both in probated wills and intestate listings (Graph 4.1.1,2). Unfortunately, there are no surviv-ing records of wills proved in the archdeaconry courts of either Suffolk or Sudbury for 1467, due either to inhibition of the lower courts or to the loss of the will registers; since the simultaneous loss of both registers is not probable, inhibition and subsequent preemption by the consistory court is most likely. In the peculiar court of Bury St. Edmunds, however, there were no perceptible increases in mortality throughout the entire year of 1467 (Graph 4.1.2,3). Thus, while the presence of an epidemic in eastern England in 1467 cannot be discounted, it cannot have been too severe in its effect.

In sum, for the protracted period of epidemic disease from spring, 1462, until autumn, 1467, one of the three major periods of almost continual epidemic disease in the half-century 1430 to 1480, the following statements can be made. First, the epidemic and ensuing heavy mortality for spring, 1462, was certainly not due to plague. The unusually short, springtime death clustering pattern was probably the result of the "pockys," which is actually reported to have taken place later in the year.[25] Severe weather conditions may have played a part in the heavy mortality also, for 1463 as well as for 1462. The pestilences reported in 1464–1465 and 1467 were probably plague, with at least the former showing heavy autumnal mortality clustering. Yet even in the case of these two epidemics, bad weather and conceivably a poor harvest could have played a major role in the high death figures, and may possibly have linked the peak mortality periods of the autumns of 1464 and 1465. Assuming that much of the high mortality in 1464–1465 was due to plague, then it appears that as in the 1430's, plague moved northward and westward through eastern England, into Norfolk.[26]

In both the testamentary and literary sources, the decade of the 1470's appears as one of almost continual national epidemics and inordinately high mortality. It was the third major period of continual epidemic disease in the years 1430 to 1480. Like the other two periods, the 1430's and the early and mid-1460's, the 1470's was a decade of bad weather. The effects of the epidemic of 1479 have already been discussed; the testamentary data show that the epidemics of 1471 and 1473 were only slightly less lethal.

In the N.C.C., in the autumn of 1471, there was a sharp, well-defined rise in numbers of both probated wills and intestate deaths (Graph 4.1.1,3). Hertfordshire too (Graph 4.1.3,3) experienced a large increase in testamentary mortality of over three times the previous year's high. In both courts, there was a slight decline during the winter, 1471–1472, and an increase again in the ensuing spring. An identical pattern can be found in the wills proved in the peculiar court of Bury St. Edmunds (Graph 4.1.2,2). Both patterns appear to be the result of bubonic plague.[27] Mortality from the archdeaconry courts of Suffolk and Sudbury (Graph 4.1.2,2) was even greater. Numbers of probates in both jurisdictions rose and reached peaks in the autumn, 1471. But unlike the clusterings of wills in the other courts, the totals for the Suffolk archdeaconries continued to rise. The archdeaconry of Sudbury showed a slight decline during the ensuing winter before reaching a spring mortality apex, but mortality from the Suffolk archdeaconry court rose steadily from the autumn, through the winter, to a fifty-year high point in the spring, 1472. All of the courts surveyed then exhibited a drop in wills probated until the next major epidemic—a mere year and a half away! To John Paston, the epidemic of 1471 was the "most universalle dethe" he had ever seen;[28] ironically enough, it appears to have been least virulent in his native Norfolk.

The national epidemic of 1473 is especially interesting because the narrative sources were so vehement in their claims that this epidemic was one of the "blody flyx," flux, or intestinal dysentery.[29] If this were correct, the historian can expect to find slightly different patterns of mortality in 1473 from those of the pestilences of 1471 and 1479, and far different patterns from the pox of 1462, with their respective autumn and spring peaks of mortality. If the epidemic were one of dysentery, then peak mortality might ordinarily be expected in the late summer, the period of highest temperatures, and thus far, lowest mortality. However, this seasonal equation must not be carried too far; epidemic diseases do change over long periods of time, and Warkworth tells us that it was "in harvist tyme" that "men fylle downe sodanly."[30]

Mortality as indicated by the testamentary sources was indeed well above normal for 1473, and the mortality peaks came predominantly in September. The only summer quarter peaks came from the wills proved in the archdeaconry court of Suffolk; and in one of the courts, the archdeaconry of Sudbury (Graph 4.1.2,2), the summer of 1473 saw the lowest number of probated wills in the five-year period of 1471–1475. But particular quarters of will clusterings aside, total crude mortality was very high. The largest individual will death toll for the fifty-year period of 1430 to 1480 for any court came from the N.C.C. for the autumn, 1473, a toll which is increased by additional intestate recordings (Graph 4.1.1,2). Testamentary mortality remained extremely high throughout the winter, 1473–1474—far higher, in fact, and less sharply defined than mortality in 1471 and 1479, apparent plague years. Both the peculiar court of B.S.E. and the archdeaconry court of Sudbury had autumn, 1473, peaks in probated wills (Graph 4.1.2,2), as did the aggregate total of all county Suffolk wills (Graph 4.1.1,2), archdeaconry of Suffolk included. In Hertfordshire, however, there is no evidence of the presence of epidemic disease at all for 1473. There were slight peaks of mortality for the archdeaconry of St. Albans as a whole during the winter, 1472–1473, and a fairly pronounced peak for the town of St. Albans during the same period (Graph 4.1.3,3), but only a very gradual rise during the ensuing spring, summer and autumn quarters. Far from seeming "epidemic," the patterns of mortality for Hertfordshire for 1473 appear to have followed the general fluctuating course of nonepidemic pre-industrial mortality.[31]

The epidemic of 1473 was different from the other outburst of infectious disease in the period 1430–1480. Probably, it was dysentery. Mortality was greatest at "harvest tyme," just as Warkworth, if not modern works on infectious disease, advised. The general patterns of mortality were considerably different from the pestilences of the 1460's and 1470's and the pox of 1462. Perhaps most significant was the absence of evidence of the flux from Hertfordshire; plague is generally far wider spread in true epidemic form than is dysentery.[32] Along with the epidemic of 1452, that of 1473 was unique among the so-called national (or in this case, regional) epidemics in that it was not found throughout the relatively small region being examined. For the flux of 1473, the descriptions of the chroniclers appear to have been quite accurate.

From about 1477, there was a decline in the number of wills registered in the archdeaconry courts of Sudbury and Suffolk (Graph 4.1.2,3), and in the wills from all Suffolk registered in the N.C.C. (Graph 4.1.1,2). This was most noticeable in the archdeaconry of Suffolk, where the registration of wills seems literally to have stopped from the winter, 1477–1478, and in the Suffolk wills in the N.C.C., where with the exception of the autumn quarter of 1479, the same thing happens from 1478. Even in the generally consistent archdeaconry court of Sudbury, there was a sharp drop in the number of registered wills from 1477 to 1480. Part, perhaps most of this drop is due to the loss or expropriation for one reason or another of the wills or will registers. But some part of the decline may be due to an actual drop in the population of the county of Suffolk. Of all the areas, Suffolk seems to be the one most frequently and most severely hit by epidemic disease. The effects of successive epidemics of 1462, 1464–1465, 1467, 1471, 1473 and 1479 have already been shown. Additionally, Suffolk appears to have suffered from yet another severe period of crisis mortality in 1477, when there were extremely large and protracted periods of probate clusterings in both archdeaconry courts in Suffolk, the peculiar court of B.S.E., and the county Suffolk wills registered in the N.C.C. Whether the 1477 crisis mortality was the result of an epidemic, as has been argued,[33] or whether it was the result of something else, is for the moment inconsequential; the fact remains that Suffolk suffered from an additional period of high, crisis-proportion mortality. Thus, in less than eighteen years, the county had at least nine years during which there existed quarters of abnormally excessive mortality. Further, in the next chapter it will be argued that several areas in Suffolk were especially susceptible to endemic disease in nonepidemic years.[34] Although fertility, among other factors, must be discussed before statements about the overall movement of Suffolk population can be made, the evidence of extremely high mortality in the county cannot be discounted.

The testamentary patterns of mortality of those epidemics which were less than national or even regional in scope are more difficult to discern, discuss aetiologically, and measure statistically. Further, with these lesser outbreaks of epidemic disease the intriguing possibility of local flareups of endemic disease exists, as suggested by John La Barba.[35] There are three reports of epidemic disease in Kent and Hertfordshire in 1431.[36] The evidence for this year is far too spare to make meaningful comments on the possibility of the presence of epidemic disease (Graph 4.1.3,1), but testamentary mortality for the archdeaconry of St. Albans does conform to the plague pattern. There was also a slight autumn peak for wills proved in the N.C.C. (Graph 4.1.1,1), and it may well be that the pestilence of 1431 was a minor outbreak of plague in parts of the region covered within this thesis.

Although there is no record of the presence of an epidemic in 1431, many of the local epidemics mentioned by the chroniclers between 1430 and 1480 were restricted by them to the city of London and its suburbs. Unfortunately, London wills used in this sample came exclusively from the P.C.C., the court with the highest registration fees, and therefore the one least representative and least sensitive to the effects of epidemic disease. Analysis of the effect of epidemic disease in London, consequently, must come from the nearby jurisdiction of the archdeaconry of St. Albans, and whatever clues the wills from the P.C.C. can give us.

According to the St. Albans chronicler Amundesham, there was an outbreak of pestilence in the city of London in 1437.[37] In the town of St. Albans (Graph 4.1.3, 1) there was an increase in probate mortality during the spring quarter, 1437, though the data are far too small to generalize upon. There is, however, more ample evidence from the N.C.C. (Graph 4.1.1,1). There, an increase in probates can be seen for the spring, 1437, although this may be attributable to the severe weather conditions of the late 1430's. In a larger sense, the local incidence of high mortality in 1437 was the beginning of a four-year upward trend in mortality which culminated in the major national epidemic of 1438–1439.

Of the local epidemics reported by the narrative sources in the period 1442–1463, four, excluding 1452, were restricted to the city of London and its immediate environs.[38] If these epidemics were anything more than local in scope, some trace of crisis-level mortality could be expected for neighboring Hertfordshire. Although again numerically very small, the archdeaconry of St. Albans testamentary patterns showed mortality peaks for spring, 1443, and winter, 1443–1444 (Graph 4.1.3,1). Since the report of *gravis pestilentia* in the parliamentary rolls came on 5 June, 1444, it is feasible that the epidemic of the early 1440's was restricted not just to London, but was present throughout eastern England, and entered London from the north. Turning to the data from the N.C.C., it can be seen that there was a small but hardly extraordinary peak in probate and intestate listings for autumn, 1444 (Graph 4.1.1,1). It is difficult to generalize on such meager evidence, but if the local epidemics of the early 1440's were in some way connected, they were probably not too widespread even in a regional sense, and probably were not too virulent.

Once again we must turn to Hertfordshire and St. Albans for an insight into the pestilence and unhealthy air which forced Parliament to flee twice from London, in 1449 and 1450. Mortality for the town of St. Albans remained basically unchanged between 1449 and 1450, but the testamentary mortality patterns for the archdeaconry as a whole, especially the southern villages and parishes, was that of plague in the autumn, 1449 (Graph 4.1.3,2). It must be noted that the Hertfordshire data, while geographically comprehensive, are numerically small. Mortality in the archdeaconry then fell through the subsequent winter and spring quarters, and rose again in the summer and autumn of 1450. But in 1449–1450, the failure of the narrative sources to mention the presence of epidemic disease outside of London and its immediate vicinity—considering parts of the archdeaconry of St. Albans to be in the London vicinity—would appear to be accurate. Of all the ecclesiastical courts in East Anglia, only the wills from the archdeaconry court of Sudbury, the jurisdiction in the diocese closest to London, and Hertfordshire showed autumnal clustering patterns for 1449 and 1450 (Graph 4.1.2,2). If there was an epidemic in East Anglia in 1449–1450, it must have been a very mild one.

John Paston wrote of a "gret pestelens" in London in late summer, early autumn, 1454.[39] There is little testamentary evidence that this epidemic spread beyond the city itself and its very immediate suburbs. Neither the town of St. Albans nor the archdeaconry as a whole showed more than a seasonal rise in their testamentary mortality (Graph 4.1.3,2). This also applies to the wills registered in the N.C.C., the archdeaconry courts of Suffolk and Sudbury, and the peculiar court of B.S.E. (Graphs 4.1.1,1; and 4.1.2,2). To the contrary, the mortality patterns throughout East Anglia for the mid-1450's seem to be patterns of stable or slightly falling death tolls. At least in comparative terms, then, with the possible exception of select early and late quarters in the 1450's, the 1440's and 1450's were epidemic-free outside of London.

Given the regional scope of the quantitative parts of this work, it is not possible to track down many of the other non-London local epidemics in the period 1430–1480 by using the testamentary sources. This is the case for the reported epidemics of 1445 in Lancashire, 1447 in Canterbury, 1448 in Oxford, 1450 in Devon, 1468 in Coventry, and 1445 and 1474 for Wales and the west country. The "grete dysesse" of 1443 and "pestelyns" of 1465 in Norfolk, however, are both traceable and apparent. Judging from the literary description and the testamentary mortality evidence, the "dyesse" of 1443 does not seem to have been an epidemic of pestilence or plague. Mortality peaked precipitously not in the fall quarter, but in the winter, for both probates and intestate listings in the N.C.C. (Graph 4.1.1,1). Although there was no mention of a severe winter in 1443, the epidemic may have been influenza or typhus. A further clue is provided by a contemporary passage from the *Journal D'Un Bourgeois De Paris*, where reference is made to *la plus terrible maladie de la verole*, which swept through France.[40] Perhaps the Norfolk epidemic was one of smallpox. The combination of literary reference from the Paston letters and mortality clustering evidence from the N.C.C. wills is of further use for the "pesteleyns" of 1465 in Norfolk. There was an enormous rise in numbers of probated wills for the autumn and winter, 1465 and 1465–1466, as has been discussed in connection with the national epidemic of 1464–1465.[41] It is probable that even the excessive mortality of 1466 was connected with the national epidemic.

One last epidemic, the French Pox of 1475, can be discussed through use of the narrative and testamentary sources. Since soldiers going on campaign overseas were often allowed to register their wills in the P.C.C.,[42] and since they were said by *The Brut* chronicler to be the victims and purveyors of this disease,[43] mortality clustering from the archbishop's court becomes particularly interesting. Little has been said thus far of the mortality patterns produced from the P.C.C. This is because these wills, when graphed, show the almost continual "unsteadiness" which is fairly typical of pre-industrial mortality, but one which appears at first glance to be almost impervious to the large, seasonal mortality clustering indicative of epidemic disease. Throughout the period 1430–1480, the wills from the P.C.C. do not cluster in the spectacular patterns of wills from all other courts, including the Prerogative Court of York.[44] The P.C.C. wills were not sensitive even to the local London epidemics, despite the fact that about 65 percent of P.C.C. testators in the sample were Londoners. Since these testators composed the very wealthiest segment of the will-registering population, the intriguing question is raised of whether or not wealth provided some degree of immunity to the ravages of epidemic disease. The link between wealth, mobility and epidemic disease will be discussed below;[45] for the moment, an investigation of the graphed testamentary data from the P.C.C. shows that the peak period of mortality came between the spring of 1474 and the spring of 1476 (Graph 4.1.3,3). Because this is the general period of the French Pox, some further discussion is necessary.

At least one historical epidemiologist has stated that the French Pox of 1475 was gonorrhea; possibly, it was part of the great epidemic of syphilis or yaws which gripped Europe toward the end of the fifteenth century and the beginning of the sixteenth century.[46] Further, it is alleged that the soldiers of Edward IV's army brought it back with them from France to England.[47] The only other mention of a pox in the fifty-year period 1430–1450 was also made in connection with a campaigning army, and the descriptions of the 1475 affliction describe in lurid detail its venereal nature.[48] Unfortunately, the testamentary evidence does not indicate a period of abnormally high mortality. First, there was no influx of wills registered in the P.C.C. from the soldiers of the French campaign, as there had been in 1419.[49] Second, and more important, the P.C.C. mortality peaks from 1474 to 1476 were not significantly larger than previous and subsequent mortality levels. The pox of 1462 brought a significant spring mortality peak, but while there were slight peaks in will probates in the spring quarters of 1474 and 1476, mortality was particularly low in the spring of 1475—if indeed a springtime mortality peak was indicative of fifteenth century syphilis or poxes at all. Further, of all the other courts surveyed, only the wills from the archdeaconry court of Suffolk and, to a lesser extent, Sudbury, showed large numbers of probated wills in the period 1474–1476, and these were in the summer and autumn of 1474. It is possible that the French Pox was not immediately lethal to those who contracted it, but the descriptions of the narrative sources would seem to indicate otherwise. One thing is certain; whatever the aetiological character and extent of the French Pox of 1475, its short-term effect on mortality was negligible.

There were virtually no mortality peaks in the testamentary evidence which are not explained and expounded upon in the narrative sources. This adds credibility to the use of the wills as a barometer of epidemic disease. The mortality graphs show considerable amounts of fluctuation in the 1440's and early 1450's, but this appears to be typical of pre-industrial mortality in periods of relatively slight incidence of epidemic disease. The only mortality peaks which do not coincide with the narrative sources' records of epidemics were those of 1477 and 1478, and as discussed above, these too may have been the results of infectious disease. Clusterings of mortality from the testamentary sources can be closely correlated with major national and regional outbreaks of epidemic disease, as reported by the literary sources. The testamentary data are somewhat less sensitive in reflecting local epidemics, although some increase in mortality in these lesser epidemics is usually evident. There were protracted periods of crisis mortality generally reflective of epidemic disease in 1433–1435, 1438–1439, 1452, 1457–1459, 1462, 1464–1465, 1471, 1473, 1477 and 1479–1480. If the will clusterings reflect demographic reality, epidemic disease was responsible, with the possible exception of 1477, for every major period of extensive, crisis mortality in the period 1430–1480. Epidemic disease, primarily plague, was the major factor controlling population in eastern England for most of this fifty-year period.

## 4.2 Season of Death

As is to be expected during a period of continual epidemics of plague, more people died in the autumn in the years 1430 to 1480 than in any other quarter. The next most frequent quarter of death was spring, the predominant pattern in industrial societies, and then winter. Fewest testators in the sample died in the summer quarter, except during purported plague years, when mortality rose in late August. But there were protracted spans of time, even in the period 1430–1480, when plague was not the major factor in mortality, and the seasonal patterns varied. Equally interesting are the questions of how different social and occupational groups responded to epidemic disease. What were the patterns of mortality for the various subgroups and subdivisions within the sample as a whole? With the aid of the computer, these questions can be raised, and perhaps answered.

The chroniclers' impressions that two decades in particular in the fifty-year period 1430–1480, the 1430's and 1470's, were decades of continual and virulent pestilence—almost certainly plague—are borne out by the computerized analysis of the testamentary data. The data are presented in Tables 4.2.1 to 4.2.6. Using the methods and permutations described in Chapter 1,[50] the sample was initially divided by decade and county. The wills from the P.C.C. were set by themselves, as well as by county when appropriate, and for this reason there is some slight, though numerically insignificant, duplication in the county samples.[51] Programs were then run for "season" for four major subdivisions, defined as follows: the entire sample; the entire male sample less priests; married males only; and the "urban" testators, with urban being defined as anyone living in London, Norwich, Ipswich, St. Albans or Bury St. Edmunds. Subsequent runs were made for different occupations and for a special division of the 1460's.

As the data in Tables 4.2.1 to 4.2.3 show, at no time in any county or in the P.C.C. wills for the first three major subdivisions of the sample was the modal figure for season of death in the 1470's anything but "4," or autumn; during the 1430's, all but one of the county divisions also showed a fall predominant mortality pattern. This was also the case, with very few exceptions, for the literally hundreds of computer runs made for the various subdivisions and occupational groups which constitute the sample for the 1430's and 1470's.[52] People died in the autumn from causes other than plague, but as the correlations between the graphed testamentary data and the narrative sources have shown, and the graphed data from the sixteenth century Bills of Mortality will show, [53] excessive autumnal mortality in pre-industrial England was almost always indicative of epidemic bubonic plague. It can also be seen that the total seasonal distribution of death was far less equal in the 1430's and especially the 1470's than it was in the other, less plague-stricken decades.

There was one consistent exception to this predominant autumnal mortality pattern of the 1430's and 1470's. This was the city of Norwich. For Norwich in both the 1430's and the 1470's, a spring pattern was the dominant one. A possible explanation of this can be offered methodologically, if not necessarily historically. The wills used for Norwich were taken primarily from the N.C.C., and to a lesser extent from the P.C.C. and the City Court; since the wills from the archdeaconry court of Norwich do not survive for most of the period 1430 to 1480, the will sample from the town is prejudiced toward the wealthier segments of its population. As can be seen from the mortality patterns of Londoners from the P.C.C.—though

*Table 4.2.1.* Season of Mortality, Entire Sample (in Percentage)*

| | n | Mode | W-1 | Sp-2 | Su-3 | F-4 |
|---|---|---|---|---|---|---|
| All 1430–80 | (14971) | 4 | 24.2 | 26.8 | 19.6 | 29.4 |
| N 1430–80 | ( 5714) | 4 | 24.0 | 27.3 | 19.2 | 28.9 |
| S 1430–80 | ( 6744) | 4 | 24.9 | 26.7 | 19.3 | 29.1 |
| H 1430–80 | ( 1335) | 4 | 24.6 | 25.9 | 20.8 | 28.5 |
| P.C.C. 30–80 | ( 1279) | 4 | 21.5 | 26.6 | 21.2 | 30.5 |
| All 1430–40 | ( 1653) | 4 | 24.7 | 26.0 | 19.6 | 28.8 |
| N 1430–40 | ( 807) | 4 | 26.3 | 24.9 | 21.1 | 27.3 |
| S 1430–40 | ( 423) | 4 | 23.4 | 29.1 | 16.8 | 30.7 |
| H 1430–40 | ( 251) | 4 | 23.9 | 25.5 | 18.7 | 31.9 |
| P.C.C. 30–40 | ( 206) | 4 | 25.2 | 23.8 | 20.4 | 30.1 |
| All 1441–50 | ( 2190) | 4 | 24.5 | 25.6 | 21.1 | 28.6 |
| N 1441–50 | ( 722) | 2 | 23.4 | 28.4 | 23.1 | 24.7 |
| S 1441–50 | ( 1031) | 4 | 25.2 | 22.8 | 21.7 | 30.2 |
| H 1441–50 | ( 248) | 4 | 25.0 | 24.2 | 16.1 | 34.3 |
| P.C.C. 41–50 | ( 198) | 4 | 26.1 | 27.5 | 16.9 | 29.6 |
| All 1451–60 | ( 2970) | 4 | 24.9 | 27.0 | 19.6 | 28.1 |
| N 1451–60 | ( 905) | 2 | 22.9 | 29.5 | 20.1 | 27.6 |
| S 1451–60 | ( 1596) | 4 | 26.3 | 25.9 | 18.8 | 29.0 |
| H 1451–60 | ( 268) | 2 | 26.1 | 26.5 | 21.6 | 25.7 |
| P.C.C. 51–60 | ( 228) | 4 | 22.8 | 27.6 | 19.3 | 30.3 |
| All 1461–70 | ( 385) | 4 | 25.1 | 27.2 | 19.0 | 28.3 |
| N 1461–70 | ( 1684) | 4 | 24.5 | 27.3 | 18.6 | 29.5 |
| S 1461–70 | ( 1611) | 4 | 27.2 | 26.6 | 18.3 | 27.9 |
| H 1461–70 | ( 221) | 2 | 21.7 | 33.9 | 24.0 | 19.9 |
| P.C.C. 61–70 | ( 350) | 4 | 18.6 | 23.7 | 24.3 | 33.1 |
| All 1471–80 | ( 4307) | 4 | 22.8 | 27.5 | 18.7 | 31.0 |
| N 1471–80 | ( 1596) | 4 | 23.6 | 26.6 | 16.6 | 33.1 |
| S 1471—80 | ( 2083) | 4 | 22.3 | 28.8 | 19.4 | 29.5 |
| H 1471–80 | ( 347) | 4 | 26.2 | 21.6 | 22.8 | 29.4 |
| P.C.C. 71–80 | ( 297) | 4 | 17.8 | 29.0 | 21.9 | 31.3 |

*Abbreviations:* N (Norfolk); S (Suffolk); H (Hertfordshire).

*Table 4.2.2.* Season of Mortality, All Male Testators Excepting Clerics
(in Percentage)

| | n | Mode | W-1 | Sp-2 | Su-3 | F-4 |
|---|---|---|---|---|---|---|
| All 1430–80 | (11483) | 4 | 24.1 | 26.5 | 19.6 | 29.7 |
| N 1430–80 | ( 4058) | 4 | 23.5 | 26.9 | 19.1 | 30.6 |
| S 1430–80 | ( 5401) | 4 | 25.1 | 26.6 | 19.4 | 20.9 |
| H 1430–80 | ( 1128) | 4 | 23.8 | 25.8 | 21.2 | 28.8 |
| P.C.C. 30–80 | ( 976) | 4 | 22.4 | 26.5 | 20.8 | 30.0 |
| All 1430–40 | ( 1100) | 4 | 24.7 | 25.0 | 20.0 | 30.3 |
| N 1430–40 | ( 493) | 4 | 25.4 | 24.1 | 22.3 | 28.2 |
| S 1430–40 | ( 283) | 4 | 24.0 | 28.3 | 16.3 | 31.4 |
| H 1430–40 | ( 202) | 4 | 23.8 | 25.2 | 18.3 | 32.7 |
| P.C.C. 30–40 | ( 145) | 4 | 26.9 | 22.1 | 21.4 | 29.0 |
| All 1441–50 | ( 1479) | 4 | 24.4 | 24.0 | 20.7 | 30.8 |
| N 1441–50 | ( 428) | 4 | 22.4 | 26.4 | 22.4 | 28.7 |
| S 1441–50 | ( 697) | 4 | 25.1 | 22.6 | 21.4 | 30.9 |
| H 1441–50 | ( 209) | 4 | 25.1 | 23.1 | 16.6 | 35.2 |
| P.C.C. 41–50 | ( 155) | 4 | 28.2 | 28.2 | 14.5 | 29.1 |
| All 1451–60 | ( 2421) | 4 | 25.8 | 26.2 | 19.8 | 28.3 |
| N 1451–60 | ( 630) | 2 | 23.3 | 29.5 | 20.7 | 26.5 |
| S 1451–60 | ( 1399) | 4 | 26.4 | 25.6 | 19.3 | 28.7 |
| H 1451–60 | ( 225) | 1 | 27.1 | 24.4 | 22.2 | 26.2 |
| P.C.C. 51–60 | ( 171) | 2 | 25.1 | 30.4 | 16.4 | 28.1 |
| All 1461–70 | ( 3024) | 4 | 25.1 | 27.3 | 19.1 | 28.3 |
| N 1461–70 | ( 1277) | 4 | 23.7 | 27.3 | 18.8 | 30.1 |
| S 1461–70 | ( 1302) | 1 | 28.2 | 27.0 | 17.7 | 27.2 |
| H 1461–70 | ( 189) | 2 | 19.0 | 34.4 | 24.9 | 21.2 |
| P.C.C. 61–70 | ( 280) | 4 | 19.3 | 23.2 | 24.6 | 32.9 |
| All 1471–80 | ( 3459) | 4 | 22.5 | 27.3 | 18.2 | 31.4 |
| N 1471–80 | ( 1230) | 4 | 23.3 | 26.2 | 16.2 | 34.4 |
| S 1471–80 | ( 1720) | 4 | 22.2 | 28.6 | 19.8 | 29.3 |
| H 1471–80 | ( 303) | 4 | 24.4 | 23.4 | 22.8 | 29.4 |
| P.C.C. 71–80 | ( 225) | 4 | 18.2 | 28.0 | 21.3 | 32.4 |

*Table 4.2.3.* Season of Mortality, All Married Males (in Percentage)

|  | n | Mode | W-1 | Sp-2 | Su-3 | F-4 |
|---|---|---|---|---|---|---|
| All 1430–80 | (8744) | 4 | 24.0 | 26.5 | 19.8 | 29.6 |
| N 1430–80 | (3165) | 4 | 23.7 | 26.8 | 19.3 | 30.2 |
| S 1430–80 | (4065) | 4 | 24.8 | 26.9 | 19.3 | 29.0 |
| H 1430–80 | ( 893) | 4 | 24.0 | 25.3 | 22.0 | 28.6 |
| P.C.C. 30–80 | ( 753) | 4 | 21.8 | 26.9 | 20.9 | 30.2 |
| All 1430–40 | ( 755) | 4 | 24.3 | 25.2 | 19.3 | 30.6 |
| N 1430–40 | ( 311) | 1 | 27.7 | 25.4 | 21.5 | 25.0 |
| S 1430–40 | ( 201) | 4 | 22.4 | 27.4 | 14.9 | 35.3 |
| H 1430–40 | ( 151) | 4 | 21.9 | 25.2 | 17.2 | 35.8 |
| P.C.C. 30–40 | ( 117) | 4 | 26.5 | 22.2 | 21.4 | 29.1 |
| All 1441–50 | (1005) | 4 | 24.7 | 23.5 | 21.8 | 29.9 |
| N 1441–50 | ( 306) | 2 | 24.2 | 26.5 | 24.5 | 24.8 |
| S 1441–50 | ( 467) | 4 | 24.2 | 22.3 | 21.6 | 31.9 |
| H 1441–50 | ( 146) | 4 | 25.4 | 21.3 | 17.8 | 35.5 |
| P.C.C. 41–50 | ( 86) | 2 | 27.9 | 30.2 | 18.6 | 23.3 |
| All 1451–60 | (1802) | 4 | 25.9 | 26.9 | 19.7 | 27.5 |
| N 1451–60 | ( 539) | 2 | 24.9 | 28.0 | 20.4 | 26.7 |
| S 1451–60 | ( 969) | 4 | 26.3 | 26.9 | 18.0 | 28.0 |
| H 1451–60 | ( 185) | 1 | 28.6 | 26.5 | 21.6 | 23.2 |
| P.C.C. 51–60 | ( 124) | 2 | 21.0 | 33.9 | 16.1 | 29.0 |
| All 1461–70 | (2339) | 4 | 25.3 | 26.7 | 19.3 | 28.7 |
| N 1461–70 | ( 998) | 4 | 23.9 | 26.6 | 18.3 | 31.2 |
| S 1461–70 | ( 973) | 1 | 28.7 | 27.5 | 17.1 | 26.7 |
| H 1461–70 | ( 151) | 2 | 18.5 | 31.1 | 29.1 | 20.5 |
| P.C.C. 61–70 | ( 236) | 4 | 19.5 | 22.0 | 26.3 | 32.2 |
| All 1471–80 | (2843) | 4 | 22.1 | 27.5 | 18.8 | 31.6 |
| N 1471–80 | (1011) | 4 | 21.7 | 26.8 | 17.3 | 34.2 |
| S 1471–80 | (1455) | 4 | 22.1 | 28.8 | 19.8 | 29.3 |
| H 1471–80 | ( 237) | 4 | 24.9 | 23.3 | 23.2 | 28.7 |
| P.C.C. 71–80 | ( 190) | 4 | 18.9 | 29.5 | 17.4 | 34.2 |

*Table 4.2.4.* Season of Mortality, Urban Testators (in Percentage)

| | n | Mode | W-1 | Sp-2 | Su-3 | F-4 |
|---|---|---|---|---|---|---|
| All 1430–80 | (2992) | 4 | 22.8 | 25.4 | 22.9 | 28.7 |
| London 1430–80 | ( 830) | 4 | 19.3 | 25.1 | 24.6 | 31.0 |
| Norwich 1430–80 | ( 694) | 2 | 22.7 | 27.8 | 21.9 | 27.3 |
| Ipswich 1430–80 | ( 245) | 4 | 26.5 | 23.7 | 18.4 | 31.4 |
| St. Albans 1430–80 | ( 571) | 4 | 24.5 | 24.5 | 23.1 | 27.3 |
| Bury St. Edmunds 30–80 | ( 652) | 4 | 24.7 | 24.5 | 23.2 | 27.6 |
| Norwich 1430–40 | ( 87) | 2 | 25.9 | 35.3 | 23.5 | 15.3 |
| 1441–50 | ( 136) | 4 | 19.1 | 23.5 | 27.2 | 29.4 |
| 1451–60 | ( 109) | 4 | 22.0 | 22.0 | 26.6 | 29.4 |
| 1461–70 | ( 164) | 2 | 22.6 | 29.3 | 19.5 | 28.0 |
| 1471–80 | ( 198) | 2 | 24.4 | 29.9 | 16.8 | 28.9 |
| Ipswich 1430–40 | ( 5) | 2 | 40.0 | 40.0 | 0.0 | 20.0 |
| 1441–50 | ( 42) | 3 | 23.7 | 21.1 | 36.8 | 18.4 |
| 1451–60 | ( 67) | 1 | 42.3 | 17.5 | 9.5 | 31.7 |
| 1461–70 | ( 69) | 4 | 24.6 | 21.5 | 16.9 | 36.9 |
| 1471–80 | ( 62) | 4 | 14.8 | 31.5 | 20.4 | 33.3 |
| St. Albans 1430–40 | ( 113) | 4 | 23.9 | 23.9 | 22.1 | 30.1 |
| 1441–50 | ( 102) | 4 | 19.0 | 27.0 | 20.0 | 33.0 |
| 1451–60 | ( 104) | 4 | 29.8 | 19.2 | 20.2 | 30.8 |
| 1461–70 | ( 110) | 2 | 21.8 | 34.5 | 25.5 | 18.2 |
| 1471–80 | ( 142) | 1 | 27.5 | 19.7 | 26.1 | 26.8 |
| Bury St. Edmunds 30–40 | ( 65) | 1 | 27.7 | 24.6 | 26.2 | 21.5 |
| 1441–50 | ( 134) | 1 | 31.4 | 18.6 | 25.7 | 24.3 |
| 1451–60 | ( 104) | 4 | 16.2 | 24.8 | 22.9 | 36.2 |
| 1461–70 | ( 133) | 2 | 27.4 | 30.4 | 22.2 | 20.0 |
| 1471–80 | ( 216) | 4 | 22.2 | 24.5 | 21.3 | 31.9 |
| London 1430–40 | ( 122) | 4 | 18.9 | 19.7 | 25.4 | 31.0 |
| 1441–50 | ( 98) | 4 | 21.3 | 28.7 | 19.1 | 30.9 |
| 1451–60 | ( 152) | 4 | 21.1 | 24.6 | 22.5 | 31.7 |
| 1461–70 | ( 240) | 4 | 17.9 | 23.0 | 27.2 | 31.5 |
| 1471–80 | ( 218) | 4 | 28.3 | 18.2 | 24.2 | 30.3 |
| Beccles 1430–80 | ( 160) | 2 | 26.3 | 33.8 | 14.4 | 25.6 |
| Bungay 1430–80 | ( 96) | 1 | 30.2 | 19.8 | 19.8 | 29.2 |
| Sudbury 1430–80 | ( 136) | 4 | 27.2 | 26.5 | 16.9 | 29.4 |
| North Hales 1430–80 | ( 46) | 2 | 17.4 | 52.2 | 8.7 | 21.7 |

*Table 4.2.5.* Season of Mortality, Occupational and Special Groups
(in Percentage)

|  | n | Mode | W-1 | Sp-2 | Su-3 | F-4 |
|---|---|---|---|---|---|---|
| Clerics 1430–80 | (1316) | 2 | 21.0 | 29.6 | 21.2 | 28.3 |
| 1430–40 | ( 334) | 4 | 25.7 | 27.2 | 19.0 | 28.1 |
| 1441–50 | ( 279) | 4 | 22.2 | 25.8 | 25.1 | 26.9 |
| 1451–60 | ( 267) | 4 | 18.7 | 29.6 | 20.6 | 31.1 |
| 1461–70 | ( 233) | 2 | 17.6 | 31.8 | 20.6 | 30.0 |
| 1471–80 | ( 203) | 2 | 19.7 | 32.5 | 21.2 | 26.6 |
| Rural Élite 1430–80 | ( 260) | 4 | 25.8 | 23.1 | 21.2 | 29.6 |
| 1430–40 | ( 49) | 1 | 34.8 | 21.7 | 21.7 | 21.7 |
| 1441–50 | ( 47) | 4 | 22.7 | 20.5 | 22.7 | 34.1 |
| 1451–60 | ( 49) | 4 | 21.3 | 29.8 | 17.0 | 31.9 |
| 1461–70 | ( 52) | 4 | 22.0 | 16.0 | 28.0 | 34.0 |
| 1471–80 | ( 63) | 4 | 26.2 | 24.6 | 18.0 | 31.1 |
| London Élite 1430–80 | ( 201) | 4 | 22.4 | 25.0 | 24.9 | 26.9 |
| Select Urban Occ. 1430–80* | ( 149) | 4 | 24.8 | 24.8 | 22.8 | 27.5 |
| Select Rural Occ. 1430–80** | ( 110) | 3 | 27.3 | 17.7 | 28.4 | 26.6 |
| All Citizens 1430–80 | ( 690) | 4 | 20.4 | 27.1 | 23.2 | 29.0 |
| All Occ. 1430–80 | (2137) | 4 | 22.4 | 25.3 | 23.2 | 28.9 |
| Female test. 1430–80 | (2128) | 4 | 26.2 | 27.4 | 18.5 | 27.4 |
| Testators with servants 1430–80 | ( 364) | 2 | 20.1 | 30.8 | 20.1 | 28.6 |

*Including bakers, barkers, barbers, butchers, carpenters, smiths, skinners and tanners.
**Including clothmakers, dyers, fullers, shearers, weavers and worsteadmen.

*Table 4.2.6.* Season of Mortality, 1460's (in Percentage)

|  | n | Mode | W-1 | Sp-2 | Su-3 | F-4 |
|---|---|---|---|---|---|---|
| 1460–63 | (1512) | 2 | 19.2 | 33.9 | 21.7 | 25.3 |
| N 1460–63 | ( 591) | 2 | 18.4 | 36.7 | 19.5 | 25.4 |
| S 1460–63 | ( 759) | 2 | 20.3 | 29.7 | 23.8 | 26.1 |
| H 1460–63 | ( 90) | 2 | 14.3 | 52.4 | 16.7 | 16.7 |
| P.C.C. 1460–63 | ( 76) | 4 | 20.8 | 25.6 | 20.8 | 34.7 |
| 1464–70 | (2753) | 4 | 27.1 | 24.4 | 18.5 | 30.0 |
| N 1464–70 | (1264) | 4 | 25.8 | 24.5 | 18.7 | 31.1 |
| S 1464–70 | (1048) | 1 | 30.6 | 24.8 | 15.6 | 28.9 |
| H 1464–70 | ( 158) | 3 | 25.9 | 23.4 | 26.6 | 23.4 |
| P.C.C. 1464–70 | ( 299) | 4 | 18.1 | 24.1 | 24.4 | 33.1 |

not to the degree of their Norwich counterparts—the wealthier segments of society were less susceptible to death in periods of crisis mortality than was the bulk of the population. More will be said about this below.[54] But the exceptional evidence from Norwich aside, it is apparent that plague was the decisive factor in controlling mortality in the 1430's and 1470's.

Plague and other epidemic diseases were a major factor in mortality in the 1440's and 1450's, though not to the degree they were in the 1430's and 1470's. Although the decennial mortality averages are still predominantly autumnal, bulk numbers of wills and intestate recordings per court indicate that gross mortality was lower in the 1440's and 1450's than in the 1430's and 1470's. The total view of seasonal mortality, especially for the 1450's, is one of far more even distribution. This more equal seasonal distribution must especially be noted for the 1440's, where a heavy autumnal pattern for Hertfordshire, indicative perhaps of the epidemics of plague in this decade in nearby London, tends to distort the decennial figures. The 1440's and 1450's were in general a period of respite, especially from plague. After the devastation of the 1430's, opportunities for acquiring more land, marrying earlier, and having children soon after marriage must have been greater than they had been since before the 1420's. As we shall see later, the population did not seem to respond during this period of remission.[55]

The 1460's were something of a transitional decade (Table 4.2.6). The first four years (in this sample the "decade" is eleven years, from 1460 to

1470) resembled the mortality patterns of the 1440's and 1450's, while the last seven years resembled the patterns of the 1430's and 1470's. Taken by decade and by county, wills from Norfolk, Suffolk and Hertfordshire reflected a modal spring mortality pattern. Part of the answer to this lies in the pox of 1462, a disease which showed an overwhelming spring mortality pattern. Perhaps more important, the years 1460 to 1463 appear to have been plague-free. From 1464, the pattern altered; the seasonal mortality distribution changed and became more autumnal with the exception of Hertfordshire, reflecting the plague patterns of the 1430's and 1470's, due to the epidemics of 1464–1465 and 1467. The population of eastern England, devastated by epidemic disease, especially plague, in the 1420's and 1430's, experienced a period of reduced epidemic activity in the 1440's, 1450's and first two years of the 1460's, only to be revisited by infectious disease on a large scale in the mid-1460's and 1470's.

There are some slight differences in mortality by county. But obviously, as will be discussed in Chapter 5, the crucial factor in mortality was not county boundary lines, but rather local geographical characteristics, such as breckland, coastland and fenland. Nevertheless, some interesting observations by county can still be made. Evidence from all counties, as well as the wills from the P.C.C., show autumnal season of death patterns, indicative of the predominant influence of plague. The evidence from the P.C.C., with its continual fall modal seasons of death is particularly noteworthy, since the graphs of seasonal mortality did not seem to indicate this (Graphs 4.1.3, 1–3). In fact, seasonal mortality for the wealthy testators of the P.C.C. was less evenly distributed in many cases than mortality for the testators from the lower courts of East Anglia and Hertfordshire. This appears to be in contradiction with the suggestion proposed earlier that great wealth may have provided a mobility which enabled the richer testators to flee from epidemics: in reality, it is not. The rich seem to have been able to avoid the severest epidemics, as shown by the graphed data. But they were not able to avoid the lesser epidemics and continual effects of endemic disease. Flight would allow a testator and his family to avoid an epidemic in a particular area at a given time, but aside from affording the opportunity not to live in one of the especially unhealthy regions, such as coastal Suffolk or the breckland, it could not permanently place him beyond the reaches of continual epidemic and endemic disease.[56] Although the wealthy were less susceptible to the ravages of epidemic disease, they were by no means immune to it.

Comparing those resident in the modern counties of Hertfordshire, Norfolk and Suffolk, we find testators from Norfolk apparently more prone to autumnal mortality than testators from the other counties, although the degree varied considerably by decade and sample. Suffolk testators also showed fall mortality patterns throughout all the various permutations, indicative perhaps of the large numbers of areas within the county itself which were continually affected by what may have been endemic plague.[57] Among the more unusual mortality patterns was the very low incidence of autumnal mortality in Hertfordshire in the 1460's, and especially the early 1460's, much of which was due to the effects of the springtime epidemics in the county in 1462 and 1463.

Urban mortality also exhibited the dominant fall mortality patterns; in fact, it was more autumnal than rural mortality. Only in the already cited exception of Norwich was there any consistent deviation from this plague-type pattern of death. The towns had no monopoly on disease, including plague, but they do seem to have been among the unhealthier areas in which to have lived in fifteenth century England, both in terms of crude mortality and fertility, if replacement ratios can be used as a barometer of the latter.[58] Migration must have been the only way in which even the smaller urban areas, such as Ipswich, could have maintained their population levels. Many of the towns, particularly in plague periods, showed a heavier than usual winter mortality pattern among their testators. As the graphs have shown, deaths in the towns during periods of plague often tended to begin in the autumn, but peak in the winter. St. Albans is an especially good example of this. Perhaps pneumonic plague, the form of plague transmittable directly from person to person—a condition facilitated by town living—but not bubonic plague, was an urban phenomenon in the fifteenth century.

It remains only to discuss comparative mortality among the various social and occupational groups which comprise the sample. As was discussed in Chapter 1, this must be done with great care, since occupations in fifteenth century England were not always what they were alleged to be. Most interesting is the mortality pattern among clerics, defined here as any testator calling himself a rector, vicar, *capallanus,* or just plain priest. Together, they comprised something under 9 percent of the entire testamentary population.[59] For the period as a whole, and for two of the three ten-year periods which have been referred to as plague decades, clerical mortality was highest in the spring, and not in the autumn. Only in the 1450's, one of the two decades least afflicted with plague, did clerics exhibit a marked fall mortality pattern. This apparent ability to avoid severe epidemics of plague was shared by certain groups of P.C.C. testators, most notably the London élite, but none of these groups appears to have been as consistently successful in escaping from heavy fall mortality as were the priests. Further, the minority of clerics who were married and listed family members in their wills showed a mortality pattern more similar to that of their nonclerical neighbors than to that of their fellow clerics.

Part of this seeming immunity of men of the cloth to the severest effects of epidemic plague lay in their wealth. The wills clearly show that the bulk of the clerics who had their wills registered were wealthier than most of their contemporaries, although this varied somewhat with the age of the individual cleric.[60] Personal wealth was further supplemented by the wealth of the church as an institution. Judging from the impressions of contemporaries, relative clerical immunity to fall mortality patterns was not due to any greater degree of personal cleanliness, nor to a greater understanding of the causes of epidemic disease. On the contrary, a spring pattern of mortality may indicate typhus, a disease always connected with personal uncleanliness, as its traditional English name, "gaol fever," suggests.[61] Possibly, through constant care of the sick and subsequent mild attacks of *pestis ambulans,* the clerical class had acquired some immunity to plague; possibly, they were not ministering to their flock as diligently as was necessary during periods of high plague mortality.

The two wealthiest groups in the sample, the London élite and the rural élite, exhibited fall-predominant mortality patterns. However, both groups had mortality distributions which were on the whole more equal and less fall-oriented than those of the rest of the sample, again indicating that wealth and mobility were of some consequence in avoiding the more serious outbreaks of plague. Of the other occupational groups selected and tested, all but one had dominant autumnal mortality patterns similar to those of the sample as a whole. These "other" groups consisted of crafts and small traders.[62] The exceptional group was the combined rural members of the textile crafts, a sample which included clothmakers (perhaps retailers in the fifteenth century, and nonintegral to this "working-class" sample), dyers, fullers, shearers (sherman), weavers, and worstedmen.[63] Unlike any of the other occupational groups, they had a summer modal death pattern, with a heavy secondary winter mortality pattern. Although there are no apparent reasons regarding epidemic disease which can be used to explain this curious phenomenon, there are several possible nonepidemic explanations.[64]

In sum, wealth and mobility were important but by no means decisive factors in providing some degree of immunity from crisis-level mortality, usually induced by epidemic plague, in fifteenth century England. Needless to say, a hazardous job, quite apart from epidemic disease, would increase individual mortality. But for the bulk of the population, whether they lived in town or country, epidemic disease, especially plague, was quite literally the decisive factor in controlling life.

## 4.3 The Bills of Mortality: A Comparative Analysis

Much has been made thus far of the plague-pattern of mortality. While it has been claimed that this is an early autumn pattern, and much indirect literary and statistical evidence has been given in support of this view, little direct statistical evidence has been offered thus far. Although there can be little question from the graphing of wills that the bulk of crisis mortality in the fifteenth century came in the autumn, especially in late September and October, and that these periods of crisis mortality invariably coincide with reports of epidemics, the wills do not tell the cause of death of the testator. For the fifteenth century, the historian can only use as much indirect evidence as possible to surmise this. For the sixteenth century, however, it is possible to state precisely what caused death for a large proportion of the population of London for several years, including periods of crisis mortality, by use of the Bills of Mortality.

A point continually stressed has been that the bacteria, protozoa and viruses which cause epidemic disease are living organisms, and therefore subject to continual biological change. Plague in the fifteenth century was not identical with plague in the sixteenth century. But some reliable statistical guide is needed to establish definitively what the plague mortality patterns so crucial to this thesis really were like. Modern data from several sources were scanned for comparative use,[65] but it was felt in the long run that whatever the statistical imperfections, data from sixteenth century England would be more accurate aetiologically and in socio-economic terms than would be statistically more sophisticated, but chronologically more remote data from a twentieth century non-European society.[66]

The Bills of Mortality for the city of London are especially complete for the period 1578–1583, years which the literary sources describe as a time of almost continual plague.[67] The origin of the Bills stems from the epidemic of 1531, which forced the royal court to move from Greenwich to Hampton Court. After a year of what appears to have been plague— from September, 1531, to September, 1532—the Royal Council asked the mayor of London to "certify how many died of plague."[68] This is apparently the earliest reference to the Bills of Mortality. They were probably kept by parish clerks, and were compiled or have survived randomly for the remainder of the century. According to Stow, it was the persistence of plague from 1577 to 1583 which convinced Elizabeth and her advisers to ensure diligent keeping of records for this period.[69] For the historical demographer, the Bills of Mortality are yet another example of the superior records, from the more complete State papers to the Parish registers, which have survived from the Tudor period onward.

The raw numbers of deaths taken from the Bills of Mortality are far greater than the numbers of deaths reported by the probated wills for 1430–1480 (Graph 4.3.1). There are several reasons for this. First, the wills reflect essentially just the adult male segment of fifteenth century society, while the Bills ostensibly record all deaths, regardless of age or sex. More important was the size of London itself. In the 1470's there were probably no more than 40,000 people living in the city; by the late sixteenth century, it had probably expanded to 150,000, an increase of nearly fourfold.[70] In 1464, a Venetian merchant commented on how, at the very height of its virulence, a pestilence was killing people at the rate of 200 per day.[71] In 1531, another Venetian observer said that even though the pestilence was waning, deaths in London were running at the rate of 400 per day.[72] Part of this increase may have been due to the comparative virulence of the epidemics in question, but it is likely that the bulk in differences of numbers was the result of the natural increase in population of England in general and of London in particular from the fifteenth century to the sixteenth century.

The possibility exists that the discrepancy in numbers was due to greater and more diligent recording in the sixteenth century. Hopefully, the arguments presented above will have allayed any lingering suspicions brought on by the large numbers of Bills of Mortality. Further, it can be argued that records from the sixteenth century have had one hundred years less opportunity to be lost or damaged than documents from the fifteenth century, as seems to have been the fate of the wills proved in the archdeaconry courts of East Anglia for 1477–1480. Finally, the reader is referred back to the arguments presented in Chapter 1; that every adult male in fifteenth century England had the opportunity to make a will, and that most men took steps to ensure that their wills would be registered in one court or another.[73] In this case, there would be little distinction as to which wills survived into the twentieth century, making the registered wills a representative demographic sample.

The Bills of Mortality were recorded in weekly intervals (I have made them over into aggregate monthly totals).[74] One of the first things that should be noted is that even though the chroniclers complained of continual plague throughout the whole period, it was only in the autumn of 1578 and the autumn of 1583, especially in September and October, that plague mortality was abnormally high (Graph 4.3.1). This should be kept in mind when considering the laments of the fifteenth century chroniclers. Although the literary sources were always quick to bemoan ex-

*Graph 4.3.1* Bills of Mortality

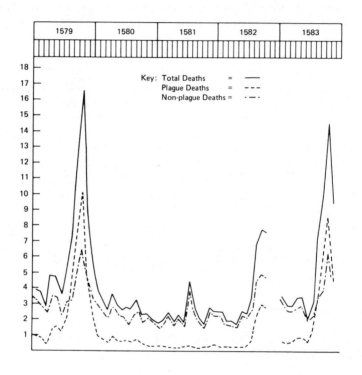

tended periods of mortality, as in 1433–1435 and 1438–1440, the clustering of mortality from the wills shows that actual crisis levels were reached generally for short periods only, in the fall, just as was the case in the sixteenth century. Another interesting point raised by the Bills of Mortality is that the peak periods of epidemic plague mortality were clearly in the autumn, in late September, October and November. This is precisely the pattern shown by the will clusterings for the fifteenth century, but is in direct contrast with the statements of many historical epidemiologists.[75]

The graphed data from the Bills of Mortality clearly show that plague was responsible for crisis mortality in the period 1578–1583. When plague mortality was high, total mortality was high. Only during crisis periods did plague mortality exceed mortality from other causes, and only during periods of high plague mortality did total mortality reach crisis proportions. Conversely, from winter, 1579, through summer, 1582, when plague mortality was almost nonexistent, total mortality was extremely low. When plague mortality increased—even ever so slightly, as in April, 1579, and more significantly in September and October, 1581— total mortality responded accordingly. Only once in the five-year period, in July, 1580, did mortality rise from nonplague causes.

Epidemic plague was the controlling factor in mortality in London from 1578 to 1583, just as epidemic disease, primarily plague, was the controlling factor in mortality in eastern England in the period 1430–1480. Epidemic plague occurred in the autumn, especially in late September and October. This was true both of mortality indicated by the Bills of Mortality for the sixteenth century and the mortality suggested by will clustering and literary evidence from the fifteenth century. Hence, when we refer to plague-type mortality, we will mean this sharp, relatively rapid and clearly defined autumnal pattern. Probably, this was bubonic plague.

## Notes

1. See above, pp. 118–121.

2. *Ibid.* Also, see N. J. T. Bailey, *Mathematical Theory of Epidemics* (London: Hafner Publishing Co., 1959).

3. See above, pp. 45–46.

4. The Peculiar Court of Bury St. Edmunds letters of administration are included in the graphs. For autumn, 1479, there were eight of these letters in the registers. This was matched only twice in the period covered—in the autumn, 1474, and, significantly, in the autumn, 1471. By comparison, for the entire period, summer, 1475, to summer, 1479, there were only six letters of administration filed.

5. See below, pp. 145–146.

6. See above, pp. 102–103.

7. *Chronicles of the Grey Friars of London,* edited by J. G. Nichols (London: Longmans, 1827), p. 22; Richard Arnold, *Customs of the City of London* (London: F. C. and J. Rivington, 1811), p. xxxvii. Arnold's description, apparently written in the early sixteenth century, appears to have been taken directly from the *Grey Friars.*

8. *Chronicle of London, 1089–1483,* edited by N. H. Nicolas (London: Longmans, 1827), p. 146; *Great Chronicles of London,* edited by A. H. Thomas (London: G. W. Jones, 1938), p. 226; *Visitations and Memorials of Southwell Minster,* edited by A. F. Leach (Westminster: Camden Society, 1891), n.s. XLVIII, p. 40.

9. Robert Fabyan, *New Chronicles of England and France,* edited by H. Ellis (London: F. C. and J. Rivington, 1811), p.666.

10. Charles Creighton, *History of Epidemics in Britain* (London: Frank Cass, 1965), I, 3rd ed., pp. 231–232.

11. Fabyan, *op. cit.,* p. 666.

12. See above, pp. 22–23.

13. See above, pp. 36–40.

14. For weather data, see above, pp. 47–50.

15. *Rot. Parl.,* V, p. 143b; V, p. 172b; Creighton, *op. cit.,* I, pp. 229–230.

16. See above, pp. 40–51.

17. The Kent wills were taken from the consistory court of Canterbury, primarily from the 1450's to 1480. There are other consistory court wills from the bishopric of Rochester, and some from the archdeaconries. The Yorkshire wills were taken from the Prerogative Court of York, primarily from 1450 to 1490.

18. For a discussion of the geographical distribution of fifteenth century epidemics, see chap. 5.

19. John Herryson, "Appendix X: Infirmarer's Roll," in T. D. Atkinson, *An Architectural History of the Benedictine Monastery of St. Etheldreda at Ely* (Cambridge: Cambridge Univ. Press, 1933).

20. For a discussion and examples of "typical" pre-industrial mortality, see E. A. Wrigley, *Population and History* (New York: McGraw-Hill, 1969), pp. 63–106.

21. Bailey, *op. cit.*

22. Fabyan, *op. cit.,* p. 653. Once again, the reader is reminded of the chronological problems concerning this reference.

23. *Calendar of State Papers and Manuscripts Relating to English Affairs: Venice,* edited by Rawdon Brown (London: H. M. Stationery Office, 1864), p. 114; *Paston Letters,* vols. I–III, edited by James Gairdner (London: Chatto and Windus, 1904), II, p. 226.

24. *Rot. Parl.,* V, pp. 618–619; *Ingulph's Chronicle of the Abbey of Croyland,* edited by H. T. Riley (London: H. G. Bohn, 1854), p. 443; John Herryson, *Abbreviata Chronica ab Anno 1377 Usque ad Annum 1469,* Caius College, Cambridge, Ms., the year 1467.

25. The disputed reference is from Fabyan, *op. cit.,* p. 653, in November.

26. See below, pp. 146–147.

27. See above, pp. 118–121.

28. *Paston Letters,* vols. I–III, edited by James Gairdner (London: Chatto and Windus, 1904), III, pp. 14–15.

29. See above, p. 44.

30. John Warkworth, *A Chronicle of the First Thirteen Years of the Reign of King Edward the Fourth*, edited by J. O. Halliwell (London: Camden Society, 1839), X, p. 23.

31. Wrigley, *op. cit.,* pp. 61–80.

32. J. F. D. Shrewsbury, *A History of Bubonic Plague in the British Isles* (Cambridge: Cambridge Univ. Press, 1971); A. H. Gale, *Epidemic Disease* (London: Penguin, 1959); and M. Burnet and D. O. White, *Natural History of Infectious Disease* (Cambridge: Cambridge Univ. Press, 1972). All discuss the virulence of the various epidemic diseases.

33. J. Tickell, *The History of the Town and County of Kingston-upon-Hull* (Hull, 1798), p. 132; J. M. W. Bean, "Plague, Population, and Economic Decline in England in the Later Middle Ages," *Ec. H. R.,* 2nd series, XV, 1962–1963, pp. 436–437.

34. See below, pp. 126–138.

35. See above, p. 64.

36. *Canterbury Cathedral Priority Obituary List,* Ms.d 12F., f. 23; *Calendar of Papal Registers,* edited by J. M. Tremlow (London: H. M. Stationery Office, 1906–1955), VIII, p. 341; John Amundesham, *Annales Monasterii S. Albani,* edited by H. T. Riley, 2 vols. (London: Longmans, 1870–1871), I, p. 62.

37. Amundesham, *op. cit.,* II, p. 127.

38. See above, pp. 39–41.

39. *Paston Letters,* I, pp. 302–303.

40. *Journal D'Un Bourgeois De Paris sous Charles VI et Charles VII,* edited by André Mary (Paris: Henri Jonquières, 1929), p. 335.

41. See above, pp. 99–100.

42. E. F. Jacob, ed., *The Register of Henry Chichele,* (Oxford: Oxford Univ. Press, 1937), II, p. xviii.

43. *The Brut: Chronicles of England,* edited by F. W. D. Brie (London: Oxford Univ. Press, 1960), II, p. 604.

44. The Prerogative Court of York (P.C.Y.) wills from the period 1460–1485 cluster in patterns similar to those from the lower courts.

45. See above, pp. 116–117.

46. Shrewsbury, *op. cit.,* p. 148.

47. *The Brut,* II, p. 604.

48. Fabyan, *op. cit.,* p. 653; *The Brut,* II, p. 604.

49. Jacob, *op. cit.,* p. xviii.

50. See above, pp. 30–36.

51. About 65% of the P.C.C. wills used in the sample were from Londoners and testators from Essex and Kent. The other 35% came from Norfolk, Suffolk and Hertfordshire, and were counted in both the P. C. C. and county samples. Thus, although the total number of wills used in the sample totaled 14,971, the tallies for the individual cohorts add up to 15,072.

52. About 250 separate computer runs were made. At one time, attempts were made to analyze each of the several hundred different occupations. Needless to say, all of this data could not be included in the text, but virtually all of the various

samples except those discussed below had autumnal modal mortality patterns.

53. See above, pp. 118–121.

54. See above, pp. 116–117.

55. See below, pp. 204–212.

56. See below, pp. 139–142.

57. See below, pp. 126–138.

58. See below, pp. 187–188.

59. For a partial statistical breakdown of the various groups within the sample, see below, p. 156.

60. For the wealth data, see below. See also, Thomas Carson, "A Socio-Economic Study of the East Anglian Clergy in the Time of Henry Despencer" (Ph.D. Dissertation: University of Michigan, 1972).

61. Among the very many discussions of historical typhus are Creighton, *op. cit.,* I, pp. 375–413; and of course, Hans Zinsser, *Rats, Lice and History* (Boston: Little Brown, 1935).

62. Each of these groups were tested separately, as well as together, but it was felt that any group having less than fifty members, as did most of the above, would be of suspect value.

63. *Ibid.*

64. Theoretically, at least, working hours were from dawn to dusk; in the summer, the working day must have been longer than it was in other seasons. Similarly, the textile workers were mostly, if not entirely, craftsmen dependent on wages. In summer, before the autumn harvest, they must have been most suscep- tible to higher bread prices, although as we have seen, a lack of foodstuffs was generally not a problem in the fifteenth century. Finally, the textile industry was not an especially healthy one to be involved with, especially as a fuller, a dyer or a shearer. In the summer, when the working day was longer, the extra time han- dling or being around the noxious elements of the industry may have been fatal. I am indebted to Prof. E. M. Carus-Wilson for her suggestions in regard to this matter.

65. Among the best sources are A. J. Coale and P. Demeny, *Regional Model Life Tables and Stable Populations* (Princeton: Princeton Univ. Press, 1973); and United Nations, Dept. of Social Affairs, Population Division, Report 17, *Methods for Population Projection by Sex and Age* (New York: United Nations, 1953).

66. For a not entirely successful attempt to use twentieth century data in comparison with fifteenth century English data, see J. C. Russell, *British Medieval Population* (Albuqerque: Univ. of New Mexico Press, 1948), especially the author's life tables and extrapolations of twentieth century Indian census data.

67. For expedience's sake, unabashed use of Creighton, *op. cit.,* chap. 6, has been made in reference to the Bills of Mortality.

68. *Ibid.,* pp. 293–297.

69. *Ibid.,* pp. 337–341.

70. Still the best discussion of the population of fifteenth century London is S. L. Thrupp, *The Merchant Class of Medieval London* (Chicago: Univ. of Chicago Press, 1948), chaps. 1 and 5. For another interpretation, see G. A. Williams, *Medieval London: From Commune to Capital,* (London: Athlone Press, 1963), pp. 315–317.

Williams claims that sons were often omitted from wills, a statement the author heartily disagrees with. Williams' evidence seems to come from seven aldermanic wills, hardly justifying his blanket statement about "quite massive evidence of omission [of children] from wills [p. 316]." Further, he appears to use later wills from the same aldermen to refute earlier *testaments.* For the population of sixteenth century London, see the estimtes of F. J. Fisher, "Development of London as a Centre for Conspicuous Consumption in the Sixteenth and Seventeenth Centuries," *Transactions of the Royal Historical Society* (T. R. H. S.), 4th series, XXX, 1948. For a less scientific assessment, see A. L. Rowse, *The Elizabethan Renaissance: The Cultural Achievement* (London: Macmillan, 1972), p. 266.

71. *Calendar . . . Venice,* I, p. 114.

72. Creighton, *op. cit.,* I, pp. 293–294.

73. See above, pp. 22–23.

74. There was some problem with weeks which fell into two separate months. The deaths were then divided proportionally into each month.

75. In particular, see Shrewsbury, *op. cit.*

# CHAPTER V

# *Patterns of Mortality, II*

## 5.1 Regions of Endemic Disease

As discussed in Chapter 3, there are many regions in the world, especially in Asia and Africa, where infectious diseases recur frequently, not only in epidemic form, but also in a permanent or semipermanent endemic form.[1] In areas of endemic plague, *pastuerella pestis* has traditionally cropped a proportion of the population in addition to the toll of epidemic plague.[2] Thus infectious disease, especially plague, may serve as a check on demographic growth not only in years of epidemic frequency, but at almost all times, via the vector of endemic disease.

The deserts and steppes of Asia and Africa, with their diverse rodent life, are far removed both geographically and zoologically from England and what is known ecologically of England in the fifteenth century.[3] Nonetheless, it is likely that endemic diseases, most notably plague,[4] were present in some virulence in fifteenth century England, and helped keep population growth in check in nonepidemic years. As we have seen, some fifteenth century texts hinted at this possibility. Endemic disease is discussed in some depth in the fifteenth century copies of John La Barba's pestilence treatise, and he believed that endemic pestilence was as great a factor in demographic limitation as were the more virulent but less frequent visitations of epidemic pestilence.[5] Several letters in the Paston collection also hint of endemic disease, and Creighton was certain that one letter in particular was a sure sign of "unhealthy infected spots" in the countryside.[6] Further, John Stourbridge, the Oxford grammarian,

126

seemed to believe that endemic disease was as much a hazard of the countryside as it was of the crowded town.[7]

It is possible that the casual attitudes which so many of the fifteenth century chronicles display toward the frequent outbreaks of pestilence, usually plague, were due to the presence of the disease in endemic form. All but the worst of the fifteenth century's numerous epidemics were described in a fatalistic, matter-of-fact manner which belied their resulting heavy mortality, as shown by the testamentary data. Further, those epidemics in the period 1430–1480 which were not plague, such as the pox of 1475, the flux of 1473, and, a bit beyond our period, the sweat of 1485, were treated by the chroniclers with much more bewilderment and in much greater detail than were even the greatest of the pestilence epidemics.[8] This was the case with the 1485 sweat despite the occurrence of major military action on English soil which resulted in a dynastic change just before its outbreak.[9] If endemic plague were a recurring hazard of everyday life, the chroniclers could hardly be expected to have expressed shock or even considerable interest at the outbreak of epidemic plague, as they appear to have done during epidemic outbreaks of other diseases.

There were regions in East Anglia, particularly in Suffolk, where testamentary mortality was especially high. Wills from fifteenth century testators survive from almost 1,300 different parishes. Judging from twentieth century gazetteers,[10] and lists of lost villages[11] and decayed churches,[12] hardly a village, hamlet, market village or town was not at some time between 1430 and 1480 represented by the wills of some of its inhabitants in one of the ecclesiastical courts. The geographical distribution of will makers throughout the period is surprisingly wide. In general, thirty to forty different parishes were represented by testators in the consistory court, and about thirty in the archdeaconry courts in any given nonepidemic quarter. During periods of crisis mortality, the numbers of parishes per quarter often increased by as much as tenfold.

There are notable individual and regional exceptions to this pattern of comprehensive will distribution by parish. Some parishes appear regularly in the will registers, in epidemic and nonepidemic quarters alike. Many of these villages appear with a frequency which seems to belie their numerical size. Further, most of these villages and parishes can be linked together into distinctive geographic regions, all of which point to the possibility of clearly delineated "unhealthy" regions of high mortality— perhaps regions of endemic disease.

To further analyze these unhealthy regions with some precision, a methodology had to be developed—something which would measure crisis mortality.[13] In pursuit of this goal, parishes were arranged by village, town, archdeaconry and modern county jurisdiction, and clustered by season of death, the latter as has been delineated in Chapter 1. [14] Any village with three or more times the mean number of testate and intestate deaths recorded in the will registers per village, in any given quarter for each archdeaconry, was considered to be a village of excess mortality. Thus, crisis mortality villages were compared with the "global" means for each archdeaconry. If the mean number of testators registered per parish in a given quarter were two, then six or more testators would signify excess or crisis mortality. It was felt that this method would take into account the considerable rise in mortality caused by epidemic disease which a fixed barometer would not. If, for example, a fixed measure of three or six deaths per village per quarter were used as the guideline for crisis mortality, this would be inadequate during epidemic quarters, when gross mortality would naturally rise. The great drawback of the method being used is that it might prejudice the sample toward the larger villages and market centers. As a precaution against this weighting of evidence toward the areas of greater population, certain large centers, aside from the obvious East Anglian urban areas—Norwich, King's Lynn, Great Yarmouth, Bury St. Edmunds and Ipswich—were not included in the endemic measure. Thus excluded were Thetford and Sudbury. The first town was omitted because of its size and because of the possibility that its will registrations might not have been complete, a problem discussed in detail below.[15] Sudbury was excluded because as the primary administrative center of the archdeaconry which bears its name, its will registration might have been abnormally high. As we shall see, Sudbury lay at the center of an "endemic" region, and the premise upon which it was rejected may not be valid.[16] Other areas of relatively large population, such as the market villages of Bungay, Beccles and Wymondham have been included within the crisis mortality sample. While it may be that these and other market centers loom prominently in the sample simply because they had more people to begin with, arguments against this view will be presented.

An important reservation must be added. Because the archdeaconry courts from the county of Suffolk are far more complete than those of Norfolk, which have large-scale will survivals from only the 1460's and 1470's, there is more opportunity for the interpretation of crisis mortality from the Suffolk wills than from their Norfolk counterparts. The wills from the archdeaconry court of Norwich, probably the most populous of the bishopric's archdeaconries, hardly survive at all, and this may explain the general absence of evidence of crisis-mortality areas within this archdeaconry. Another qualifying test given to a village or a town before it was classified as a possible region of endemic disease was that it had to exhibit crisis mortality more than once. At one time or another in the 200 seasonal quarters between 1430 and 1480, over 15 percent of the several hundred parishes studied experienced at least a single quarter of excessive, crisis mortality. It is the recurrence of high mortality, especially during nonepidemic quarters, which is the principal factor under consideration.

It is of course possible that the areas described as unhealthy or endemic regions—the areas of high and frequent elevated mortality—were simply the regions of highest population. Studies of the *Domesday Book* have shown that East Anglia was one of the most densely populated areas in England in the late eleventh century,[17] and the returns from the Poll Tax of 1377 indicate that this situation persisted even after the Black Death and the subsequent epidemics of 1361–1362, 1369, and the epidemics of the 1370's.[18] It has been stated that southeastern, south-central, and eastern Norfolk, and northeastern Suffolk were the most populous areas in England throughout the later Middle Ages.[19] This factor, and the factors discussed above must be considered when trying to convert crisis mortality in nonepidemic years into a test for endemic disease.

With these reservations in hand, the analysis may begin. Tables 5.1.1, 5.1.2 and 5.1.3 show the incidence of crisis mortality in the villages and market centers of the archdeaconries of Suffolk, Sudbury and Norfolk. Table 5.1.4 shows the incomplete tabulations from the archdeaconry of Norwich. The villages are placed in direct order of the number of crisis mortality quarters that they experienced from 1430 to 1480. From a geographical plotting of these villages, certain distinct regions of high frequency of crisis mortality can be mapped out (Map 2).

Most prominent among these unhealthy regions was a long coastal strip extending from Great Yarmouth (if this urban area can be included, for even from the wills of its testators registering in the N.C.C. alone, it had over a dozen quarters of crisis mortality), in Norfolk, to Aldeburgh in Suffolk. The heart of this region seems to have extended from Lowestoft to Dunwich. Geographically, it is separated from much of the rich farmlands of eastern Suffolk by Aldewood Forest, and is distinguished by low, marsh and fenlike areas. Because of the proximity of these marshlands, the possibility of malaria as an important control on the population as well as endemic plague, must be considered. England is said by several authorities to have suffered quite severely from malaria during the later Middle Ages.[20]

Foremost in this coastal region among the villages of high mortality was North Hales, or Covehithe, as it is alternatively called. By all accounts a fairly small and undistinguished village in the fifteenth century, North Hales nonetheless experienced fourteen quarters of crisis mortality in the period 1430–1480, a frequency greater than any of the larger villages as

*Table 5.1.1.* Villages of Crisis Mortality, Archdeaconry of Suffolk*

| | |
|---|---|
| North Hales (14) | F-51;Su-52;W-57;F-58;Sp-59;F-59;F-60;<br>Su-61;F-64;F-65;W-66;Sp-72;F-73;Sp-77. |
| Beccles (13) | Sp-47;W-54;Sp-54;W-57;Sp-60;F-63;<br>Sp-65;W-66;F-74;F-75;F-76;W-77;F-79. |
| Bungay (10) | Sp-49;F-58;Sp-60;F-61;Su-62;F-64;<br>Su-69;Su-71;W-74;W-78. |
| Pakefield (5) | W-47;Sp-53;Su-53;W-59;F-73. |
| Southwold (4) | Sp-57;F-71;F-74;Sp-75. |
| Kessingland (3) | Sp-53;Sp-55;W-77. |
| Reydon (3) | F-58;W-62;F-73. |
| Dunwich (2) | Sp-62;Sp-66. |
| Lowestoft (2) | W-49;Su-69. |
| Pettistree (2) | Sp-34;Sp-72. |
| Sutton (2) | Sp-52;Sp-54. |
| Woodbridge (2) | F-48;W-59. |

*In order of village, numbers of crisis mortality quarters, and individual listing of the quarters.

*Table 5.1.2.* Villages of Crisis Mortality, Archdeaconry of Sudbury

| | |
|---|---|
| Mildenhall (10) | Su-34;Su-35;Sp-37;F-43;W-62;Su-72;F-72;<br>Sp-74;Su-74;Sp-77. |
| Lavenham (7) | F-47;F-52;Sp-57;Sp-76;W-77;Su-77;Sp-70. |
| Stoke-Nayland (6) | F-52;W-58;W-73;Sp-76;W-80;Su-80. |
| Soham (3) | Sp-60;Su-65;Su-74. |
| Barnham (2) | F-73;Sp-77. |
| Burwell (2) | W-72;Sp-76. |
| Drinkestone (2) | Su-58;F-64. |
| Elmswell (2) | Sp-57;Su-51. |
| Eye (2) | W-52;Sp-70. |
| Long Melford (2) | Sp-57;Su-80. |
| Snailwell (2) | F-44;Sp-62. |
| Stow Market (2) | Sp-53;Sp-62. |
| Thornden (2) | Sp-57;F-58. |
| Walsham-le-<br>  Willows (2) | W-70;Sp-77. |

*Table 5.1.3.* Villages of Crisis Mortality, Archdeaconry of Norfolk

| | |
|---|---|
| Wymondham (9) | Sp-60;Sp-65;Su-65;F-65;F-66;F-67; F-76;W-79;F-79. |
| Shipdham (8) | F-60;Sp-61;Su-62;F-65;Su-67;F-79; W-80;Su-80. |
| East Dereham (7) | W-38;W-57;W-62;Sp-62;Sp-69;W-69;W-64. |
| Hingham (7) | F-39;F-60;Sp-66;Sp-71;F-67;W-70;F-71. |
| Buckenham (3) | F-66;F-79;W-80. |
| Necton (3) | Sp-58;W-63;Sp-60. |
| North Walsham (3) | W-66;W-74;F-79. |
| Walsingham (3) | F-44;S-55;F-73.* |
| Attleborough (2) | Su-60;F-66. |
| Catfield (2) | Su-60;Su-68. |
| Diss (2) | Sp-59;W-70. |
| Ellingham Magna (2) | Su-76;Su-77. |
| Upwell (2) | Su-62;F-71. |
| Worsted (2) | Sp-60;F-79. |

*Combined totals from Little Walsingham and Great Walsingham.

*Table 5.1.4.* Villages of Crisis Mortality, Archdeaconry of Norwich (as taken from the N.C.C. only)

| | |
|---|---|
| Beeston-Mar (2) | Su-31;F-65. |
| Blofield (2) | F-32;F-38. |
| Upton (2) | F-65;F-79. |
| Wiggenhall (2) | Sp-47;F-52. |

measured by the probated wills and intestate listings, and greater even than the crisis mortality frequency of towns like Great Yarmouth and King's Lynn, as taken from the N.C.C. registers. Kessingland and Pakefield were other villages in this coastal strip particularly marked by crisis mortality, as were Southwold, Dunwich, Blythburgh and Reydon. With the possible exception of Southwold, none, of these villages was particularly large or flourishing, or at least large enough to have been capable of sustaining high mortality by virtue of its own population under normal fifteenth century conditions. Oddly enough, on the basis of the testamentary evidence, the port town of Lowestoft does not seem to have had the frequency of crisis mortality one would expect in relation to its size. Only in the winter of 1449 and the summer of 1469 did mortality reach crisis levels, although this may be partly attributable to mechanical problems in the source materials.[21] If the definition of crisis mortality is extended to include parishes in which crisis mortality levels were reached once, then the villages of Wangford, Walberswick, Aldeburgh, Westleton, Wrentham, Benacre, South Cove, Henstead, Gisleham, Carlton-Colville, Gunton, Corton and Blundeston would also be included—in effect, a coastal strip containing most of the villages from Yarmouth, through North Hales, to at least Dunwich, and perhaps to Aldeburgh.

It is important to note that most of these coastal villages had their mortality clustering in purportedly nonepidemic quarters. In the case of North Hales, only three of the protracted periods of crisis mortality came in quarters which can clearly be identified as epidemic. In the case of Southwold, Reydon and Pakefield, only one of the crisis quarters coincided with a season of national or regional epidemics; and in the case of Kessingland and Dunwich, none of the crisis seasons came in a period of national epidemic disease. This gives somewhat more credence to the assertions of the literary sources about high-mortality endemic disease, and their connection with certain unhealthy rural areas.

It may be argued that a lowland region such as the Yarmouth to Aldeburgh strip, covered in some areas with marshland, and perhaps on a road from Ipswich and Stow Market north through Lowestoft to Great Yarmouth was almost by definition an area naturally susceptible to the ravages of disease. This is precisely the point being forwarded. Perhaps the endemic disease which afflicted the region most severely was not plague, but malaria or tuberculosis, even though crisis mortality is generally weighted to the autumn quarters. The fact remains that infectious diseases, epidemic and endemic, plague, dysentery, smallpox, influenza or malaria appear to have been the major factor in determining mortality in fifteenth century East Anglia, and probably in England as a whole.

There were other areas of high incidence of crisis mortality in the county of Suffolk. One of them was a border region with Norfolk, along the Waveney, from Beccles to Bungay, close to and dissecting the previously described Norfolk-Suffolk coastal region toward the north (Map 2). Both Beccles and Bungay appear to have been busy and fairly prosperous market villages in the fifteenth century, and Beccles had a will-registering population which approached that of Ipswich, the east Suffolk county center and archdeaconry seat.[22] Both villages were on major roads, and would have been more susceptible to disease brought by wayfarers than would be smaller, more isolated villages. Yet as with the coastal Suffolk region, the high mortality is not explicable in terms of epidemic disease and size alone. Beccles, with a frequency of thirteen crisis mortality quarters, and Bungay, with a frequency of ten, each had crisis quarters with a low proportion of coincidence with national or regional periods of epidemics—only one in the case of Beccles and two for Bungay. Further, although the percentage of daughters per family in both of these market villages was approximate to the levels of the sample as a whole, the percentage of sons was far below the norm.[23]

There are further distinct regions of high, crisis-type mortality in both the county Suffolk archdeaconries. In the archdeaconry of Suffolk, there is a kidney-shaped area extending from Sutton in the southeast, through Woodbridge and possibly Ufford, to Pettistree and Wickham Market in the north (Map 2). Aldewood Forest lies to the east of this region. Like Bungay and Beccles, Woodbridge and Wickham Market were market centers, and the possibility that their sheer size accounted for the high will mortality must be considered. Also, the area lies on a main road from Ipswich to the coastal towns of eastern East Anglia. But as with Beccles and Bungay, there is little correlation between the incidence of national epidemics as reported by the chroniclers and demonstrated from the will data as a whole. Furthermore, most of the quarters of high mortality in this region occur in the relatively epidemic free 1440's and 1450's.

The archdeaconry of Sudbury, in the western half of Suffolk, had several regions of frequent crisis mortality. The largest of these was an area centered around Sudbury, the archdeaconry's nominal seat. As viewed from the testamentary data, Sudbury does not seem to have been much larger than a medium-sized market village, and was probably not as populous as Beccles. It certainly was not as important economically as Ipswich or Great Yarmouth, and was smaller than its rival center in west Suffolk, Bury St. Edmunds.[24] Yet taking this into account, and considering that as the archdeaconry seat the will registration must have been especially good (the reason it is not included in Table 5.1.2), Sudbury still had a very high frequency of crisis mortality quarters. Aside from Sudbury itself, the region sprawls in no certain geographic pattern save its orientation to Sudbury itself, from Stoke-by-Nayland in the southeast, northwest through Great Cornard and Sudbury to Long Melford. It also includes Lavenham, one of the unhealthiest towns of all, judging from mortality clustering,[25] and possibly the villages of Thorpe Morieux, Kersey and Glemsford, all of which experienced a single quarter of crisis mortality from 1430 to 1480 (Map 1). Stoke-Nayland and Lavenham, both fair-sized and seemingly prosperous villages, suffered with frequent crisis-level mortality, but rarely did these crisis quarters coincide with national epidemics. And although this was a populous region, close to the Stour, and it can be argued once again that the larger parishes are simply reflecting their bulk size, it is important to note that other large villages close to but not within the area, such as Hadleigh, Haverhill and Felixstowe, do not reflect the same high mortality figures in the distinctive clustering patterns.[26] If size alone were responsible for the high figures reflecting what has been called crisis mortality, especially in nonepidemic years, then it would follow that all large villages and market centers would be equally represented, rather than particular villages at particular times, as is the case.

There are other regions of crisis-level mortality in the archdeaconry of Sudbury. One small area lies between the market villages of Eye and Thornden, and spills over the county boundary to include Diss in Norfolk. Another larger, L-shaped area lies west of the Eye-Thornden area, encompassing Stow Market—as the name implies, a large market village[27]—on the river Orwell to the southeast, and running through Drinkstone and Elmswell to Walsham-le-Willows in the north (Map 2). Neither of these two regions appears to have had as frequent occurrences of crisis mortality as did the Sudbury or coastal Suffolk regions; nevertheless, the familiar pattern of high frequency of crisis mortality in nonepidemic years again appears.

There is a large area in western Suffolk and in those parts of Cambridgeshire which fell under the jurisdiction of the bishopric of Norwich which had as high a frequency of crisis mortality as did the Sudbury and coastal Suffolk regions. This western area runs in a rough circle from Mildenhall to Soham to Burwell, and through the small parish of Snailwell. Geographically, it borders on the breckland and fenlands (Map 2), both unhealthy areas. Even today the breckland remains wild; in the fifteenth century it was mostly unwooded as well, with the trees of Thetford Forest being the results of twentieth century plantations.[28] It suffers from a pronounced lack of rainfall, and is one of the few places in England which has been described as "steppelike."[29] Further, it harbors a large and varied wild rodent and rabbit population. Thus, in the breckland are to be found now and perhaps even more so in the fifteenth century some of the geograhical and zoological conditions which in other countries have produced regions of endemic plague. The fenlands are an unhealthy, disease-ridden area, in which malaria was bred in the view of many historical epidemiologists, and with a climate which can cause tuberculosis.[30]

Testamentary mortality clustering shows these insalubrious climatic conditions. Mildenhall, albeit one of England's larger parishes,[31] suffered especially from continual periods of crisis mortality, with only North Hales and Beccles registering more frequently. As with the other areas and villages of high crisis mortality, Mildenhall suffered most frequently not during quarters of national epidemics, but in periods of purported normality. The same may be said of Burwell, Soham and tiny Snailwell. The villages in this area were very far apart by East Anglian standards, reflecting not only the poor climatic conditions, but also infertile soil. The wide distances between these villages throws further doubt on the Shrewsbury thesis of the spread of bubonic plague in fifteenth century England.[32]

Because the records of the archdeaconry courts of Norfolk are less comprehensive for the fifteenth century than those of Suffolk, it is more difficult to identify regions of crisis mortality, and perhaps endemic disease, within their jurisdictions. Yet by using wills from only the N.C.C., and when possible from the two archdeaconry courts, certain areas can still be singled out. The coastal area extending north from Aldeburgh in Suffolk to Great Yarmouth has already been discussed, as has the area between Thornden and Diss. Another distinct region, lying in the heavily populated area between Norwich and Yarmouth, can also be mapped out, even by using wills from the N.C.C. only. This area is within the jurisdiction of the archdeaconry of Norwich. One of the most densely settled regions in eleventh, fourteenth, and apparently fifteenth century England,[33] it was bounded by Upton in the north, Acle in the east, Buckenham in the south (which is actually in the archdeaconry of Norfolk; and this "extra" coverage is probably why it, of all the villages in this crisis-mortality zone, has the highest individual frequency of crisis mortality), and Blofield in the west (Map 2). As with the areas in Suffolk, crisis mortality clustered distinctly in years without epidemics. The villages in this zone lay on or about what may have been a main road from Norwich to Yarmouth.

In the county of Suffolk, the two archdeaconries were divided into integral, geographic units of approximately equal size and wealth. In the county of Norfolk, this was not so (Map 1); the archdeaconry of Norwich contained all the richest areas in the county and all the major boroughs, apparently because it was thought to have been the senior archdeaconry. Yet for at least parts of the 1460's and 1470's the wills from the more rural, poorer, and less populated archdeaconry of Norfolk have survived, and this may be the reason that more regions of frequent crisis-level mortality can be found within the jurisdictions of this archdeaconry than in the archdeaconry of Norwich. It is also possible that the lack of archdeaconry court wills is not the reason for fewer endemic disease regions in the wealthier archdeaconry; rather, it may have been that the wealthier areas were wealthier because they lacked the continual presence of endemic disease, and were in effect healthier.

The most important of the crisis-mortality zones in the archdeaconry of Norfolk was a large area west of the city of Norwich, stretching from Wymondham in the east, to East Dereham in the north, to Necton in the west, and Attleborough in the south. This was a fairly fertile area in the fifteenth century, and was well settled, judging from the Poll Tax returns.[34] Other villages within the area which experienced frequent and severe crisis mortality were Shipdham, Great Ellingham and Hingham. Wymondham,[35] Shipdham, East Dereham and Hingham, all market centers on major roads, suffered very heavily—as a group, more heavily and more frequently than any other collection of villages in East Anglia. Again it may be argued that they loomed large in the scheme of crisis mortality because of their size alone, but it is curious that none of the other surrounding large market centers and villages, most notably Swaffham and East Harling, suffered from crisis mortality at all. And as was the pattern for the Suffolk villages, most of these quarters of crisis mortality do not coincide with the quarters of national or regional epidemic disease.[36]

Two other districts of crisis mortality can be distinguished in Norfolk. One lies in the northeast of the county, a region of poorer soils, and extends from North Walsham, through Worstead, to Catfield (Map 2). North Walsham was a large market village, and the district as a whole lies on the road from Yarmouth to the villages of the Cromer Ridge. Worstead was the center of an area of rural textile manufacture. The other district, not particularly a geographical unity, was in the fenlands, in the western part of the county. It included Thorpland, Wiggenhall[37] and Upwell. These villages appear to have been relatively small in the fifteenth century, but as with all the other regions, most of the quarters of crisis mortality do not coincide with periods of high national mortality.

There were a few isolated villages with frequent high-crisis mortality. One was Walsingham, with a shrine popular among pilgrims, and thus a large transient population. Another was Laxfield, a market center in the northern part of the archdeaconry of Suffolk, in the heart of a rich farming area. Finally, there was Barnham, in the archdeaconry of Sudbury, and fairly close to the breckland and Thetford. Thetford itself, because of its size and because it fell mostly under the jurisdiction of the archdeaconry court of Norwich, has not been included in the survey of crisis mortality. However, judging from partial mortality evidence of the wills from the N.C.C., it appears to have had several quarters of crisis mortality, and probably was part of the breckland-fenland endemic region. It is possible that Thetford's decline in the later Middle Ages was due in part to endemic disease.[38] Walsingham, Laxfield and Barnham were the only three villages which could not be geographically grouped together with other similarly afflicted villages into districts of crisis mortality, and perhaps endemic disease.

In sum, certain hypotheses can be advanced about epidemic and endemic disease. Judging from the frequency of crisis mortality in seasons and years in which national and regional epidemics were *not* reported as having taken place, endemic disease, or, as John La Barba called it, "unhealthiness," played an important and possibly major role in checking population growth in certain well-defined areas. The decline of particular local districts may even be explicable in part by endemic as well as by epidemic disease. The areas which suffered most had several things in common besides high incidences of crisis mortality in nonepidemic quarters. First, all of them had one or more market villages. Second, most of the areas lay near or on major roads between urban centers. Finally, many of the areas lay near distinct geographical regions, such as the breckland, extensive (by relative standards) woodlands, fenlands, or coastal areas, places which may not have contained East Anglia's richest farmland, but which could have housed the wildlife known to purvey many diseases which exist in endemic form.

Patterns of mortality clustering by village and region caused by epidemic disease indicate that almost all villages and towns exhibited crisis mortality, rather than a select few, as was the case with endemic disease. Thus the high, total mortality reflected by epidemic disease was not the result of protracted crisis mortality in a few villages, towns or districts, but, on the contrary, high, if not always crisis-level mortality in almost all villages, and increased urban mortality, a phenomena discussed in section 5.2. Epidemic disease in the fifteenth century appears to have affected most villages in a blanket fashion, perhaps not with the virulence of the plague epidemics of the fourteenth century, but comprehensively nonetheless. Endemic disease, on the other hand, appears to have afflicted only particular villages and regions, but affected them very frequently.

Finally, an important question posed earlier and throughout the text must be answered: could crisis mortality not be crisis mortality at all, but rather, just a reflection of particular large villages and towns, or merely an extraordinarily diligent local clerk? The distinct geographical clustering of almost all the villages and towns which exhibit crisis mortality, and the lack of isolated cases, is sufficient response to the latter doubt; and the answer to the first part of the question would also appear to be no. True enough, certain large villages like Beccles, East Dereham and Soham had more than their share of crisis mortality, but then so did many villages of

very modest size, such as Snailwell, North Hales and Upton. More important, many large market villages such as Hadleigh, Felixstowe and Leiston
would not be reflecting their true late medieval sizes if crisis mortality
clustering were used as a demographic standard, or as a guide to comparative densities of settlement. Something must have been responsible
for unusually high and closely bunched mortality in distinct regions
during nonepidemic years. A definitive answer can not be given on the
basis of the testamentary data alone, but a strong probability is endemic
disease.

## 5.2 Town and Country: The Urban and Rural Patterns of Mortality Contrasted

It has frequently been assumed that plague was primarily an urban
phenomenon in fifteenth century England.[39] Part of this conception may
come from the frequency with which the wealthy and powerful members
of society are advised and advise each other to flee from urban areas,
especially London, in time of plague. This is a misconception. Many of the
traditional ideas about epidemics being restricted to urban areas may stem
from a misreading of the narrative sources. The only real urban area of
any size in fifteenth century England was London, and most of the
admonitions of flight concern or are connected with it.[40] There is no
justification for extending these warnings to the lesser urban centers.
Norwich, Ipswich, St. Albans and Bury St. Edmunds, the urban areas
discussed in this section, were all quite small in both physical area and
population throughout the fifteenth century, as were York, Bristol,
Coventry, Exeter, Southampton and other towns.[41] They can be considered urban by virtue of their functions as economic, social, educational,
ecclesiastical and administrative centers, rather than by their size.
Further, simply because inward-looking urban chroniclers mention that
people were fleeing from a town, the modern historian cannot assume
that the entire countryside was epidemic-free. Certain rural areas were as
unhealthy as the capital city; urban rats did not have a monopoly of fleas
carrying *pastuerella pestis*.

For purposes of this sample, London, Norwich, Ipswich, Bury St.
Edmunds and St. Albans were considered to be urban areas. Three other
centers within the geographical borders of this study which might be
considered as urban—King's Lynn, Great Yarmouth and Thetford—
could not be used for lack of records. Lynn and Yarmouth both had
peculiar court jurisdictions, and although wills survive from both towns
from the fourteenth century, none survive from the period 1430–1480.

Thetford was part of the archdeaconry of Norwich, whose wills also do not survive in great detail from the period under consideration. Wills from townsmen from all three towns were also registered in the N.C.C., however, and these wills have been included in the sample.

Mortality in urban areas has already been briefly discussed in Chapter 4.[42] As described there, all towns but Norwich showed predominant, autumnal plague-type mortality patterns; and London, based on the wills from the P.C.C.—an admittedly incomplete, upper-class sample—showed one of the heaviest fall mortality patterns of all. In fact, it appears from the testamentary evidence (Tables 4.2.1–4.2.6) that London suffered more heavily from epidemics in the fifteenth century than did most of the rest of the country. In the plague-filled decades of the 1430's and 1470's, the wealthiest Londoners showed massive autumnal mortality patterns; and even in the 1440's, 1450's and 1460's, Londoners wealthy enough to have had their wills registered in the P.C.C. showed fall predominant patterns of mortality. While this is not surprising in light of the literary evidence, it is on the surface quite different from the graphed results discussed in Chapter 4. Since the graphed results were taken from the same data as the computerized results, this is an apparent contradiction. On one hand, we have mortality graphs showing few pronounced fall-mortality peaks, and none of the dramatic peaks of concerted mortality indicative of epidemic disease in general at any time. On the other hand, a thorough investigation of all deaths for all seasons from every year between 1430 and 1480, as opposed to the more spectacular though briefer mortality patterns of the graphs, shows a more consistently autumnal pattern for the 830 wealthy Londoners than for any other group in the entire sample. What can be said now about wealth and the ability to flee from epidemics? More important, how can these apparently contradictory results be explained, if they can be explained at all?

A possible answer lies in the relationship of endemic disease and epidemic disease, and the fact that the London sample used was an upper-class one. During the most severe epidemics, Londoners wealthy enough to have had their wills registered in the P.C.C. would almost certainly have been wealthy enough to have fled from the city. Yet this could not be done all the time in a half century of recurring epidemic disease, to say nothing of endemic disease. It would have been most difficult for a merchant or craftsman to flee from his work about every other year in a fifty-year period for a protracted length of time and expect to maintain his business or craft. Further, in London, England's only true metropolis in the later Middle Ages, plague must have been endemic. The sixteenth century Bills of Mortality show that there were deaths from plague almost every week in the period 1578–1583, regardless of reports of its presence in epidemic form.[43] The wealthy could and did flee from the most severe epidemics, but flight from a condition which existed at almost all times was not practical, and probably not possible. Flight certainly was the expedient resorted to in the most dire years, such as 1438–1439, 1464 and 1479, and no doubt this is the reason for the lack of pronounced peaks in the graphs. In other epidemic years, wealthy Londoners must have stayed in the city; and although they probably avoided the most protracted mortality patterns exhibited by the poorer segments of society, they could not avoid epidemics entirely. There are slight autumnal peaks of mortality discernable from the graphs, and these slight peaks and the constant fall-mortality caused by continual endemic plague are responsible for the heavy autumn-mortality patterns shown by the computer. It would be foolish to stretch this point too far. There is evidence which indicates that the poorer groups in society also fled during severe epidemic years. But with all that has been said about particular rural areas and their apparent unhealthiness, London must have been the unhealthiest area of them all.[44]

If London was a repository for epidemic and endemic disease, especially plague, it is by no means certain that the smaller towns were. The city of Norwich sample used in this study is also weighted toward the wealthier members of society.[45] The wealth standards of the Norwich testators, while far lower than those of the Londoners, were higher than the levels of the testators of the surrounding countryside, and those of the sample as a whole. Yet the situation of the city was exactly the opposite of that of London. There are sharp mortality peaks which coincide with the severest national epidemics, but a general pattern of spring, rather than fall, mortality is found. In this respect, Norwich was unique, not only in the urban sample, but in the entire survey. Further, it is only in the purportedly epidemic free decades of the 1440's and 1450's that Norwich shows any decennial fall-type mortality patterns; in other decades covered, the city has a distinctly spring-death pattern. Certainly, epidemic disease did not bypass Norwich, but the town may have been relatively immune from at least one disease, plague. The area surrounding the city contained some of the richest farmland and densest population in fifteenth century England.[46] At risk of calling Norwich comparatively clean and healthy, it does not appear to have suffered from the continual and chronic patterns of autumn mortality that so many other areas, especially London, did. Without trying to pursue this topic beyond the limits that the source materials allow, it can be said that at least endemic plague was primarily a local affliction, not common to all parts of the country, while epidemic plague was a bane common to all. While the large city London appears to have suffered from virtually everything, the small city Norwich did not.

Like London, Bury St. Edmunds, Ipswich and St.Albans had fall-predominant mortality patterns; unlike London, they did not have them in extreme, and showed considerable decennial variation. St. Albans even had a slight winter-mortality pattern for the 1470's, the only major sub-sample to have such. None of the above areas was epidemic-free. All showed pronounced mortality peaks in the reported periods of national and regional epidemics; but none showed the overwhelming autumnal patterns of London, nor the seeming endemic-plague immunity of Norwich. These patterns, and those discussed for the crisis-mortality regions, reinforce the idea that while epidemics on a national scale affected most areas, smaller scale epidemics and endemic infectious diseases were not just urban problems, but afflictions of particular regions and areas, rural and urban, dependent upon local conditions.

In all the cities, with the sole exception of one group, the very wealthy London élite, replacement ratios were lower than in rural areas.[47] Even in Norwich, the town which had the lowest frequency of crisis mortality and a springtime pattern of seasonal mortality, replacement ratio levels for males were not equal to their agrarian counterparts in the archdeaconry. In all cases, for all decades, the urban replacement ratios were lower than those of the rural equivalents. These "fertility" nadirs were especially depressed in Bury St. Edmunds and Ipswich; further, the Bury results are particularly interesting because the sample is such a good one, coming from a peculiar court, and from a town which was far wealthier per testator than the bulk of the surrounding villages in west Suffolk, and the sample as a whole. Although great individual wealth and numbers of children were related for the entire sample, this was less so for the urban segment. Interestingly enough, this situation of apparently lower fertility per testator exists in spite of the fact that marriage and remarriage ratios were generally as high or higher in urban areas. Remarriage in the towns was fairly common, especially among the wealthier segments of society. Thus the lower urban fertility takes on further importance in light of higher urban-marriage ratios.[48]

In sum, it cannot be said that epidemic or endemic disease, especially plague, was an urban phenomena in the fifteenth century. It cannot even be said in general terms that urban areas were more prone to epidemic disease than rural areas. Certainly London was one of the unhealthiest places of all, subject to both epidemic disease and chronic endemic disease. But the next largest city studied, Norwich, did not suffer as frequently as London or the sample as a whole; and the other three urban areas, St. Albans, Bury St. Edmunds and Ipswich, were afflicted in approximate proportion with the rest of the sample. And of all the urban areas, only London had as high a frequency of crisis mortality in proportion to its population as did selected rural districts of protracted crisis mortality. No particular area, town or country, had a monopoly of epidemic or endemic disease, especially plague, by virtue of its pattern of settlement. If population density were a key factor in the transmission of infectious diseases, only London appears to have had one high enough to make a significant difference in the incidence of disease. Rather, special geographical circumstances and location, such as proximity to the fens or breckland, and the local animal population, seem to have been most crucial.

## 5.3 The Dissemination of Epidemic Disease

It has been suggested that particular areas were subject to crisis-mortality patterns in nonepidemic years as well as in epidemic years, and we have chosen to call these areas regions of endemic disease. London, coastal Suffolk, the breckland, the areas around Aldewood Forest and Sudbury, and central Norfolk seem to have been especially unhealthy. At the same time, almost all areas were infected during the many periods of large-scale outbreaks of epidemic disease. Did epidemics begin in the endemic regions and then spread outward? Did diseases follow major roads and routes of communication? Or did they appear spontaneously in many different areas, without apparent pattern? These are the questions to which answers will be attempted in this section.

As the worst epidemic of plague to strike England in recorded history, the Black Death of 1348–1349 made a large impact on contemporaries, and as a result, can be followed across parts of England.[49] However, even if a model of dissemination for plague can be constructed, there are problems in applying it to the fifteenth century. First, in this study there are regional limitations in the tracing of epidemics. Further, East Anglia, if not Hertfordshire, is at an "end" of England; traveling from the south or the west, the only land approaches, one would probably not be passing through East Anglia, but rather going to some place within it. Finally, epidemic diseases change aetiologically, especially over a century. Nevertheless, it will be helpful to establish the path of the Black Death, and attempt to use it as a model for charting the path of epidemic disease in the fifteenth century.

Most of the fourteenth century narrative sources agree that the Black Death first entered England through one of the western or southwestern ports.[50] Although contemporary scholarly opinion seems to favor Melcombe Regis on the coast of Dorset, there are fourteenth century chroniclers and twentieth century historians who say that Bristol, Exeter and even Southampton were among the likely points of entry.[51] The dates of initiation vary also, ranging through the summer and autumn of 1348.[52] The Black Death spread through the west country, probably by way of main routes of communication, as it appears to have struck major urban centers such as Bath and Gloucester before it reached the more remote regions of the western countryside.

By the spring of 1349, the plague was appearing throughout the country, having abandoned the generally geographical pattern followed in the previous autumn and winter. Probably this was due to its simultaneous introduction in many ports. This certainly was the case in East Anglia, with its many havens in close proximity and contact with the continent, for the Black Death appeared in Norfolk and Suffolk before Cambridgeshire. In the west, the plague advanced from Bristol into Oxfordshire by the spring of 1349, and then into Berkshire by the summer and Buckinghamshire by summer and autumn. In the south, it spread from Southampton northward into Hampshire, Wiltshire and Surrey in the winter, and then into London. The plague probably entered the capital by more routes than just the Southampton one, as many chronicles suggest,[53] and conceivably from the city's own port facilities. It may have been present in London as early as the autumn, 1348.

In Hertfordshire, the Black Death entered from the south, on the major routes from London. Its presence in and around St. Albans has been studied thoroughly by A.E. Levett.[54] Although she believes that the effects were not as severe for Hertfordshire as other scholars have claimed them to be for the bulk of the country, Levett does subscribe to the widespread nature of the disease, believing that it struck most of the villages in the archdeaconry of St. Albans.[55] It appears to have been disseminated in a logical pattern, via the major routes of communication, just as it initially passed through the west country. Thus, at least one manner in which plague spread in the fourteenth century was a comparatively slow diffusion, by means of major roads, in a thorough and relentless fashion.

The East Anglian experience was different from that of Hertfordshire. The Black Death was more severe there than anywhere else except London, and it seems to have spread rather haphazardly, in defiance of geographical direction and predictability.[56] Most accounts have the plague first entering East Anglia no later than the spring of 1349, and not from the west country, but independently from the continent by way of the ports, especially King's Lynn and Yarmouth. Through the course of spring and summer, 1349, immediately following its introduction, the records indicate that the Black Death appeared throughout Norfolk and Suffolk almost at random, and almost everywhere. Several regions, especially urban areas, were struck severely. Blomefield felt that Norwich never regained its position as second city in the kingdom after the devastation of 1349—if indeed it had ever held it—and Russell too believed that the city suffered greatly.[57] Grimwood claimed that Sudbury never recovered from the Black Death,[58] and there is little doubt that King's Lynn and Yarmouth were devastated also. Ipswich, where the bishop of Norwich chose to spend most of his time during the epidemic, may have been more fortunate than the other East Anglian towns, but was by no means left unaffected. Specific nonurban areas such as the breckland and the Goodsand and Greensand regions of Norfolk were hit hard while the fenlands seem to have been less harshly afflicted.

Two guiding factors may be taken from the great plague of 1348–1350. First, it was England's most severe plague epidemic, and one of pneumonic and septicemic as well as bubonic plague. In this sense, it must be at least partially different in aetiological nature from the plagues of the fifteenth century, most of which were bubonic. This difference is especially important in regard to seasonal frequencies, and should be kept in mind as we proceed to the second factor, patterns of dissemination. On one hand, the Black Death traveled in a systematic pattern, via main routes of communication, striking large settlements, especially market villages, before it hit more remote, rural areas. This was probably the pattern for Hertfordshire, into which the plague was introduced from London. On the other hand, the Black Death made its way into other areas from many different points, and spread almost without logic, appearing erratically in geographically remote places before it appeared n major villages and towns closer to the points of its entrance. These two manners of transmission of plague will be the models which will be tested for fifteenth century epidemic disease.

Three epidemics of fifteenth century pestilence—in these cases, almost certainly plague—those of 1464–1465, 1471 and 1479, will be examined, rather than all the pestilence epidemics from 1430 to 1480. For comparative purposes, the pox of 1462 and the flux of 1473 will also be charted. These epidemics were chosen to the exclusion of the equally virulent epidemics of the 1430's because of the superior testamentary data from the 1440's onward. Once again, we shall start with the pestilence of 1479, the most virulent epidemic of the century. The literary sources give useful dates for its onset and conclusion. Brushing aside the report of its commencement in 1478, the earliest reliable record of its presence come from Southwell, in Nottinghamshire in the summer, and from East Anglia in the late summer. In London, the pestilence was said to have "dured" from September through October, but Worcestre claimed that his stepson died from it there in January, 1480.[59] From the use of the literary sources alone, then, it would seem that the epidemic began in the north country or north Midlands, came south, and passed through East Anglia and into London. The testamentary evidence provides further clues. Most of the mortality peaks for the East Anglian courts were in the autumn of 1479 and the winter of 1479–1480, although there were slight summer peaks in the N.C.C. Several of the Paston Letters show that the summer references are to the deaths of various family members, but not explicitly to their causes, while the earlier references in the same collection were to the diseases which caused such deaths. If the pestilence of 1479 did follow a distinct path, the mode of dissemination of the first of the plague models, and did make its initial East Anglia appearance in the summer, it does not seem to have become virulent until the autumn. This suggests the possibility that a new strain of pestilence was introduced into East Anglia in the second half of 1479, but had to combine with the ever-present strains of endemic disease to produce the severe outbreak which eventually occurred—just as was suggested by John La Barba!

The graphed mortality results for 1479 provide us with further information. In the archdeaconry of St. Albans, the mortality rise began not in the autumn, but in the summer. The town of St. Albans, on a major road to and from London, would logically be affected before London itself if the pestilence came solely from the north, and mortality there did reach a peak in the summer quarter. While mortality in the archdeaconry as a whole peaked in the fall, there was heavy late summer and early autumn crisis-level mortality in several parishes north of the town, including Hexton and Codicote.

Mortality clustering for individual parishes in East Anglia provide further indications as to the course of the pestilence of 1479. No Norfolk villages exhibited crisis mortality in the spring or summer of 1479. In the ensuing autumn, however, there was extensive crisis mortality; more impressive, it was spread throughout a very large number of parishes. Mortality was up all over the county, with over 100 villages showing a significant upturn in numbers of registered wills of their inhabitants. In Suffolk, the testamentary data for 1479 are incomplete, but the excellent peculiar court of Bury St. Edmunds likewise shows a significant increase in probate mortality for all the town's parishes. Further, both the towns of Norwich and B.S.E. showed mortality increases at the same time during the autumn, indicative of simultaneous rather than systematic spread of the epidemic throughout East Anglia. The only exception to this random pattern was the winter mortality peak in the archdeaconry of Sudbury, the bishopric's most southwesterly district, and this may have been due as much to incomplete data as to the path of the epidemic.

Thus, in 1479, the fifteenth century's most severe outbreak of epidemic disease, as in 1348–1350, the fourteenth century's most severe outbreak, the path of pestilence, almost certainly plague, appears to have been twofold: both along the major highways of communication and simultaneously from within a particular area itself. On one hand, the pestilence appears to have started somewhere in the north, and proceeded slowly south, by way of St. Albans, to London. On the other hand, it seems to have spread haphazardly and quickly throughout East Anglia. Quite possibly, a new, virulent strain of infectious disease was introduced and combined with an already present variety. In 1348–1350, the apparently random, seemingly spontaneous outburst of plague in far-flung and geographically remote areas was due to multiple points of introduction and the very virulence of the new infectious disease itself; in 1479, the random outbursts in East Anglia may have been due to the ignition of endemic strains "left behind."

In contrast to the epidemic of 1479, the pestilence of 1464–1465 appears to have followed an orderly progression through East Anglia, as well as through the rest of England. The first literary reference to this epidemic comes from London, in the autumn of 1464, and is one of the fullest and most descriptive from the period. It claimed that the pestilence was strongest in the city between late September and October. The next dated literary reference to an epidemic comes from Norfolk, in the late summer of 1465. From these two references alone, little else can be said; as discussed above, the East Anglian experience may not even have been connected aetiologically with the epidemic of 1464.[60] It is necessary to turn to the testamentary evidence for further answers.

Mortality peaked in the fall of 1464 in both the town and archdeaconry of St. Albans. There is no evidence that the pestilence lingered on after the fall. In Suffolk, there was also a pronounced autumn-1464 mortality peak. Further, this peak began first in the parishes of the archdeaconry of Sudbury, the area of Suffolk nearest to Herfordshire, and moved gradually eastward into the archdeaconry of Suffolk, with autumn, winter and spring peaks in mortality. Thus, judging from the wills of the Norfolk courts, there does seem to be a link between the literary source record of pestilence in London in 1464 and that in Norfolk in 1465. There was a slight Norfolk testamentary peak in the autumn of 1464, a dormant period through the winter and spring of 1464–1465, a slight rise in mortality in the summer, and a dramatic and extensive mortality peak in fall, 1465. It seems that the epidemics of 1464 and 1465 were connected then, if only in the introduction of a new, virulent strain of pestilence into Norfolk. Obviously, more must be known about mortality patterns in Essex before definitive statements can be made.[61] But it is probable that the epidemic of 1464–1465 moved from London through Hertfordshire, into western Suffolk, and then east toward coastal Suffolk. The epidemic then moved north into Norfolk, and was present there in the autumn of 1464, but did not reach severe conditions until the autumn of 1465. There was almost no mortality clustering by parish in Norfolk in the autumn of 1464; there was extensive mortality clustering in the autumn of 1465. As in 1479, it was quite comprehensive geographically, covering villages in all regions of both Norfolk county archdeaconries. Like the pestilence of 1479, that of 1464–1465 must have come to East Anglia from other areas in England and perhaps from local sources and not from abroad, as in 1348–1350. None of the major port towns of Norfolk, including King's Lynn and Great Yarmouth (taking just the wills from the N.C.C.), show heavy patterns of mortality, in contrast to the inland towns and villages of the county. But unlike the 1479 East Anglian experience, the epidemic of 1464–1465 seems to have been most heavily dependent for its introduction upon other areas of England. Without totally precluding the possibility of an exacerbated local strain of endemic pestilence playing a major role, it is most likely that this epidemic came into East Anglia through major routes of communication in a slow, generally orderly fashion. The inland market villages on major routes were most severely affected, and the random, simultaneous spread of epidemic disease probably played only a small role in its mode of dissemination. It followed the west country pattern of 1348–1349.

One final outbreak of pestilence, the epidemic of 1471, will be examined. There is no dated mention of the epidemic's presence in London, but there are two precise chronological references to it, from Southwell Minster in Nottinghamshire, and from the *Paston Letters.* Both fix the date in late summer, early autumn. The graphed testamentary data indicate that this epidemic proceeded across East Anglia and Hertfordshire suddenly and without any precise, well-defined patterns. In all courts, mortality rose sharply and quickly in the autumn of 1471, in the pattern of bubonic plague. Only in the archdeaconries of Suffolk does heavy mortality linger on past the fall of 1471; and even within this county, the mortality peak in the B.S.E. peculiar court was limited to the autumn. Crisis-mortality clustering confirms this picture of haphazard spontaneity. Clustering was high and widespread, as it always was during epidemic periods, but was present in a wide array of villages, and not concentrated in market villages or towns along major roads. Villages like Kettlebergh, Barford, West Bradenham and Sutton (the last two near zones of excessive mortality; see Map 2), all fairly small and somewhat out of the way, experienced their sole quarter of crisis mortality from 1430 to

1480 in the autumn of 1471. The pestilence of 1471 was more random and more rapidly disseminated than that of 1465, in the pattern of the epidemic of 1479 in East Anglia.

Of the three virulent epidemics of pestilence, probably plague, in the period 1430–1480 which can be traced through the testamentary data, one, that of 1464–1465, seems to have followed the slow, steady, geographical pattern of dissemination of the Black Death of 1348–1350 in the west country, following the main routes of communication, and reaching major centers before it reached areas more inaccessible though closer to its point of initiation. Another, that of 1471, seems to have been far more sudden and spontaneous than that of 1464–1465, much like the Black Death of 1348–1350 in East Anglia, following no logical or geographic patterns, but sweeping across the infected areas very quickly. The greatest epidemic of the fifteenth century, that of 1479, followed both models—just like the Black Death itself—depending upon region. While it appears to have traveled geographically from the north country into London, it also swept across East Anglia with no apparent regard to geographical or chronological regularities. Thus, plague could and did spread in the fifteenth century by either method, and could spread by either method over the same area at different times, or by different methods in different areas at the same time.

To see if the model forwarded for the dissemination of pestilence holds for other types of epidemic disease, it is necessary to examine two distinctly nonplague epidemics of the period, the pox of 1462 and the flux of 1473. There is only a single reference to the pox; it came late in the autumn of 1462, while Edward IV was on campaign against the Scots. The literary sources give no clues as to its identity, although smallpox is probably the best guess,[62] and there are no autumn peaks in any of the courts studied. But while there were no fall, 1462, peaks, there were, without exception, very severe and pronounced spring, 1462 peaks in probate mortality. In the archdeaconry of Norfolk, registered wills reached their highest levels ever. In all courts, mortality rose to an apex very suddenly, and then declined with the same rapidity, dissipating by the summer. Only in the archdeaconry of St. Albans was there another mortality peak within a two-year period, and that was for the spring of 1463, and was probably not connected in any way with the spring, 1462, pox. The graphs, then, can tell us very little about the path of this mysterious epidemic, except that it was very rapid in arriving, and equally quick to depart. It must have been extremely contagious, a criterion which fits smallpox. However, the speed with which the epidemic spread through Hertfordshire and East Anglia suggests the possibility of influenza.

Although mortality clustering shows the widespread nature of the pox, no clear path of diffusion can be discerned from this method of investigation either. A wide variety of fairly obscure villages, such as Snailwell, East Bergholt, Thurlow and Easton-Suffolk, as well as the larger market villages such as Bungay, experienced crisis mortality in the spring of 1462. The rapidity and spontaneity of this epidemic are similar to the pestilence epidemic of 1471,with its high but relatively brief period of mortality.

The flux of 1473 is reported by the literary sources as having occurred at "hervist tyme," and has been identified with some confidence as intestinal dysentery.If the epidemic were one of dysentery, it would probably have been less widespread then plague, or smallpox or influenza, if either of the latter two were the identity of the pox of 1462. The 1473 flux was indeed geographically limited. There were no mortality peaks whatsoever for either the town or the archdeaconry of St. Albans; and despite the severe death toll in East Anglia, there is no surviving mention of its presence in London. From the start, it is clear that the flux was territorially different from the other infectious diseases—a major epidemic in terms of crude mortality, but one which nevertheless was regional even within the limited areas of this study. Further, the graphed data tell us that the effects of the flux were geographically restricted even within East Anglia. It was far more virulent in Norfolk than it was in Suffolk. Within the latter county, the eastern parishes were struck more severely than were the western parishes; and in the archdeaconry of Suffolk, there was a genuine dysenterylike late-summer mortality peak. In Norfolk too the mortality distribution was not uniform across the county, but was more severe in the parishes of the archdeaconry of Norwich than in those of the archdeaconry of Norfolk. Towns were hit especially hard, with Norwich, Thetford, Great Yarmouth and the large village of Walsingham[63] suffering heavy mortality. Some distinct geographical districts appear to have been affected more harshly than others, as well. Among them were a coastal region around Walsingham, Great Ryburgh and Weybourne in north Norfolk, and a large area running from Cawston and Wymondham, through Norwich, and east to Great Yarmouth. In effect, a comparatively small district, primarily in the archdeaconry of Norwich, bore the brunt of the flux epidemic. This was a far smaller area than was affected by virtually any of the other epidemics studied. The flux does not appear to have followed a consistent geographical progression in its mode of dissemination, and was neither rapid and sudden nor particularly short-lived in those areas which it afflicted. Mortality was highest in the autumn of 1473 and the winter of 1473–1474; the epidemic ran its course quickly only in the city of Norwich, and there it did so at great cost in human lives.

In sum, four of the five major epidemics studied followed the model patterns of the spread of epidemic disease: either a slow, geographical procession along major roads and through the principal towns and villages first, and then to outlying precincts; or quickly and suddenly, oblivious to any geographic boundaries or restraints. The fifth epidemic, probably dysentery, was much more restricted geographically. It was, however, as lethal, if possibly not as contagious, as almost any other major epidemic in the period 1430–1480.

# Notes

1. F. G. Clemow, *Geograhy of Epidemic Disease* (Cambridge: Cambridge Univ. Press, 1903); J-N. Biraben, *Les Hommes et la peste* (The Hague: Mouton, 1975). Also, see above, pp. 81–90.

2. *Ibid.*

3. There are few worthwhile geographic descriptions which have survived from the fifteenth century. Perhaps the best is William of Worcestre, *Itinerum,* Corpus Christi College, Cambridge, Unique Ms. 210. In his edition, John Harvey (Oxford: Clarendon, 1969), calls it "ecological." The author does not go quite so far. Among the better modern studies on the geography of fifteenth century England are: A.R.H. Baker and R. A. Butlin, eds., *Studies of Field Systems in the British Isles* (Cambridge: Cambridge Univ. Press, 1973); and H. C. Darby, ed., *Historical Geography of England before 1800* (Cambridge: Cambridge Univ. Press, 1973).

4. Many historical epidemiologists believe that endemic malaria was a major health hazard in fifteenth century East Anglia. See M. Burnet and D. O. White, *Natural History of Infectious Disease* (Cambridge: Cambridge Univ. Press, 1972); and William MacArthur, "A Brief Study of English Malaria," *British Medical Bulletin,* 8, 1951–1952.

5. See above, p. 64.

6. As reported in Charles Creighton, *A History of Epidemics in Britain,* (Cambridge: Cambridge Univ. Press, 1894), I, p. 226n. The quotation reads as follows: "And forasmuch as there was a child dead at Asteleys, and one other like to be dead in the same place, what time I rode out about my little livelihood, my lady and I both thought pity on my mistress your wife to see her abide there, and desired her to come to my poor house, unto such time as you should otherwise be advised." Needless to say, the validity of Creighton's statement must be held in some doubt.

7. See above, pp. 76–77.

8. A notable exception to this is the "pockys" of 1462.

9. There are few detailed modern accounts of the 1485 sweat. See Creighton, *op. cit.,* I, pp. 237–281; A. H. Gale, *Epidemic Diseases* (London: Penguin, 1959), pp. 42–50; and M. B. Shaw, "A Short History of the Sweating Sickness," *Annals of Medical History,* V, 1933.

10. See, for example, Oliver Mason, *The Gazetteer of England,* 2 vols. (Newton

Abbot: David and Charles, 1972); and Frank Smith, *A Genealogical Gazetteer of England* (Baltimore: Genealogical Publishing Co., 1968).

11. Maurice Beresford, *Deserted Medieval Villages* (London: Lutterworth Press, 1968).

12. C. J.W. Messent, *Parish Churches of Norfolk and Norwich* (Norwich: H. W. Hunt, 1936).

13. For a different use of the concept of crisis mortality, see R. S. Schofield, "Crisis Mortality," *Local Population Studies*, 9, 1972. The author is aware of the mechanical shortcomings of the method used. However, an additional test for seasonality was run. With the epidemic years 1439, 1452, 1462, 1464, 1465, 1471, 1473 and 1479 eliminated, the endemic villages and the rest of the villages were tested for season of death. While both groups had modal figures of 4, or autumn, the endemic group had a mean of 2.61, and the rest of the sample had 2.47. A less global measure was also needed. The annual seasonal means were taken for ten of the forty-four suspected endemic villages, from 1460 to 1480, with the epidemic years of 1462, 1464–1465, 1471, 1473 and 1479–1480 programmed out. The sample mean was 2.50. The means for the crisis mortality villages were as follows: North Hales, 2.72; Beccles, 2.65; Bungay, 2.59; Southwold, 2.60; Mildenhall, 2.70; Lavenham, 2.61; Snailwell, 2.54; Wymondham, 2.62; East Dereham, 2.63; and Blofield, 2.52.

14. See above, pp. 28–31.

15. See above, p. 133.

16. See above, pp. 129–136.

17. H. C. Darby, "Domesday Geography of Norfolk and Suffolk," *Geographical Journal*, LXXXV, 1935; also, "Domesday England," in H. J. Darby, *Historical Geography of New England before 1800* (Cambridge: Cambridge Univ. Press, 1973).

18. R. A. Pelham, "Fourteenth Century England," in *Historial Geography.* The author has worked through much of the 1377, 1379, and 1381 Poll Tax data to see if they could be used comparatively with the fifteenth century data. This proved to be impossible. For 1377, the assessment was made at 4d per head for all adults over age fourteen, and most historians agree that the degree of evasion was quite low. The subsequent assessments were at varying rates not fully known, and evasion was widespread. Thus, only the 1377 assessment could be used, when returns for particular parishes were available. Data from series P.R.O. E. 359 and P.R.O. E. 179 were used. Unfortunately, only partial returns exist for both Norfolk and Suffolk, and very few records from the designated "crisis mortality" villages survive. There are much fuller data, especially for Suffolk from 1381, but even this is incomplete, and not usable on a county-wide scale. The 1381 Suffolk returns are reprinted in Edgar Powell, *The Rising in East Anglia* (Cambridge: Cambridge Univ. Press, 1896). A good, descriptive account of all three poll taxes can be found in M. Beresford, *The Lay Subsidies* (Cambridge: Phillimore, 1963). In those few cases where it is feasible to use the 1377 data, reference will be made. It may be possible to use the Lay Assessments of 1523–1524 and 1524–1525. Although the precise levies are at times uncertain, the village by village coverage for Norfolk and Suffolk is quite good. See John Sheail, "The Regional Distribution of Wealth in England as Indicated in the 1524–1525 Lay Subsidy Returns" (D.

Phil. thesis: University of London, 1968). The author hopes to do this work in the near future.

19. See especially the articles by R. A. Donkin, R. F. Glasscock, and A. R. H. Baker in *New Historical Geography*. The 1377 Poll Tax data from the P.R.O. series E. 179 and E. 359, though slightly different, both show Norfolk and Suffolk as being among the most populous and densely settled counties in England. These figures have been edited and printed by J. C. Russell, *British Medieval Population* (Albuquerque: Univ. of New Mexico Press, 1948), although the author's calculations were arithmetically different than Russell's. Apparently, Russell used only the E 359 figures, and not those in E 179/180/50 (Suffolk), and E 179/149/61 (Norfolk).

20. See above, footnote 4.

21. Perhaps the lack of crisis mortality quarters in Lowestoft was due to the presence of a city court in which many of the local wills were proved, and which has not survived into the twentieth century. There were city or peculiar courts in Norwich, Bury St. Edmunds, King's Lynn, Great Yarmouth and Ely. But the neighboring port of Yarmouth, whose city court wills do not survive for the fifteenth century, shows very many years of crisis mortality in the Norwich Consistory Court (N.C.C.) wills alone.

22. Between 1430 and 1480, Beccles testators left wills registered in the archdeaconry and consistory courts. For some of the vital statistics, see Chapter 7.

23. See below, pp. 192, 200.

24. For the numbers, see below, p. 156.

25. It is possible that the textile industry played a role in the high number of crisis mortality quarters in Lavenham. See below, pp. 194–195. The relevant volumes of the *Victoria History of the Counties of England* (V.C.H.) occasionally provide valuable textual and bibliographic information on particular parishes.

26. Hadleigh is listed in the Poll Tax returns of 1381, P.R.O. E. 179/180/34. It had 265 taxpayers, by my count, with as many as 100 additional possible taxpayers partially illegible. This compares with 398 completely visible taxpayers from Mildenhall.

27. Stow Market, P.R.O. E. 179/180/45, had at least 179 taxpayers in 1381, and the list is clearly incomplete.

28. See the report of the Forestry Commission, *The East Anglian Forests* (London: H. M. Stationery Office, 1972), pp. 4–14.

29. *Ibid.*

30. See H. C. Darby, *The Medieval Fenland* (Newton Abbot: David and Charles, 1974).

31. As stated above, Mildenhall had 398 taxpayers in 1383.

32. See Appendix C.

33. See above, footnote 22. Also, see Pelham, *op. cit.*

34. *Ibid.*

35. There was a monastery in Wymondham, and this and the poor who were attracted to it may have swelled the crisis-mortality lists.

36. It should be noted that there were two parishes in Wymondham, and five in East Dereham.

37. There were four Wiggenhall parishes scattered along the Ouse: Wiggenhalls St. Germans, St. Mary Magdalen, St. Mary the Virgin, and St. Peter. Because of problems of omission in the wills, the parish is not specified in the text. It is probable that the crisis Wiggenhall was Wiggenhall St. Germans. In any case, all four parishes were close enough together so as to conform to the endemic regions thesis, and all in the fen region.

38. In the Little Domesday Book, Thetford was one of the largest boroughs in East Anglia. In 1334, it was not even among the sixteen boroughs assessed for the lay subsidy of that year. See the articles by Darby and Glasscock in *New Historical Geography*.

39. See above, Chapter 2, footnote 114. Another historian who limits the role of plague in the fifteenth century to urban areas is A. R. H. Baker, "Changes in the Later Middle Ages," in *New Historical Geography*, pp. 243–244.

40. For a discussion of flight from medieval London, see S. L. Thrupp, *Merchant Class of Medieval London* (Chicago: Univ. of Chicago Press, 1948), pp. 226–227; and "Aliens in and Around London in the Fifteenth Century," in A. E. J. Hollaender, ed., *Studies in London History* (London: Hodder and Stoughton, 1969).

41. For a discussion of late medieval York, see J. N. Bartlett, "Expansion and Decline of York in the Later Middle Ages," *Ec.H.R.*, 2nd series, XII, 1959–1960. For Exeter and Bristol, see E. M. Carus-Wilson, *Expansion of Exeter at the Close of the Middle Ages* (Exeter: Exeter University Press, 1963); and his *Medieval Merchant Venturers* (London: Methuen, 1954). For Southampton, see Olive Coleman, "Trade and Prosperity in the Fifteenth Century: Some Aspects of Trade in Southampton," *Ec.H.R.*, 2nd series, XVI, 1963–1964; and Colin Platt, *Medieval Southampton* (London: Routledge and Kegan Paul, 1974). For Coventry, see C. V. Phythian-Adams, *Coventry in Crisis, 1518–1525* (Leicester: Leicester University Press, 1969); and his "Ceremony and Citizen: The Communal Year at Coventry, 1450–1550," in Peter Clark and Paul Slack, eds., *Crisis and Order in English Towns, 1500–1700* (London: Routledge and Kegan Paul, 1972). M. M. Postan discusses the overall picture in two very important articles: "The Fifteenth Century," *Ec.H.R.*, VIII, 1939; and "Some Agrarian Evidence of Declining Population in the Later Middle Ages," *Ec.H.R.*, 2nd series, II, 1950.

42. See above, pp. 108, 114–115.

43. See above, pp. 118–121.

44. What is needed is an analysis of the poor and middle-class Londoners' mortality patterns, perhaps from the wills of the commissary court. When the wills of these lesser members of London society are analyzed it may be that the dramatic clusterings of the autumnal mortality in epidemic years, so evident for the provincial towns and rural districts, will appear for the city of London also.

45. See above, p. 108.

46. See Glasscock, *op. cit.*

47. See below, pp. 187–203.

48. See below, pp. 175–183.

49. Among the contemporary or near contemporary chronicles which discuss it are: Robert of Avesbury, *Continuato Chronicarum*, edited by E. M. Thompson (London: Eyre and Spottiswoode, 1889); Thomas Walsingham, *Historia Anglicana*,

edited by H. Riley (London: Longmans, 1863); Ranulph Higden, *Polychronicon,* edited by J. R. Lumby (London: Longmans, 1865); John Capgrave, *The Chronicle of England,* edited by F. Hingeston (London: Longmans, 1858); Henrici Knighton, *Chronicon,* edited by J. R. Lumby (London: Eyre and Spottiswoode, 1889); Galfridi Le Baker, *Chronicon,* edited by E. M. Thompson (Oxford: Clarendon Press, 1889); and "A Fourteenth Century Chronicle from the Grey Friars at Lynn," edited by A. Granson, *English Historical Review,* LXXII, 1957.

50. For a good summary of the progression of the Black Death, see Philip Ziegler, *The Black Death* (New York: Harper and Row, 1969), pp. 117–186.

51. *Ibid.,* pp. 114–117.

52. *Ibid.*

53. *Ibid.,* pp. 146–155.

54. A. E. Levett, *Studies in Manorial History* (Oxford: Clarendon Press, 1936), chap. 6.

55. *Ibid.*

56. Augustus Jessopp, "The Black Death in East Anglia," in his *The Coming of the Friars and other Essays* (London: T. F. Unwin, 1889), pp. 200–238.

57. F. Blomefield, *History of the County of Norfolk,* vol. III (London, 1806); Russell, *op. cit.,* p. 228.

58. As cited by Ziegler, *op. cit.,* in reference to C. G. Grimwood, *History of Sudbury* (Sudbury, 1952), p. 86.

59. For references to all literary sources, see Chapter 2.

60. See above, pp. 89–100.

61. A good collection of Essex wills survives in the commissary court of London registers for much of the fifteenth century.

62. Yet again, the reader is reminded of the questionable nature of the 1462 reference. The existence of the epidemic is based on the testamentary mortality data, which is overwhelming, rather than the isolated literary reference.

63. Because of problems of specification in the wills, Great and Little Walsingham testamentary data have been aggregated.

# CHAPTER VI

## The Demographic Composition of the Will-Registering Population

### 6.1 Facts and Figures

It is essential to find out precisely who composed the will-making population, and in this and the next chapter, we shall move away from the gruesome topic of mortality and examine the demographic constitution of the sample population. For reasons proposed and discussed in Chapter 1, it has been assumed that the will-registering population was generally representative of adult male, fifteenth century English society, save perhaps the poorest 25–30 percent.[1] Discussion in this chapter will be limited strictly to the will makers themselves—that is, adults only. The offspring of the testators will be covered in detail in Chapter 7.

Eighty-six percent of the will-registering population were males (Table 6.1.1). The proportion was highest in the archdeaconry courts, and a bit lower in the consistory and prerogative courts. About 10 percent of the male population were secular clergy. Because of the bureaucratic rules, described in detail in Chapter 1, very few of the clergy had their wills proved in the archdeaconry courts, using instead the consistory court, and, to a lesser extent, the prerogative and peculiar courts. The Prerogative Court of York, not used statistically in this thesis, contained more clerical wills, ranging as high as 15 percent in certain years in the latter half of the fifteenth century.[2]

Of the male population, about two-thirds claimed to be or to have been married at one time in their lives. If the male population less clerics, a few

*Table 6.1.1.* Basic Data Breakdown of the Testator Population

|  | Totals | Percentage* |
|---|---|---|
| Total number of probated wills | 14971 | |
| Intestates, probates only, and letters of administration | 5114 | |
| Total sample, less London, Kent, and Essex P.C.C. testators** | 13793 | |
| Norfolk testators | 5714 | 38.2 |
| Suffolk testators | 6744 | 45.0 |
| Hertfordshire testators | 1335 | 8.9 |
| P.C.C. testators (including provincials) | 1279 | 8.6 |
| Urban testators (London, Norwich, Bury St. Edmunds, Ipswich, St. Albans) | 2992 | 20.0 |
| London testators | 830 | 27.7 of above |
| Norwich | 694 | 23.0 of above |
| Ipswich | 245 | 8.2 of above |
| Bury St. Edmunds | 652 | 21.8 of above |
| St. Albans | 571 | 19.0 of above |
| Breakdown by decade: | | |
| 1430–1440 | 1653 | 11.0 |
| 1441–1450 | 2190 | 14.6 |
| 1451–1460 | 2970 | 19.8 |
| 1461–1470 | 3851 | 25.7 |
| 1471–1480 | 4307 | 28.7 |
| Males | 12843 | 85.7 |
| Females | 2128 | 14.2 |
| Clerics | 1316 | 8.8 |
| Males less Clerics | 11527 | 89.7 of males |
| Married Males | 8744 | 68.0 |
| Widows | 810 | 38.0 of fem. |
| Citizens | 690 | 4.6 |
| Testators listing status other than cleric, "armigerous," yeoman, or husbandman | 1447 | 9.7 |
| Testators with at least one child, either sex | 7498 | 50.0 |
| Testators with at least one child of each sex | 2823 | 18.8 |
| Rural élite testators | 260 | 1.7 |

*All percentages are taken from the total number of wills probated, unless otherwise specified.

**All totals refer only to probated wills, and not intestate listings.

of whom were married, is taken, this marriage ratio rises to about three-quarters of the total male, nonclerical population. This figure would increase by another 10 percent if males who mentioned children and not wives, but who were probably married at some time in the past, were included.[3] Of the males who claimed to be married, about one in five were widowers.

About 14 percent of the sample were females, though many more women than this made original wills.[4] About 38 percent of the entire female sample were widows, and about 40 percent called themselves or indicated that they were "single" women. The rest had husbands alive or children but no husbands at the time the will was made. The predominance of women without living consorts is shown in Table 6.3.4.

Urban testators, with "urban" as defined in Chapter 5, constituted 20 percent of the total sample. Because testators from London have been included, this proportion is higher than it could have been in the nation as a whole. Much depends on how urban is defined for the fifteenth century. If rural market centers are included, the proportion rises to almost 45 percent of the total population. If Londoners and nonresident P.C.C. testators are excluded, the approximate percentage of the urban testators to the total was about 16 percent. In Norfolk, urban testators made up about 13 percent of the entire will-registering population, excluding testators from either Great Yarmouth or King's Lynn; if the total will-registering populations from either of these towns were known, it is probable that this figure would rise to about 18 percent.[5] In Suffolk, urban testators constituted approximately 13 percent of the population; and in Hertfordshire—here the archdeaconry of St. Albans—about 43 percent of the population, a figure disproportionately enlarged by the town of St. Albans.[6]

Of the will-registering sample, only about 10 percent of the testators, most of whom were urban, listed an occupation.[7] It is by no means assured, however, that the other 90 percent of the testator population were clerics, gentry, yeomen or peasants, or that the craftsmen among the occupation listers lived solely in the towns. The variance in occupation groups was enormous, with almost three hundred different occupations being listed. "Professional" men, including medical doctors, lawyers and jurists, notaries, and *doctori theologici;* an enormous variety of craftsmen, including brewers, chandlers, caulkers, cutlers, masons and wheelwrights, as well as more common millers and smiths; merchants and craftsmen from the textile industry; and the great merchants of London—all proved wills in the ecclesiastical courts. Among the more surprising of the occupations listed by the will makers, at least in the context of the fifteenth century, were cooks, gardeners, gravediggers and herdsmen. A complete record is provided in Appendix B.

About half of those testators who listed occupations in their wills also called themselves citizens of the towns that they inhabited. These citizen testators proved to be demographic special cases. Foremost among them were the citizen mercers, grocers, drapers and fishmongers of London, or the London élite. They married and remarried earlier and more often, were wealthier and older, and had more sons and daughters than did the rest of the sample. This was probably the function of their earlier age of marriage, and will be discussed in some detail below.[8] While the London élite and the other London citizens, next to the gentry, were the wealthiest and apparently most fecund group in the entire will testamentary population, the citizens of the provincial towns also appear to have been wealthier and to have had more children than was average for the rest of the sample.[9]

The rural élite—gentlemen, esquires, knights and on up—represented about 2 percent of the male will-registering population. Like the clerics, they were not supposed to have had their wills proved in the archdeaconry courts, and very few did. The bulk of their wills were registered in the consistory and prerogative courts. Surprisingly few of the rural élite called themselves anything other than gentleman or esquire, even in the P.C.C., and the overwhelming bulk of these testators were gentry, rather than nobility, as it is more strictly defined.[10] Like the citizens, they had higher marriage ratios, far higher remarriage ratios, and many more sons and daughters.

About 2 percent of the testators mentioned or bequeathed goods to servants.[11] Servants probably had a low priority of inclusion in the wills, for the total number of testators employing help must have been greater than 2 percent.[12] Those testators mentioning servants were on the average wealthier than the generality of the sample population. They had higher ratios of first-time marrige and remarriage, and more sons and daughters than the sample as a whole.[13] Widows and older unmarried women testators, the group which might be expected to have had a relatively high proportion of household servants, had fewer than was the sample norm.

Finally, there is the population breakdown by county and decade. More testators came from Suffolk than from the other two counties surveyed, Norfolk and Hertfordshire. They made up 45 percent of the probate sample. Next came testators from Norfolk, who made up about 38 percent of the probate sample. This was not because Suffolk was more heavily populated than was Norfolk; to the contrary, it is probable that the opposite was true. The reason is the relative completeness of the records of the archdeaconry courts in Suffolk from 1450 onward, and the survival of the wills of the peculiar court of Bury St. Edmunds. If the wills from the archdeaconry court of Norwich, perhaps the most populous of the Norwich diocese's four archdeaconries, and from the archdeaconry court of Norfolk survived in greater detail, and the wills from the city courts of Norwich, King's Lynn and Great Yarmouth survived at all,[14] the numerical positions of the two counties might be reversed. Hertfordshire wills, represented only by the registrations of the archdeaconry of St. Albans, constituted about 8.9 percent of the total sample, and the wills from the P.C.C. from London, Kent and Essex about 8.1 percent. Including provincial testators from Norfolk, Suffolk and Hertfordshire, the P.C.C. testators comprised about 8.6 percent of the total sample.

The breakdown by decade shows the incompleteness of the will-registering population of the 1430's, and comparative incompleteness of the 1440's. The steady decennial rise in numbers of wills from 1450 to 1480 may have been due in part to increasing population, in part to the survival of some county Norfolk archdeaconry courts wills only for the 1460's and 1470's, and in part to the ever-increasing virulence of epidemic disease, which in turn produced several quarters of crisis mortality.

## 6.2 Age and Wealth

Age and wealth, and their relationship to mortality, fertility and marriage are key demographic elements. Although definitive figures can never be given for either of these two factors by use of the testamentary data alone, reasonably accurate suppositions can be made. As briefly alluded to in Chapter 1, further methods had to be developed in order to adapt the raw will data into functional variables. The age format was based essentially on whether or not testators had children. An unfortunate consequence of this was that about half of the will-registering population could not be classified for age at all. Age Group 1 consisted of all testators who mentioned living parents in their wills. In an attempt to broaden this group, early efforts were made to include any testators who mentioned ascendant generation relatives. However, it was eventually decided that aunts and uncles could be of virtually any age in relation to the testators, while parents were by definition one generation older than their children, and the ascendant generation scheme was not used.

It is probable that living parents were almost always included by testators in their wills; this was even more likely if the testator was not married, and approximately two-thirds of those in Age Group 1 were not.[15] Piety and perhaps even personal affection toward parents were

*Table 6.2.1.* Age (in percentage)

| | | 1 | 2 | 3 | 99 |
|---|---|---|---|---|---|
| *By County* | | | | | |
| All | 1430–80 | 1.3 | 30.8 | 19.5 | 48.4 |
| N | 1430–80 | 1.3 | 27.4 | 21.5 | 49.8 |
| S | 1430–80 | 1.1 | 35.9 | 15.6 | 47.5 |
| H | 1430–80 | 1.3 | 22.8 | 25.1 | 50.9 |
| P.C.C. | 1430–80* | 2.8 | 27.1 | 26.5 | 43.6 |
| *By Decade* | | | | | |
| 1430–40 | | 1.9 | 18.2 | 20.0 | 59.8 |
| 1441–50 | | 1.2 | 24.8 | 21.0 | 53.0 |
| 1451–60 | | 1.2 | 30.2 | 18.7 | 49.9 |
| 1461–70 | | 1.2 | 34.4 | 18.3 | 46.2 |
| 1471–80 | | 1.4 | 35.2 | 20.3 | 43.1 |

*Abbreviations:* N (Norfolk; S (Suffolk); H (Hertfordshire); P.C.C. (Prerogative Court of Canterbury).
*The P.C.C. figures are for all counties; therefore, there is some slight duplication.
1=parents alive; testators probably under 25 years of age.
2=children under age; testators 25–50.
3=married children; children of age; grandchildren; godchildren with children; testators 50 years and over.
99=nonclassifiable.

shown by the very large numbers of testators who had masses sung for the souls of those who had borne them. Living parents do not appear on the average to have been older than their fifties,[16] and most of them were named as will executors by their offspring. Further, almost all of the married testators who listed parents had no children.[17] Of those very few who did, none had more than one. Very few testators had both parents alive at the time of the will, and mothers were far more common in the wills (and, one assumes, alive) than were fathers. For all these reasons, most especially because so few of the testators who named parents were married, and because among these practically none had children, it has been assumed that testators in Age Group 1 were under twenty-five years of age.[18]

Age Group 2 consists of all testators who had children under age, but not living parents. The inclusion of testators mentioning sibling generation relatives into Group 2 was considered, but not used. As was the case with the aunts and uncles of ascendant generation considered for Age Group 1, it was decided that brothers and sisters and cousins could be of virtually any age in relation to the testators. Since this age category is totally dependent on children, and up to 50 percent of the testators mention no children, a great many of the "middle" age group testators could not be included in it. It is probable that the bulk of the unclassifiable will-makers would fall into this category. Testators in Age Group 2 are considered to have been between the ages of twenty-five and forty-five, and perhaps fifty, at oldest.

Age Group 3 consists of all testators with married children or with children of age, thus completing the three-tiered system of the age variable. As with the "middle" age group, Age Group 3 is heavily dependent upon the testators having had children. As with the previous two age groups, a scheme involving the inclusion of testators who mentioned descendent generation relatives (in this case primarily nieces and nephews) was tried and eventually rejected. However, one additional measure was used to broaden Age Group 3; any testators who listed godchildren—a very frequent inclusion in the wills—who themselves had children were added to this group.[19] Also included were testators who listed grandchidren, but whose own children had predeceased them. All testators in this age category were considered to be over fifty years of age.

Because of the childbearing qualifications necessary for a testator to be included in one of the three age groups, a nonclassifiable "99" category had to be established. Although the percentage of the sample which composed Age Group 99 varied through time, the category generally hovered at around 50 percent of the total sample. The reader is reminded, therefore, that all percentages in Table 6.2.1 are based on about half the testator population. There is of course the question as to where the unclassifiable 99's would fall. Judging from the information we have from the wills as to the ages of majority,[20] it is unlikely that many of the unclassifiables would fall into Age Group 1, if their numbers could somehow be reclassified on another basis. It is probable that the figures for Age Group 1 are accurate for the sample as a whole. It is more difficult to reapportion the unclassifiables into the second and third age categories. For reasons to be discussed below, there are indications that most of Age Group 99 belongs in Age Group 2. But a definitive answer cannot be given, and it may be that the 99's would divide themselves equally into the second and third age groups.

As to trends of change, Age Group 99 decreases somewhat by decade, reflecting the rising number of families with children, or at least children as recorded in the wills. The smaller number of unclassifiables in the P.C.C. group reflect the smaller number of childless families there, as well. Except for the decade of the 1430's, the ten-year period of least will reliability as a demographic source, the data from Age Groups 1 and 3 are fairly regular in pattern. For the 1430's, the numbers of the youngest category are well up, the numbers of the middle category well down. Part of this is due to the larger number of unclassifiables, but it is important to note that the figure for the oldest category, Age Group 3, remains fairly steady, indicating that the bulk of the unclassifiables would fall not equally into Age Groups 2 and 3, but most heavily into Age Group 2. Further investigation does show that Age Group 2 rises in total in indirect relationship with the falling figures of Age Group 99. In general, however, there seem to have been no major changes in the testator population pyramid by decade over the period 1430–1480, and especially between 1440 and 1480. There are no significant increases or decreases in either Age Group 1 or Age Group 3, and the numbers of progeny aside, the adult population appears neither to have aged nor to have grown younger to any large degree throughout the period. This in turn may indicate that any growth in overall population in the period 1440–1480 would have had to come in the latter decades—that is, in the second generation, in the 1460's and 1470's. This new generation would then appear as testators in Age Groups 1 and 2 in wills proved in the 1480's and 1490's. After this point, an aging will-making population might well be expected. This conforms to a great degree with the replacement ratio data to be presented in Chapter 7.[21]

There were no great differences of age by county; only the wealthy P.C.C. testators, regardless of county, stand apart in this respect. There were more young adults (Age Group 1) from the P.C.C. than from any of the provincial courts. Equally, there were a larger number of older persons (Age Group 3) for the P.C.C., although the middle category of age (Age Group 2) is fairly close to the lower court's average. In effect, then, the additional number of classifiables for the P.C.C. went equally into the younger and older age groups at the expense of the unclassifiable category. This in turn raises the intriguing question of a correlation between age and wealth. A bivariate correlation was conducted, and the results can be seen in Table 6.2.2. They indicate that the bulk of the classifiable testators for the entire sample fell into the middling categories of age and wealth; needless to say, these are the modal categories. Yet in both of the categories, the old and the young tended to fall somewhat toward the extremes of wealth. There seems especially to have been a higher than normal incidence of wealthy old and poor old, as opposed to old in the

*Table 6.2.2.* Crosstabulation of Wealth by Age

| WEALTH | AGE COUNT ROW PCT COL PCT TOT PCT | 1.00 | 2.00 | 3.00 | 99.00 | ROW TOTAL |
|---|---|---|---|---|---|---|
| 1.00 | | 1 | 11 | 12 | 13 | 42 |
| | | 2.4 | 26.2 | 28.6 | 42.9 | 0.3 |
| | | 0.6 | 0.3 | 0.5 | 0.3 | |
| | | 0.0 | 0.1 | 0.1 | 0.4 | |
| 2.00 | | 0 | 34 | 26 | 67 | 131 |
| | | 0.0 | 28.0 | 19.8 | 51.1 | 0.9 |
| | | 0.0 | 0.9 | 1.0 | 1.0 | |
| | | 0.0 | 0.3 | 0.2 | 0.5 | |
| 3.00 | | 14 | 454 | 273 | 623 | 1364 |
| | | 1.0 | 33.3 | 20.0 | 45.7 | 9.8 |
| | | 8.4 | 10.5 | 10.3 | 9.2 | |
| | | 0.1 | 3.3 | 2.0 | 4.5 | |
| 4.00 | | 16 | 502 | 319 | 321 | 1658 |
| | | 1.0 | 30.3 | 19.2 | 49.5 | 11.9 |
| | | 9.6 | 11.6 | 12.1 | 12.1 | |
| | | 0.1 | 3.6 | 2.3 | 5.9 | |
| 5.00 | | 38 | 1017 | 647 | 1490 | 3192 |
| | | 1.2 | 31.9 | 20.3 | 46.7 | 22.9 |
| | | 22.9 | 23.5 | 24.5 | 21.9 | |
| | | 0.3 | 7.3 | 4.5 | 10.7 | |
| 6.00 | | 73 | 1715 | 968 | 2753 | 5509 |
| | | 1.3 | 31.1 | 17.6 | 50.0 | 39.5 |
| | | 44.0 | 35.7 | 26.6 | 40.5 | |
| | | 0.5 | 12.3 | 6.9 | 19.8 | |
| 7.00 | | 5 | 183 | 86 | 418 | 692 |
| | | 0.7 | 26.4 | 12.4 | 60.4 | 5.0 |
| | | 3.0 | 4.2 | 3.3 | 6.1 | |
| | | 0.0 | 1.3 | 0.6 | 3.0 | |
| 99.00 | | 19 | 403 | 313 | 612 | 1347 |
| | | 1.4 | 29.9 | 23.2 | 45.4 | 9.7 |
| | | 11.4 | 9.3 | 11.8 | 9.0 | |
| | | 0.1 | 2.9 | 2.2 | 4.4 | |
| COLUMN TOTAL | | 166 | 4323 | 2644 | 6802 | 13935 |
| | | 1.2 | 31.0 | 19.0 | 48.8 | 100.0 |

middle stratum of wealth. There is a similar correlation between wealth and youth. For the very wealthy testators of the P.C.C., there was a longer life span and perhaps an earlier age of majority than for the less wealthy.[22] For the bulk of the middling and the lower middling testators of Norfolk, Suffolk and Hertfordshire, there was far less correlation between age and wealth. Testators from the provinces from all three classifiable categories of age fell more evenly into all seven categories of wealth, with the modal figure lying in the middle age column and the second lowest wealth row.

The age data for Norfolk and Hertfordshire are quite similar, and surprisingly so since the wills come in one instance primarily from a consistory court and in the other instance almost exclusively from an archdeaconry court. Both counties show low numbers of younger testators, and about equal numbers of testators in the middle and older age groups. The Suffolk figures differ somewhat. There were significantly larger numbers in the middle age group for Suffolk, and a sharp decrease in the older category. This may reflect the strong archdeaconry court dominance in the Suffolk will sample, but in light of the Hertfordshire results, nothing definitive can be said. More significantly, it may reflect the relatively large number of high mortality districts to be found in county Suffolk.

In general, the following things can be said about the age characteristics of the testamentary population. Almost all testators were over twenty-five years of age. If the age of majority can be defined as ranging from about sixteen through twenty-five, depending upon region and wealth, it was likely to be closer to twenty-five for all but the richest groups in the society. Old age, youth and great wealth were connected. Generally, there was little change in the age structure of the will-registering population between 1440 and 1480; if there was an age-specific change during this period, it probably came in the nonadult segment of the population in the 1470's, as we shall see in Chapter 7. As will be discussed, population growth in the fifteenth century must have come from either an increase in fertility or a dramatic aetiological change in epidemic diseases.

New techniques had to be devised for determining the wealth of the will-registering population, just as they had to be devised for age. They have been based on the omnipresent system of bequest to the high altar of the church of burial of the testators in lieu of tithes forgotten. Eight categories of wealth were devised. The first contained all testators who bequeathed over one pound to the high altar; the second, one mark or greater; and the third, 10 shillings or over. Because the numbers from the first three categories were comparatively few, they have been combined and reclassified as wealth category A. Wealth category 4 (or B) consists of all testators who bequeathed between 6 shillings and 10 shillings; category

5 (or C), 2 shillings to 6 shillings; category 6 (or D), 5 pence to 20 pence; and category 7 (or E) consisted of bequests from 1 penny to 4 pence. Any testator who left a bequest in forms of kind other than grain or livestock, who left no bequest at all, or whose bequest was obviously not in accordance with the mobile wealth left throughout the rest of the will, was classified as unknown, or 99.

The results of the wealth survey can be seen in Table 6.2.3. When taken by county, the modal wealth of the testators invariably falls in category 6 (or D), with the next most common bequest in category 5 (or C). Thus, while the will-registering population was by no means destitute, the wealth survey does show that the conceptions held by some scholars that the fifteenth century will-making and registering populations were only upper and middle class are invalid.[23] Well over two-thirds of the testators in the wealth divisions gave less than five shillings to the high altar for tithes forgotten.

Of all counties, testators from those parts of Hertfordshire surveyed were poorest. Further, Table 6.2.3 shows that St. Albans was the poorest of the "urban" centers. In light of previous studies which indicated that the archdeaconry of St. Albans was the wealthier of the Hertfordshire archdeaconries, it becomes evident that this county was one of the poorer areas in generally wealthy eastern and southeastern England in the fifteenth century.[24] Despite the predominance of consistory court wills in the county, Norfolk does not appear to have been richer in terms of testator wealth than was Suffolk, although it did have the highest proportion of unclassifiable testators. East Anglia seems to have been a very wealthy area, in any case.[25]

By decade, the wealth tables show more interesting results. There are greater numbers of unclassifiable bequests in the high crisis-mortality decades of the 1430's and 1470's than in the other three decades. In the 1470's, this was indicative of a growing if still relatively small segment of the testamentary population who were leaving nothing at all to the high altar, or whose bequests were considerably below the levels of mobile wealth that they portrayed in their wills. Pious bequests were lower in the 1470's, and the friars—more so the Dominicans than the Franciscans—seem to have been the primary bequest losers. The figures for wealth by decade indicate that the will-registering population was probably getting broader from the 1430's to the 1470's. There was a steady decline of numbers in categories 1, 2, and 3, and a corresponding rise in numbers in the lower categories. These were regular, secular trends. Probably this steady progression toward the lower wealth categories does not mean that the population was as a whole getting poorer but rather that the will-registering population was getting even broader.

*Table 6.2.3.* Wealth (in percentage)

|  |  | 1 | 2 | 3 | A 4 | B 5 | C 6 | D 7 | E 99 |
|---|---|---|---|---|---|---|---|---|---|
| **By County** | | | | | | | | | |
| All | 1430–80 | 0.3 | 0.9 | 9.8 | 11.0 | 11.9 | 22.9 | 39.5 | 5.0 | 9.7 |
| N | 1430–80 | 0.4 | 0.9 | 9.3 | 10.6 | 11.8 | 23.8 | 38.5 | 3.3 | 12.1 |
| S | 1430–80 | 0.2 | 1.1 | 10.2 | 11.5 | 12.4 | 23.3 | 40.4 | 4.9 | 7.0 |
| H | 1430–80 | 0.4 | 0.5 | 9.7 | 10.6 | 7.9 | 16.7 | 40.5 | 12.2 | 11.9 |
| **By Decade** | | | | | | | | | |
| 1430–40 | | 0.6 | 1.1 | 11.3 | 13.0 | 14.4 | 21.8 | 33.7 | 2.8 | 14.3 |
| 1441–50 | | 0.2 | 1.1 | 11.3 | 12.6 | 15.6 | 23.0 | 35.3 | 3.3 | 10.1 |
| 1451–60 | | 0.3 | 1.1 | 12.1 | 13.5 | 12.2 | 23.2 | 38.2 | 4.2 | 8.7 |
| 1461–70 | | 0.3 | 9.8 | 8.5 | 9.6 | 11.4 | 24.6 | 42.3 | 5.6 | 6.4 |
| 1471–80 | | 0.2 | 0.8 | 8.2 | 9.2 | 9.4 | 21.6 | 42.0 | 6.5 | 11.2 |
| **Urban Areas** | | | | | | | | | |
| All 1430–80 | | 0.3 | 0.7 | 12.9 | 13.9 | 14.6 | 20.3 | 35.9 | 5.3 | 10.0 |
| Norw. 30–80 | | 0.6 | 1.6 | 19.0 | 21.2 | 18.3 | 21.1 | 21.1 | 2.0 | 16.3 |
| Ipsw. 30–80 | | 0.8 | 2.0 | 11.8 | 14.6 | 19.6 | 21.2 | 30.6 | 3.7 | 10.2 |
| St. Alb. 30–80 | | 0.2 | 0.5 | 6.5 | 7.2 | 9.6 | 14.4 | 42.7 | 13.3 | 12.8 |
| B.S.E. 30–80 | | 0.0 | 0.6 | 12.0 | 12.0 | 12.9 | 23.9 | 47.4 | 2.0 | 1.2 |

1 = bequests in pounds
2 = marks
3 = 10/ - up          1,2,3, together = A
4 = 6/ - 9/           1,2,3, together = B
5 = 2/ - 5/           1,2,3, together = C
6 = 5d - 20d          1,2,3, together = D
7 = 1d - 4d           1,2,3, together = E
99 = nonclassifiable

Urban wealth, using the established criterion of what was urban, was greater than that of corresponding rural wealth; when the Londoners and provincial urban testators from the P.C.C. can be included, it becomes far greater than that of the countryside. Urban wealth patterns were far more varied, as well. In the city of Norwich, the modal category, incredibly, was A, even if only barely so. At the same time, Norwich had the largest segment of unclassifiable testators, while Bury St. Edmunds had the smallest for the entire sample. Urban wealth in categories A, B, C, and D was in general more evenly distributed in the cities than in the rural areas, also. St. Albans and Bury St. Edmunds had the poorest urban-area testators. The case of St. Albans has already been discussed; both the county and archdeaconry around it appear to have been among the poorest in fifteenth century southern England. In Bury St. Edmunds, the reason for the large numbers in category D is probably attributable to the diligent efforts of the peculiar court sacrist and his agents in getting townsmen to register their wills.[26]

Individual wealth had an effect on the demographic characteristics of the community, as Tables 6.2.4–6.2.9 show. There was little relationship between wealth and first-marriage, but a strong connection between wealth and remarriage, which only the very rich achieved with any significant frequency. The relationship between wealth and children is more difficult to put into perspective. Even after the connection, if any, between the two variables has been found, the very nature of the source of the data, the wills, leads to further questions. Does wealth, simply and with no qualifications, mean more children? Or, as has been found for other pre-industrial societies, does wealth bring on an increasing sense of awareness and knowledge which in turn may lead to some sort of family limitation?[27] And even after the answers to these questions are formulated, further problems must be considered. Perhaps a lack of wealth had no effect on the actual numbers of children a testator produced, but only limited the numbers of children he could afford to provide for and hence include in the will. Perhaps some offspring were provided for before the will was made, or perhaps the wealthy testator could simply afford to include all his progeny in the will, and hence appear more fertile to the historian five centuries later. All these factors must be considered in light of the data.

In the bivariate crosstabulations conducted with and without clerical testators and always without the rural elite and the testators from the P.C.C., the wealthiest segment of the will-registering population, there was a fairly even distribution of numbers of sons among the testators of various levels of wealth. In the data presented in Tables 6.2.4 to 6.2.8, it can be seen that there was no monopoly on one or multiple sons, based on

*Table 6.2.4.* Crosstabulation of Wealth by Spouse

| | | SPOUSE | | | | | | ROW |
|---|---|---|---|---|---|---|---|---|
| | COUNT ROW PCT COL PCT TOT PCT | 0.0 | 1.00 | 2.00 | 3.00 | 4.00 | 7.00 | TOTAL |
| WEALTH | | | | | | | | |
| | 1.00 | 17 | 23 | 1 | 1 | 0 | 0 | 4 |
| | | 40.5 | 54.8 | 2.4 | 2.4 | 0.0 | 0.0 | 0. |
| | | 0.4 | 0.3 | 0.5 | 9.1 | 0.0 | 0.0 | |
| | | 0.1 | 0.2 | 0.0 | 0.0 | 0.0 | 0.0 | |
| | 2.00 | 56 | 71 | 4 | 0 | 0 | 0 | 13 |
| | | 42.7 | 54.2 | 3.1 | 0.0 | 0.0 | 0.0 | 0. |
| | | 1.2 | 0.2 | 1.9 | 0.0 | 0.0 | 0.0 | |
| | | 0.4 | 0.5 | 0.0 | 0.0 | 0.0 | 0.0 | |
| | 3.00 | 482 | 847 | 32 | 3 | 0 | 0 | 136 |
| | | 35.3 | 62.1 | 2.3 | 0.2 | 0.0 | 0.0 | 9. |
| | | 10.3 | 9.4 | 14.8 | 27.3 | 0.0 | 0.0 | |
| | | 3.5 | 6.1 | 0.2 | 0.0 | 0.0 | 0.0 | |
| | 4.00 | 612 | 1016 | 27 | 2 | 1 | 0 | 165 |
| | | 36.9 | 61.3 | 1.6 | 0.1 | 0.1 | 0.0 | 11. |
| | | 13.1 | 11.2 | 12.5 | 18.2 | 25.0 | 0.0 | |
| | | 4.4 | 7.3 | 0.0 | 0.0 | 0.0 | 0.0 | |
| | 5.00 | 1028 | 2109 | 53 | 3 | 0 | 0 | 319 |
| | | 32.2 | 66.0 | 1.7 | 0.1 | 0.0 | 0.0 | 22. |
| | | 22.0 | 23.3 | 24.5 | 27.3 | 0.0 | 0.0 | |
| | | 7.8 | 18.1 | 0.4 | 0.0 | 0.0 | 0.0 | |
| | 6.00 | 1767 | 2671 | 67 | 1 | 2 | 1 | 5509 |
| | | 32.1 | 66.6 | 1.2 | 0.0 | 0.0 | 0.0 | 39. |
| | | 37.9 | 60.6 | 31.0 | 9.1 | 50.0 | 100.0 | |
| | | 12.7 | 36.3 | 0.5 | 0.0 | 0.0 | 0.0 | |
| | 7.00 | 232 | 455 | 5 | 0 | 0 | 0 | 69 |
| | | 33.5 | 55.9 | 0.7 | 0.0 | 0.0 | 0.0 | 5. |
| | | 5.0 | 5.0 | 2.2 | 0.0 | 0.0 | 0.0 | |
| | | 1.7 | 3.3 | 0.0 | 0.0 | 0.0 | 0.0 | |
| | 99.00 | 470 | 848 | 27 | 1 | 1 | 0 | 134 |
| | | 34.9 | 63.0 | 2.0 | 0.1 | 0.1 | 0.0 | 9. |
| | | 10.1 | 9.4 | 12.5 | 9.1 | 25.0 | 0.0 | |
| | | 3.4 | 6.1 | 0.2 | 0.0 | 0.0 | 0.0 | |
| | COLUMN TOTAL | 4664 | 2039 | 215 | 11 | 4 | 1 | 13935 |
| | | 33.5 | 64.9 | 1.6 | 0.1 | 0.0 | 0.0 | 100.0 |

*Table 6.2.5.* Crosstabulation of Wealth by Spouse, Excepting Clerics

| | SPOUSE | | | | | | ROW TOTAL |
|---|---|---|---|---|---|---|---|
| COUNT<br>ROW PCT<br>COL PCT<br>TOT PCT | 0.0 | 1.00 | 2.00 | 3.00 | 4.00 | 7.00 | |
| WEALTH | | | | | | | |
| 1.00 | 5 | 22 | 1 | 1 | 0 | 0 | 29 |
| | 17.2 | 75.9 | 3.4 | 3.4 | 0.0 | 0.0 | 0.2 |
| | 0.1 | 0.2 | 0.5 | 10.0 | 0.0 | 0.0 | |
| | 0.0 | 0.2 | 0.0 | 0.0 | 0.0 | 0.0 | |
| 2.00 | 30 | 71 | 4 | 0 | 0 | 0 | 105 |
| | 28.6 | 67.6 | 3.8 | 0.0 | 0.0 | 0.0 | 0.8 |
| | 0.9 | 0.8 | 1.9 | 0.0 | 0.0 | 0.0 | |
| | 0.2 | 0.6 | 0.0 | 0.0 | 0.0 | 0.0 | |
| 3.00 | 278 | 845 | 32 | 3 | 0 | 0 | 1158 |
| | 24.0 | 73.0 | 2.8 | 0.3 | 0.0 | 0.0 | 9.1 |
| | 7.9 | 9.4 | 15.0 | 30.0 | 0.0 | 0.0 | |
| | 2.2 | 6.6 | 0.3 | 0.0 | 0.0 | 0.0 | |
| 4.00 | 351 | 1017 | 26 | 2 | 1 | 0 | 1392 |
| | 25.2 | 72.7 | 1.9 | 0.1 | 0.1 | 0.0 | 10.9 |
| | 10.0 | 11.2 | 12.1 | 20.0 | 25.0 | 0.0 | |
| | 2.7 | 7.9 | 0.2 | 0.0 | 0.0 | 0.0 | |
| 5.00 | 764 | 2104 | 53 | 2 | 0 | 0 | 2923 |
| | 26.1 | 72.0 | 1.8 | 0.1 | 0.0 | 0.0 | 22.9 |
| | 21.7 | 23.3 | 24.8 | 20.0 | 0.0 | 0.0 | |
| | 6.0 | 16.5 | 0.4 | 0.0 | 0.0 | 0.0 | |
| 6.00 | 1545 | 3669 | 67 | 1 | 2 | 1 | 5295 |
| | 29.2 | 69.4 | 1.3 | 0.0 | 0.0 | 0.0 | 41.4 |
| | 43.9 | 40.7 | 31.3 | 10.0 | 50.0 | 100.0 | |
| | 12.1 | 25.7 | 0.5 | 0.0 | 0.0 | 0.0 | |
| 7.00 | 213 | 455 | 5 | 0 | 0 | 0 | 673 |
| | 31.6 | 67.6 | 0.7 | 0.0 | 0.0 | 0.0 | 5.3 |
| | 6.1 | 5.0 | 2.3 | 0.0 | 0.0 | 0.0 | |
| | 1.7 | 3.0 | 0.0 | 0.0 | 0.0 | 0.0 | |
| 99.00 | 332 | 841 | 26 | 1 | 1 | 0 | 1201 |
| | 27.6 | 10.0 | 2.2 | 0.1 | 0.1 | 0.0 | 9.4 |
| | 9.4 | 9.3 | 12.1 | 10.0 | 25.0 | 0.0 | |
| | 2.6 | 6.6 | 0.2 | 0.0 | 0.0 | 0.0 | |
| COLUMN TOTAL | 3518 | 9019 | 214 | 10 | 4 | 1 | 12766 |
| | 27.6 | 70.6 | 1.7 | 0.1 | 0.0 | 0.0 | 100.0 |

*Table 6.2.6.* Crosstabulation of Wealth by Male Progeny

|  | | MALES | | | | | | | | | | |
|---|---|---|---|---|---|---|---|---|---|---|---|---|
| WEALTH | COUNT<br>POW PCT<br>COL PCT<br>TOT PCT | 0.0 | 1.00 | 2.00 | 3.00 | 4.00 | 5.00 | 6.00 | 7.00 | 8.00 | 9.00 | ROW<br>TOT |
| 1.00 | | 21 | 11 | 5 | 4 | 1 | 0 | 0 | 0 | 0 | 0 | 4 |
| | | 50.0 | 26.2 | 11.9 | 9.5 | 2.4 | 0.0 | 0.0 | 0.0 | 0.0 | 0.0 | 0. |
| | | 0.3 | 0.3 | 0.3 | 0.7 | 0.6 | 0.0 | 0.0 | 0.0 | 0.0 | 0.0 | |
| | | 0.2 | 0.1 | 0.0 | 0.0 | 0.0 | 0.0 | 0.0 | 0.0 | 0.0 | 0.0 | |
| 2.00 | | 74 | 39 | 11 | 6 | 1 | 0 | 0 | 0 | 0 | 0 | 13 |
| | | 56.5 | 29.9 | 8.4 | 4.6 | 0.8 | 0.0 | 0.0 | 0.0 | 0.0 | 0.0 | 0. |
| | | 0.9 | 1.1 | 0.7 | 1.1 | 0.6 | 0.0 | 0.0 | 0.0 | 0.0 | 0.0 | |
| | | 0.5 | 0.3 | 0.1 | 0.0 | 0.0 | 0.0 | 0.0 | 0.0 | 0.0 | 0.0 | |
| 3.00 | | 743 | 339 | 191 | 68 | 19 | 3 | 1 | 0 | 0 | 0 | 136 |
| | | 54.5 | 24.9 | 14.0 | 5.0 | 1.4 | 0.2 | 0.1 | 0.0 | 0.0 | 0.0 | 9. |
| | | 9.2 | 9.7 | 11.5 | 12.5 | 11.5 | 6.3 | 9.1 | 0.0 | 0.0 | 0.0 | |
| | | 5.3 | 2.4 | 1.4 | 0.5 | 0.1 | 0.0 | 0.0 | 0.0 | 0.0 | 0.0 | |
| 4.00 | | 950 | 366 | 216 | 85 | 27 | 10 | 2 | 0 | 0 | 0 | 165 |
| | | 57.8 | 22.1 | 13.1 | 5.1 | 1.6 | 0.6 | 0.1 | 0.0 | 0.0 | 0.0 | 11. |
| | | 11.8 | 10.5 | 13.4 | 15.8 | 16.4 | 20.8 | 18.2 | 0.0 | 0.0 | 0.0 | |
| | | 6.8 | 2.6 | 1.6 | 0.6 | 0.2 | 0.1 | 0.0 | 0.0 | 0.0 | 0.0 | |
| 5.00 | | 1770 | 607 | 405 | 148 | 47 | 9 | 3 | 1 | 1 | 1 | 319 |
| | | 55.5 | 25.3 | 12.7 | 4.8 | 1.5 | 0.3 | 0.1 | 0.0 | 0.0 | 0.0 | 22. |
| | | 22.8 | 23.2 | 25.0 | 27.2 | 28.5 | 18.0 | 27.3 | 33.3 | 50.0 | 100.0 | |
| | | 12.7 | 5.8 | 2.9 | 1.1 | 0.3 | 0.1 | 0.0 | 0.0 | 0.0 | 0.0 | |
| 6.00 | | 2280 | 1444 | 560 | 155 | 48 | 17 | 3 | 2 | 0 | 0 | 550 |
| | | 59.5 | 26.2 | 10.2 | 2.8 | 0.9 | 0.3 | 0.1 | 0.0 | 0.0 | 0.0 | 39. |
| | | 40.7 | 41.5 | 34.5 | 28.5 | 29.1 | 35.4 | 27.3 | 66.7 | 0.0 | 0.0 | |
| | | 23.4 | 10.4 | 4.0 | 1.1 | 0.3 | 0.1 | 0.0 | 0.0 | 0.0 | 0.0 | |
| 7.00 | | 473 | 155 | 50 | 12 | 1 | 0 | 1 | 0 | 0 | 0 | 69 |
| | | 68.4 | 22.4 | 7.2 | 1.7 | 0.1 | 0.0 | 0.1 | 0.0 | 0.0 | 0.0 | 5 |
| | | 5.9 | 4.5 | 3.1 | 2.2 | 0.6 | 0.0 | 9.1 | 0.0 | 0.0 | 0.0 | |
| | | 3.4 | 1.1 | 0.4 | 0.1 | 0.0 | 0.0 | 0.0 | 0.0 | 0.0 | 0.0 | |
| 99.00 | | 751 | 317 | 181 | 66 | 21 | 9 | 1 | 0 | 1 | 0 | 134 |
| | | 55.8 | 23.9 | 13.4 | 4.9 | 1.6 | 0.7 | 0.1 | 0.0 | 0.1 | 0.0 | 9 |
| | | 9.3 | 9.1 | 11.2 | 12.1 | 12.7 | 18.8 | 9.1 | 0.0 | 50.0 | 0.0 | |
| | | 5.4 | 2.3 | 1.3 | 0.5 | 0.2 | 0.1 | 0.0 | 0.0 | 0.0 | 0.0 | |
| COLUMN<br>TOTAL | | 4062 | 3478 | 1621 | 544 | 165 | 48 | 11 | 3 | 2 | 1 | 1399 |
| | | 57.9 | 25.0 | 11.6 | 3.9 | 1.2 | 9.3 | 0.1 | 0.0 | 0.0 | 0.0 | 100. |

*Table 6.2.7.* Crosstabulation of Wealth by Male Progeny, Excepting Clerics

| WEALTH | MALES<br>COUNT<br>ROW PCT<br>COL PCT<br>TOT PCT | 0.0 | 1.00 | 2.00 | 3.00 | 4.00 | 5.00 | 6.00 | 7.00 | 8.00 | 9.00 | ROW<br>TOT |
|---|---|---|---|---|---|---|---|---|---|---|---|---|
| | 1.00 | 9 | 11 | 5 | 4 | 0 | 0 | 0 | 0 | 0 | 0 | 29 |
| | | 31.0 | 37.9 | 17.2 | 13.8 | 0.0 | 0.0 | 0.0 | 0.0 | 0.0 | 0.0 | 0.2 |
| | | 0.1 | 0.3 | 0.3 | 0.7 | 0.0 | 0.0 | 0.0 | 0.0 | 0.0 | 0.0 | |
| | | 0.1 | 0.1 | 0.0 | 0.0 | 0.0 | 0.0 | 0.0 | 0.0 | 0.0 | 0.0 | |
| | 2.00 | 49 | 38 | 11 | 6 | 1 | 0 | 0 | 0 | 0 | 0 | 105 |
| | | 46.7 | 36.2 | 10.9 | 5.7 | 1.0 | 0.0 | 0.0 | 0.0 | 0.0 | 0.0 | 0.8 |
| | | 0.7 | 1.1 | 0.7 | 1.1 | 0.6 | 0.0 | 0.0 | 0.0 | 0.0 | 0.0 | |
| | | 0.4 | 0.3 | 0.1 | 0.0 | 0.0 | 0.0 | 0.0 | 0.0 | 0.0 | 0.0 | |
| | 3.00 | 541 | 335 | 191 | 68 | 19 | 3 | 1 | 0 | 0 | 0 | 1158 |
| | | 46.7 | 28.9 | 16.5 | 5.9 | 1.6 | 0.3 | 0.1 | 0.0 | 0.0 | 0.0 | 9.1 |
| | | 7.8 | 9.7 | 11.9 | 12.6 | 11.7 | 6.5 | 9.1 | 0.0 | 0.0 | 0.0 | |
| | | 4.2 | 2.6 | 1.5 | 0.5 | 0.1 | 0.0 | 0.0 | 0.0 | 0.0 | 0.0 | |
| | 4.00 | 631 | 365 | 216 | 83 | 27 | 8 | 2 | 0 | 0 | 0 | 1392 |
| | | 49.0 | 26.2 | 15.5 | 5.0 | 1.9 | 0.6 | 0.1 | 0.0 | 0.0 | 0.0 | 10.9 |
| | | 10.0 | 10.5 | 13.4 | 15.3 | 16.7 | 17.4 | 18.2 | 0.0 | 0.0 | 0.0 | |
| | | 5.9 | 2.9 | 1.7 | 0.7 | 0.2 | 0.1 | 0.0 | 0.0 | 0.0 | 0.0 | |
| | 5.00 | 1507 | 404 | 402 | 148 | 47 | 9 | 3 | 1 | 1 | 1 | 2923 |
| | | 51.6 | 27.5 | 13.8 | 5.1 | 1.6 | 0.3 | 0.1 | 0.0 | 0.0 | 0.0 | 22.9 |
| | | 21.8 | 28.3 | 25.0 | 27.4 | 28.0 | 19.6 | 27.3 | 33.3 | 50.0 | 100.0 | |
| | | 11.8 | 6.3 | 3.1 | 1.2 | 1.4 | 9.1 | 0.0 | 0.0 | 0.0 | 0.0 | |
| | 6.00 | 1067 | 1443 | 560 | 155 | 48 | 17 | 3 | 2 | 0 | 0 | 5285 |
| | | 57.8 | 27.3 | 10.6 | 2.9 | 0.9 | 0.3 | 0.1 | 0.0 | 0.0 | 0.0 | 41.4 |
| | | 44.2 | 41.6 | 34.8 | 28.7 | 29.6 | 37.0 | 27.3 | 66.7 | 0.0 | 0.0 | |
| | | 23.9 | 11.3 | 4.4 | 1.2 | 0.4 | 0.1 | 0.0 | 0.0 | 0.0 | 0.0 | |
| | 7.00 | 454 | 155 | 00 | 12 | 1 | 0 | 1 | 0 | 0 | 0 | 673 |
| | | 67.5 | 23.0 | 7.4 | 1.8 | 0.1 | 0.0 | 0.1 | 0.0 | 0.0 | 0.0 | 5.3 |
| | | 6.6 | 9.6 | 3.1 | 2.2 | 0.6 | 0.0 | 9.1 | 0.0 | 0.0 | 0.0 | |
| | | 1.6 | 1.2 | 0.4 | 0.1 | 0.0 | 0.0 | 0.0 | 0.0 | 0.0 | 0.0 | |
| | 99.00 | 614 | 316 | 176 | 65 | 19 | 9 | 1 | 0 | 1 | 0 | 1201 |
| | | 51.1 | 26.3 | 14.7 | 5.4 | 1.6 | 0.7 | 0.1 | 0.0 | 0.1 | 0.0 | 9.4 |
| | | 8.9 | 9.1 | 10.9 | 12.0 | 11.7 | 19.6 | 9.1 | 0.0 | 50.0 | 0.0 | |
| | | 4.8 | 2.5 | 1.4 | 0.5 | 0.1 | 0.1 | 0.0 | 0.0 | 0.0 | 0.0 | |
| | COLUMN<br>TOTAL | 5922 | 3467 | 1611 | 541 | 162 | 46 | 11 | 3 | 2 | 1 | 12766 |
| | | 54.2 | 27.2 | 12.6 | 4.2 | 1.3 | 0.4 | 0.1 | 0.0 | 0.0 | 0.0 | 100.0 |

*Table 6.2.8.* Crosstabulation of Wealth by Female Progeny

| FEMALES | | | | | | | | | | |
|---|---|---|---|---|---|---|---|---|---|---|
| COUNT ROW PCT COL PCT TOT PCT | 0.0 | 1.00 | 2.00 | 3.00 | 4.00 | 5.00 | 6.00 | 7.00 | 8.00 | ROW TOT |
| WEALTH | | | | | | | | | | |
| 1.00 | 27 | 7 | 4 | 3 | 0 | 1 | 0 | 0 | 0 | 4 |
|  | 64.2 | 16.7 | 9.5 | 7.1 | 0.0 | 2.4 | 0.0 | 0.0 | 0.0 | 0. |
|  | 0.3 | 0.3 | 0.4 | 0.9 | 0.0 | 3.8 | 0.0 | 0.0 | 0.0 | |
|  | 0.2 | 0.1 | 0.0 | 0.0 | 0.0 | 0.0 | 0.0 | 0.0 | 0.0 | |
| 2.00 | 38 | 15 | 12 | 4 | 2 | 0 | 0 | 0 | 0 | 13 |
|  | 74.8 | 11.5 | 9.2 | 3.1 | 1.5 | 0.0 | 0.0 | 0.0 | 0.0 | 0. |
|  | 1.0 | 0.7 | 1.2 | 1.1 | 2.5 | 0.0 | 0.0 | 0.0 | 0.0 | |
|  | 0.7 | 0.1 | 0.1 | 0.0 | 0.0 | 0.0 | 0.0 | 0.0 | 0.0 | |
| 3.00 | 955 | 233 | 121 | 40 | 3 | 5 | 0 | 1 | 0 | 136 |
|  | 10.0 | 17.5 | 8.9 | 2.9 | 0.1 | 0.4 | 0.0 | 0.1 | 0.0 | 9. |
|  | 9.2 | 11.0 | 11.9 | 11.4 | 3.7 | 19.2 | 0.0 | 33.3 | 0.0 | |
|  | 6.9 | 1.7 | 0.9 | 0.3 | 0.0 | 0.0 | 0.0 | 0.0 | 0.0 | |
| 4.00 | 1133 | 257 | 150 | 51 | 15 | 1 | 1 | 0 | 0 | 165 |
|  | 71.4 | 15.5 | 9.0 | 3.1 | 0.9 | 0.1 | 0.1 | 0.0 | 0.0 | 11. |
|  | 11.5 | 11.8 | 14.8 | 14.5 | 18.5 | 3.8 | 25.0 | 0.0 | 0.0 | |
|  | 8.5 | 1.8 | 1.1 | 8.4 | 0.1 | 0.0 | 0.0 | 0.0 | 0.0 | |
| 5.00 | 2336 | 475 | 253 | 97 | 24 | 4 | 2 | 0 | 1 | 319 |
|  | 73.2 | 14.9 | 7.9 | 3.0 | 0.8 | 0.1 | 0.1 | 0.0 | 0.0 | 22. |
|  | 22.7 | 21.8 | 25.0 | 27.6 | 29.6 | 15.4 | 50.0 | 0.0 | 100.0 | |
|  | 16.8 | 3.4 | 1.8 | 0.7 | 0.2 | 0.0 | 0.0 | 0.0 | 0.0 | |
| 6.00 | 75.6 | 15.8 | 6.1 | 1.9 | 0.5 | 0.1 | 0.0 | 0.0 | 0.0 | 39. |
|  | 40.5 | 40.0 | 33.1 | 29.1 | 32.1 | 26.9 | 25.0 | 66.7 | 0.0 | |
|  | 29.9 | 6.3 | 2.4 | 0.7 | 0.2 | 0.1 | 0.0 | 0.0 | 0.0 | |
| 7.00 | 545 | 80 | 36 | 10 | 1 | 0 | 0 | 0 | 0 | 69 |
|  | 81.6 | 11.6 | 5.2 | 1.4 | 0.1 | 0.0 | 0.0 | 0.0 | 0.0 | 5. |
|  | 5.5 | 3.7 | 3.6 | 2.8 | 1.2 | 0.0 | 0.0 | 0.0 | 0.0 | |
|  | 4.1 | 0.6 | 0.3 | 0.1 | 0.0 | 0.0 | 0.0 | 0.0 | 0.0 | |
| 99.00 | 948 | 235 | 182 | 44 | 10 | 8 | 0 | 0 | 0 | 134 |
|  | 70.4 | 17.4 | 7.6 | 3.3 | 0.7 | 0.0 | 0.0 | 0.0 | 0.0 | 9. |
|  | 9.2 | 10.8 | 10.1 | 12.5 | 12.3 | 30.8 | 0.0 | 0.0 | 0.0 | |
|  | 6.8 | 1.7 | 0.7 | 0.3 | 0.1 | 0.1 | 0.0 | 0.0 | 0.0 | |
| COLUMN TOTAL | 10275 | 2180 | 1014 | 351 | 81 | 26 | 4 | 3 | 1 | 1393 |
|  | 73.7 | 15.4 | 7.3 | 2.5 | 0.6 | 0.2 | 0.0 | 0.0 | 0.0 | 100.0 |

*Table 6.2.9.* Crosstabulation of Wealth by Female Progeny, Excepting Clerics

FEMALES

| WEALTH | COUNT ROW PCT COL PCT TOT PCT | 0.0 | 1.00 | 2.00 | 3.00 | 4.00 | 5.00 | 6.00 | 7.00 | 8.00 | ROW TOT |
|---|---|---|---|---|---|---|---|---|---|---|---|
| | 1.00 | 15 | 7 | 4 | 2 | 0 | 1 | 0 | 0 | 0 | 29 |
| | | 51.7 | 24.1 | 13.8 | 6.9 | 0.0 | 3.4 | 0.0 | 0.0 | 0.0 | 0.2 |
| | | 0.2 | 0.3 | 0.4 | 0.6 | 0.0 | 3.8 | 0.0 | 0.0 | 0.0 | |
| | | 0.1 | 0.1 | 0.0 | 0.0 | 0.0 | 0.0 | 0.0 | 0.0 | 0.0 | |
| | 2.00 | 72 | 15 | 12 | 4 | 2 | 0 | 0 | 0 | 0 | 105 |
| | | 68.6 | 14.3 | 11.4 | 3.8 | 1.9 | 0.0 | 0.0 | 0.0 | 0.0 | 0.8 |
| | | 0.8 | 0.7 | 1.2 | 1.1 | 2.5 | 0.0 | 0.0 | 0.0 | 0.0 | |
| | | 0.6 | 0.1 | 0.1 | 0.0 | 0.0 | 0.0 | 0.0 | 0.0 | 0.0 | |
| | 3.00 | 751 | 237 | 121 | 40 | 3 | 5 | 0 | 1 | 0 | 1158 |
| | | 64.9 | 20.5 | 10.4 | 3.5 | 0.3 | 0.4 | 0.0 | 0.1 | 0.0 | 9.1 |
| | | 8.2 | 10.9 | 12.0 | 11.5 | 3.3 | 19.2 | 0.0 | 33.3 | 0.0 | |
| | | 5.9 | 1.9 | 0.9 | 0.3 | 0.0 | 0.0 | 0.0 | 0.0 | 0.0 | |
| | 4.00 | 921 | 253 | 150 | 51 | 15 | 1 | 1 | 0 | 0 | 1392 |
| | | 66.2 | 18.2 | 10.8 | 3.7 | 1.1 | 0.1 | 0.1 | 0.0 | 0.0 | 10.9 |
| | | 10.1 | 11.7 | 14.9 | 14.6 | 18.8 | 3.8 | 25.0 | 0.0 | 0.0 | |
| | | 7.2 | 2.0 | 1.2 | 0.4 | 0.1 | 0.0 | 0.0 | 0.0 | 0.0 | |
| | 5.00 | 2010 | 474 | 251 | 97 | 24 | 4 | 2 | 0 | 1 | 2923 |
| | | 70.8 | 10.2 | 8.0 | 3.3 | 0.8 | 0.1 | 0.1 | 0.0 | 0.0 | 22.9 |
| | | 22.7 | 21.8 | 24.9 | 27.8 | 30.0 | 15.4 | 50.0 | 0.0 | 100.0 | |
| | | 16.2 | 3.7 | 2.0 | 0.8 | 0.2 | 0.0 | 0.0 | 0.0 | 0.0 | |
| | 6.00 | 3939 | 872 | 326 | 192 | 26 | 7 | 1 | 2 | 0 | 5285 |
| | | 74.5 | 16.5 | 6.4 | 1.9 | 0.5 | 0.1 | 0.0 | 0.0 | 0.0 | 41.4 |
| | | 43.2 | 40.2 | 33.3 | 23.2 | 32.5 | 26.9 | 25.0 | 66.7 | 0.0 | |
| | | 30.9 | 6.8 | 2.6 | 0.8 | 0.2 | 0.1 | 0.0 | 0.0 | 0.0 | |
| | 7.00 | 516 | 00 | 36 | 10 | 1 | 0 | 0 | 0 | 0 | 673 |
| | | 81.1 | 11.9 | 5.3 | 1.5 | 0.1 | 0.0 | 0.0 | 0.0 | 0.0 | 5.3 |
| | | 0.0 | 8.7 | 3.6 | 2.9 | 1.3 | 0.0 | 0.0 | 0.0 | 0.0 | |
| | | 4.0 | 0.6 | 0.8 | 0.1 | 0.0 | 0.0 | 0.0 | 0.0 | 0.0 | |
| | 99.00 | 810 | 233 | 98 | 43 | 9 | 8 | 0 | 0 | 0 | 1201 |
| | | 67.4 | 19.4 | 8.2 | 3.6 | 0.7 | 0.7 | 0.0 | 0.0 | 0.0 | 9.4 |
| | | 8.9 | 10.7 | 9.7 | 12.3 | 11.3 | 30.8 | 0.0 | 0.0 | 0.0 | |
| | | 6.3 | 1.8 | 0.8 | 0.3 | 0.1 | 0.1 | 0.0 | 0.0 | 0.0 | |
| | COLUMN TOTAL | 2124 | 2171 | 1008 | 348 | 83 | 26 | 4 | 3 | 1 | 12766 |
| | | 71.9 | 17.0 | 7.9 | 2.7 | 0.6 | 0.2 | 0.0 | 0.0 | 0.0 | 100.0 |

factors of wealth alone. Generally, it was categories C and D of wealth in which most of the multiple-son families were found. When one considers that there was a strong correlation between frequency of marriage and remarriage and wealth, the large number of multiple sons among testators of middling and poorer wealth takes on even further significance, since they had a lower rate of marriage. As will be discussed in Chapter 7, there was a direct relationship between the very richest of the sample's groups, the rural elite and the P.C.C. testators, and numbers of sons.[28] But for those just a bit wealthier than the average, those of middling wealth, and those who were poorer and poorest, numbers of sons and personal riches do not appear to have been connected.

How then is this seeming lack of correlation between sons and wealth in all but the most extreme instances of the latter to be interpreted, in light of the questions posed above? In the heir-starved and disease-ridden fifteenth century, it is not likely that anyone, wealthiest or poorest, practiced deliberate limitation of births. In this epidemic century of abundant and comparatively easily obtained land, all sons must have been welcomed, at least until well into the 1480's. Because of the direct relationship between the wealthiest segment of society and numbers of sons, however, the possibility of an aberration in the source must be considered. Did the rural and urban élite actually have more children, or just the resources which enabled them to include more children in their wills? Unfortunately, on the basis of the testamentary data alone, a definitive answer cannot be given. But as argued in Chapter 1, it is the contention of this thesis that at least one living son was without exception always included in the wills; and because the very wealthy testators had on average both more sons and a lower frequency of no sons than did the rest of the sample, it is probable that the relationships between wealth levels and numbers of sons as shown in Tables 6.2.2 and 6.2.7 and presented in Chapter 7, are natural ones, and not peculiarities of the source. Thus, between the wealthy—but not the wealthiest, who are not included in the bivariate correlations—middling and poorest-level testators, there was little difference in numbers of sons. As we shall see in Chapter 7, this distinction does not hold when dealing with society's economic élite.[29] Only the very wealthiest were able to provide the shelter and mobility necessary to protect, to some degree, their children from the greatest factor in fifteenth century mortality, epidemic disease.

Further evidence to support these views comes from the relationship between wealth and numbers of daughters included in the wills. As can be seen from Tables 6.2.8 and 6.2.9, the connection between wealth and daughters was a strong one. This is almost certainly due to mechanical factors. As has been discussed, daughters were the nuclear family members most likely to be left out of the wills, and it is only in the very wealthy segments of the will-registering population that their will numbers approach anything like what they must have been in the fifteenth century. Put simply, more money meant more daughters—but most important in regard to the data presented within, greater wealth meant more to be distributed to the progeny within the will, and hence more room to include daughters. This was not the case with male children, whose will numbers probably reflect accurately their true numbers in society.

## 6.3 Marriage

The figures presented for marriage are not rates of marriage in the modern sense. Rather, they are a reflection of the numbers of spouses directly mentioned in the wills, be they dead or alive. It was decided to employ this method, which is true to the sources, rather than to attempt extrapolation into demographically more useful but historically less certain modern ratios of marriage. Tables 6.3.1 through 6.3.4 are literal recordings of the numbers of spouses directly mentioned in each will. Dead spouses, usually present in the wills because of money provided to say masses for their souls or because a testator desired to be buried next to his or her deceased consort, and remarriages have been included in the ratios. Statistically, as can be seen in each of the data tables, remarriage, except among the testators of the P.C.C. was insignificant. It had little effect on the ratios as a whole. The addition of dead spouses—the inclusion of widows and widowers—in the ratios added up to 10 percent in the number of living spouses in some of the tabulations.

The decision to include deceased spouses and remarriages was taken because of the nature of the sources. It was felt that there were enough uncertainties in dealing with wills demographically without adding statistical complications which would compound the problem even further. More important, an effective "counterpart" peculiarity was found in the wills which served to decrease the percentage of marriage almost as effectively as the above measure inflated it. In certain wills, a testator with children who were obviously legitimate did not list a spouse. Following the strict guidelines set down in determining "spouse," they could not be included in the spouse ratio, since they were not explicitly mentioned, even though it is almost certain that they were married at one time or another. Programs were run to assess quantitatively the effects of the additive elements, remarriage and the inclusion of dead consorts, and the subtractive element, the failure to count unnamed parents of well-documented children. In all cases, the additive effect dominated, adding

*Table 6.3.1.* Spouse Ratios, Entire Sample

| | R.R. | Mode | %Test. Not Married | % Remarriage |
|---|---|---|---|---|
| All 1430–80 | .69 | 1.0 | 33.2 | 2.2 |
| N 1430–80 | .63 | 1.0 | 38.4 | 1.6 |
| S 1430–80 | .71 | 1.0 | 30.5 | 1.5 |
| H 1430–80 | .77 | 1.0 | 26.3 | 2.7 |
| P.C.C. 30–80 | .79 | 1.0 | 31.1 | 8.5 |
| All 1430–40 | .55 | 1.0 | 47.4 | 1.6 |
| N 1430–40 | .47 | 0.0 | 54.3 | 1.1 |
| S 1430–40 | .53 | 1.0 | 47.5 | 0.7 |
| H 1430–40 | .67 | 1.0 | 33.1 | 0.4 |
| P.C.C. 30–40 | .72 | 1.0 | 35.9 | 6.8 |
| All 1441–50 | .64 | 1.0 | 38.0 | 1.6 |
| N 1441–50 | .55 | 1.0 | 46.8 | 2.2 |
| S 1441–50 | .66 | 1.0 | 34.2 | 0.6 |
| H 1441–50 | .80 | 1.0 | 23.2 | 2.1 |
| P.C.C. 41–50 | .72 | 1.0 | 35.2 | 7.0 |
| All 1451–60 | .68 | 1.0 | 33.8 | 2.0 |
| N 1451–60 | .60 | 1.0 | 41.3 | 1.1 |
| S 1451–60 | .71 | 1.0 | 30.9 | 2.9 |
| H 1451–60 | .80 | 1.0 | 25.0 | 2.9 |
| P.C.C. 51–60 | .73 | 1.0 | 36.8 | 9.2 |
| All 1461–70 | .73 | 1.0 | 30.0 | 2.3 |
| N 1461–70 | .71 | 1.0 | 30.5 | 1.4 |
| S 1461–70 | .71 | 1.0 | 30.8 | 1.6 |
| H 1461–70 | .81 | 1.0 | 24.0 | 5.0 |
| P.C.C. 61–70 | .82 | 1.0 | 26.9 | 8.0 |
| All 1471–80 | .74 | 1.0 | 28.7 | 2.6 |
| N 1471–80 | .69 | 1.0 | 33.1 | 2.1 |
| S 1471–80 | .76 | 1.0 | 25.9 | 1.8 |
| H 1471–80 | .77 | 1.0 | 26.2 | 2.9 |
| P.C.C. 71–80 | .87 | 1.0 | 24.9 | 10.5 |

*Table 6.3.2.* Spouse Ratios, All Male Testators Excepting Clerics

| | R.R. | Mode | % Test. Not Married | % Remarriage |
|---|---|---|---|---|
| All 1430–80 | .78 | 1.0 | 24.2 | 2.0 |
| N 30–80 | .76 | 1.0 | 26.1 | 1.3 |
| S 30–80 | .77 | 1.0 | 23.9 | 1.2 |
| H 30–80 | .82 | 1.0 | 20.5 | 2.4 |
| P.C.C. 30–80 | .89 | 1.0 | 21.8 | 9.5 |
| All 1430–40 | .71 | 1.0 | 31.3 | 2.3 |
| N 30–40 | .65 | 1.0 | 37.3 | 1.2 |
| S 30–40 | .71 | 1.0 | 29.7 | 0.7 |
| H 30–40 | .75 | 1.0 | 25.7 | 0.5 |
| P.C.C. 30–40 | .88 | 1.0 | 22.1 | 8.3 |
| All 1441–50 | .77 | 1.0 | 25.0 | 1.8 |
| N 41–50 | .73 | 1.0 | 29.0 | 2.1 |
| S 41–50 | .75 | 1.0 | 25.6 | 0.5 |
| H 41–50 | .88 | 1.0 | 15.1 | 2.5 |
| P.C.C. 41–50 | .86 | 1.0 | 24.5 | 9.1 |
| All 1451–60 | .77 | 1.0 | 24.6 | 1.7 |
| N 51–60 | .74 | 1.0 | 27.0 | 1.1 |
| S 51–60 | .77 | 1.0 | 24.2 | 1.0 |
| H 51–60 | .87 | 1.0 | 18.2 | 3.1 |
| P.C.C. 51–60 | .82 | 1.0 | 28.1 | 9.4 |
| All 1461–70 | .80 | 1.0 | 23.0 | 2.1 |
| N 61–70 | .79 | 1.0 | 22.0 | 1.0 |
| S 61–70 | .77 | 1.0 | 25.3 | 1.7 |
| H 61–70 | .83 | 1.0 | 20.1 | 3.2 |
| P.C.C. 61–70 | .93 | 1.0 | 18.2 | 9.7 |
| All 1471–80 | .80 | 1.0 | 22.4 | 2.1 |
| N 71–80 | .77 | 1.0 | 24.4 | 1.7 |
| S 71–80 | .80 | 1.0 | 21.5 | 1.1 |
| H 71–80 | .81 | 1.0 | 21.6 | 2.6 |
| P.C.C. 71–80 | .94 | 1.0 | 18.2 | 10.2 |

*Table 6.3.3.* Spouse Ratios, All Urban Testators

| | R.R. | Mode | %Test. Not Married | % Remarriage |
|---|---|---|---|---|
| All 1430–80 | .78 | 1.0 | 27.7 | 5.3 |
| London 30–80 | .85 | 1.0 | 27.3 | 10.2 |
| Norwich 30–80 | .73 | 1.0 | 31.6 | 4.1 |
| Ipswich 30–80 | .73 | 1.0 | 30.6 | 2.4 |
| St. Albans 30–80 | .79 | 1.0 | 25.0 | 3.7 |
| B.S.E. 30–80 | .77 | 1.0 | 25.5 | 2.4 |
| London 1430–80 | .85 | 1.0 | 27.3 | 10.2 |
| 1430–40 | .84 | 1.0 | 29.5 | 10.7 |
| 1441–50 | .72 | 1.0 | 35.1 | 6.4 |
| 1451–60 | .79 | 1.0 | 34.5 | 12.7 |
| 1461–70 | .89 | 1.0 | 22.6 | 9.8 |
| 1471–80 | .92 | 1.0 | 21.7 | 11.6 |
| Norwich 1430–80 | .73 | 1.0 | 31.6 | 4.1 |
| 1430–40 | .71 | 1.0 | 30.6 | 1.2 |
| 1441–50 | .71 | 1.0 | 32.4 | 2.9 |
| 1451–60 | .73 | 1.0 | 32.1 | 5.5 |
| 1461–70 | .75 | 1.0 | 29.3 | 4.3 |
| 1471–80 | .72 | 1.0 | 33.5 | 5.1 |
| Ipswich 1430–80 | .73 | 1.0 | 30.6 | 2.4 |
| 1430–40 | .60 | 1.0 | 40.0 | 0.0* |
| 1441–50 | .61 | 1.0 | 39.5 | 0.0* |
| 1451–60 | .65 | 1.0 | 36.5 | 1.6 |
| 1461–70 | .88 | 1.0 | 20.0 | 6.1 |
| 1471–80 | .73 | 1.0 | 31.5 | 1.9 |
| St. Albans 30–80 | .79 | 1.0 | 25.0 | 3.7 |
| 1430–1440 | .70 | 1.0 | 30.1 | 0.0* |
| 1441–50 | .72 | 1.0 | 30.0 | 2.0 |
| 1451–60 | .80 | 1.0 | 25.0 | 2.9 |
| 1461–70 | .90 | 1.0 | 16.4 | 6.4 |
| 1471–80 | .84 | 1.0 | 22.5 | 6.3 |
| B.S.E. 1430–80 | .77 | 1.0 | 25.5 | 2.4 |
| 1430–40 | .67 | 1.0 | 32.3 | 0.7 |
| 1441–50 | .68 | 1.0 | 32.9 | 0.7 |
| 1451–60 | .84 | 1.0 | 18.1 | 1.9 |
| 1461–70 | .76 | 1.0 | 24.4 | 0.7 |
| 1471–80 | .83 | 1.0 | 23.1 | 5.5 |
| Bungay 1430–80 | .64 | 1.0 | 39.6 | 2.0 |
| Beccles 1430–80 | .68 | 1.0 | 33.1 | 1.3 |
| Sudbury 1430–80 | .79 | 1.0 | 22.8 | 1.5 |

*Poor data

Table 6.3.4. Spouse Ratios, Occupational and Special Groups
for All Testators

| | R.R. | Mode | % Test. Not Married | % Remarriage |
|---|---|---|---|---|
| Rural Élite 30–80 | .90 | 1.0 | 19.6 | 8.5 |
| 1430–40 | 85 | 1.0 | 21.7 | 6.5 |
| 1441–50 | .96 | 1.0 | 13.6 | 9.1 |
| 1451–60 | .81 | 1.0 | 25.5 | 6.4 |
| 1461–70 | .92 | 1.0 | 24.0 | 12.0 |
| 1471–80 | .94 | 1.0 | 14.8 | 8.2 |
| London Élite 30–80 | 1.06 | 1.0 | 11.9 | 14.9 |
| 1430–40 | 1.19 | 1.0 | 9.4 | 18.8 |
| 1441–50 | 1.04 | 1.0 | 12.0 | 12.0 |
| 1451–60 | 1.02 | 1.0 | 12.8 | 15.4 |
| 1461–70 | 1.02 | 1.0 | 14.0 | 14.0 |
| 1471–80 | 1.12 | 1.0 | 7.1 | 16.7 |
| Select Urban Occ. 1430–80* | .87 | 1.0 | 14.8 | 2.0 |
| Select Rural Oc. 1430–80** | .91 | 1.0 | 12.7 | 3.8 |
| All Citizens 1430–80 | 1.01 | 1.0 | 11.7 | 10.7 |
| Non-citizen Occ. 1430–80 | .86 | 1.0 | 19.3 | 4.6 |
| All Occ. 1430–80 | .93 | 1.0 | 15.7 | 7.5 |
| Female Test. 1430–80 | .63 | 1.0 | 41.9 | 4.1 |
| Testators with servants 30–80 | .82 | 1.0 | 25.0 | 5.5 |

*All urban bakers, barbers, barkers, tanners, butchers, carpenters, skinners, smiths, tailors who were not citizens of their towns.
**All rural clothmakers, dyers, fullers, shermans, weavers, worsteadmen.

between 2 and 5 percent to the total spouse figures. This is a significant but not distorted figure, and certainly one which does not effect the general viability of the data. The stated purpose of the thesis has been to assess changes and responses to changes in the demographic composition of fifteenth century society, and not to proffer concrete statistical figures, something not possible by the use of the wills alone. With these reservations in mind, we can look at the data.

Marriage was very common among the will-registering population. Even in the sample run for the entire set—that is, including clerics—the mean figures for marriage were comparatively high. In a period of easily obtainable land, there must have been relatively few restraints on marriage. Table 6.3.2 shows the data for marriage for all adult males except clerics. Ratios of marriage are consistently high, almost always exceeding 75 percent of the totals. Remarriage, however, does not seem to have been frequent. Remarriage ratios exceed 10 percent only for the P.C.C.; as described above, there was a direct correlation between remarriage and individual wealth. Yet the higher ratio of remarriage for the P.C.C. testators should not be seen as the sole contributing element to the larger marriage factor in general for the P.C.C. The percentage of testators from this court who did not marry at all, at least according to the testamentary data, was consistently lower than that of Norfolk and Suffolk, and close to that of Hertfordshire in all decades but the 1440's. Thus, not only did the wealthy will makers of the P.C.C. remarry more frequently than did their provincial counterparts, but they married more frequently a first time.

Marriage ratios were surprisingly high for Hertfordshire, as represented by the wills from the archdeaconry of St. Albans, or at least surprisingly high in view of the very low child-replacement ratios for the archdeaconry.[30] Equally curious was the fact that Hertfordshire was the poorest county covered in the survey. Despite this, remarriage was higher than in correspondingly more wealthy and more fertile East Anglia, and first-marriage was at the highest levels of the sample. Yet remarriage was usually under 5 percent, and it was a high proportion of first-marriages which gave Hertfordshire its high overall marriage ratios. Thus, in the wealthiest segment of the sample, the P.C.C. testators, both marriage and remarriage were high; in the poorest segment of the sample, testators from the archdeaconry of St. Albans, first-time marriage was very frequent, and remarriage, if not frequent by P.C.C. standards, was more usual than it was in wealthy East Anglia.[31]

With a few exceptions, there were no significant trends in the marriage ratios in the period 1430–1480 for the cleric-less table. The data for the 1430's tends to be somewhat lower than that of the sample as a whole, but as described in Chapter 1, this is probably due to flaws in the pre-1440 will evidence. There are some exceptions to the apparent lack of secular trends in the marriage data. In urban areas, there was a tendency toward lower marriage percentages in the middle decades of the period—that is, the period of least epidemic virulence. In the P.C.C., there was a significant rise in remarriage through the period, a rise which became quite pronounced in the 1470's. Remarriage in general rose significantly in the decades of most severe virulence and most frequent visitation of epidemic disease. It was significantly higher in the 1430's, 1460's and 1470's than it was in the 1440's and 1450's. There must surely have been a greater need and opportunity for remarriage after a period of concerted mortality.[32]

A key question is, what were the average ages of marriage for males and females? Hajnal has proposed a theory about a prototype European marriage pattern and age, and when it first became widespread.[33] While it is not possible to assess definitively the average age of first-marriage of all testators, approximations can be made. Most interesting are the marriage ratios for those testators in Age Group 1, the group which had parents living at the time the wills were originally made, and whose members appear to have been under twenty-five years of age. As indicated above, the will data are most complete for males. The ratios of marriage are quite low for the testators of Group 1, hovering at about one-third, almost the precise inverse of the average ratio of the sample as a whole. Further, a disproportionate share of this one-third comes from the wealthiest segment of the under-twenty-fives, the gentry and the P.C.C. testators.[34] A closer look at the individual married will-registerers in Group 1 would seem to indicate that they were closer to the upper age limits of the group—that is, around twenty-four or twenty-five—than they were to the lower limits, at around eighteen to twenty. It is probable that the average age of first marriage for males in the middle decades was over twenty-five, even for the wealthiest segments of society; and the scantier evidence for female testators indicate that this was the case for them as well.[35] In the depopulated fifteenth century, this is surprisingly low. At the same time, it extends Hajnal's European age of marriage back into the fifteenth century, a century which he chose to leave as a murky never-never land between medieval and modern Europe.[36]

Marriage patterns as indicated by the wills varied in different geographical areas and between different occupational groups within the sample. Marriage was more frequent in the urban areas than it was in rural areas. In light of the dismal child replacement ratios for urban areas, this contrast takes on greater interest: while first-marriages and remarriages were greater in the towns than in the country, rural male replacement ratios were far higher.[37] In two large market villages surveyed,

Beccles and Bungay, both in the heart of a district which has been designated as one of crisis-mortality, marriage ratios were lower than they were in the defined urban areas, but about the same as they were in the rural areas. At the same time, fertility in these market centers, intermediate in size between the cities and the rural villages, was well below that of the countryside.[38] Conceivably, the low market-village figures for both marriage and child-replacement ratios are reflective of an unmarried, highly transient segment of the population. It has been stated that a large number of unmarried persons flock to urban areas, even in pre-industrial societies.[39] Many of these urban transients, if they did indeed exist in the provincial towns, may have failed to make or have their wills registered, although the wealth data for Bury St. Edmunds and St. Albans would argue against this point of view.

Within the urban sample, certain groups had particularly high ratios of marriages. Foremost among these were the London élite. Especially high was their percentage of remarriage, which was the largest for the entire sample. At the same time, the percentage of London merchants not marrying was very low. Thus, the group's high marriage ratio was the result not only of a larger than normal frequency of remarriage, but also a higher percentage of first-marriages, and a low number of nonmarrieds. Conversely, when the marriage ratios for Londoners fell during the 1440's and 1450's, the drop was due to both a fall in remarriage and a fall in first-marriages. There was a strong connection between the ratios of marriage and the occurrence of periods of crisis mortality; immediately after bad times, the marriage ratios rose. As with the London élite, marriage and remarriage were higher than the norm for the sample's other major wealthy subgroup, the rural élite. The patterns were almost identical to those of the wealthy Londoners: remarriage was at its lowest and nonmarriage at its highest in the relatively disease-free decades of the 1440's and 1450's, and vice versa.

Among urban dwellers in general, marriage was higher among citizens than unenfranchised craftsmen. Yet taken as a whole, testators mentioning some sort of occupation or craft affiliation had slightly higher first-marriage and remarriage ratios than did the nonoccupation claiming and presumably primarily agricultural bulk of the sample. In the other major occupational groups surveyed, the unenfranchised urban craftsmen and the rural textile workers, the percentage of first-marriages was also higher than that of the sample as a whole. Remarriage, however, was very slight in both groups.

Among others, clerics overwhelmingly reported themselves as not married. Although in all cases the figures were slight, the clerical marriage figures were lower in proportion to the rest of the sample than the clerical child-replacement ratios. Put simply, more clerics report children than report wives, a relationship in direct contrast with the rest of the sample.[40] The group with the lowest percentage of marriage were female testators. About 42 percent of the female will-registering population were not married, by the standards established above, and this does not include widows, who were counted in the married sample.

In sum, frequency of marriage was connected with great wealth, but there was little correlation between all other wealth groups and first-marriage. Remarriage, on the other hand, was directly related to the wealth assessment of the testator. Marriage ratios were higher in urban than in rural areas, and urban craftsmen tended to marry more often than their rural counterparts of approximate wealth. The frequency of marriage and especially remarriage was directly linked with epidemic disease, but otherwise there were few long-term trends in either of the two variables. Finally, marriage took place for most of the male population after the age of twenty-five, and was on the average probably over twenty-five for even the wealthiest segments of will-registering society.

## Notes

1. See above, Chapter I, footnote 27.

2. In 1466, a random sampling of wills from the P.C.Y. showed 15.6% of the testators were clerics. In 1467, 15.2% of testators were clerics.

3. For a discussion of the method used to determine the marriage ratios, see pp. 175–176.

4. See above, pp. 22–28.

5. It is not possible to estimate the will-registering populations of either town from the consistory court wills alone. The King's Lynn testators in particular seem to have been considerably underenumerated. In 1377, Yarmouth had 1,941 taxpayers, Lynn had 3,127, and Norwich 3,952.

6. St. Albans' regional importance was diminished by proximity of London. But the town had 571 testators, almost all from the archdeaconry court, placing it well ahead of the East Suffolk regional urban center, Ipswich, which had only 245 will registers. It was the fourth largest center in the will sample.

7. This does not include clerics, the rural élite, yeomen, or those testators calling themselves husbandmen.

8. See above, pp. 180–183.

9. At first, it appeared that the franchise was broader in the provincial towns than in London. This was not so. Rather, only the wealthiest testators—that is, those registering wills in the P.C.C.—were included from London. The majority of provincial citizens had their wills registered in the consistory courts, and there the range of citizen occupations was broader.

10. There were only about a dozen titled peers, the most illustrious being John, Duke of Bedford, brother of Henry V.

11. There were about twenty testators who were themselves servants. They were generally in the employ of the very wealthiest testators, and showed about the same demographic features, including levels of wealth, as did the sample as a whole.

12. Only about 55 wills listed *famuli* and other farm workers, rather than "domestic" servants.

13. The low percentage of testators with servants may not have been entirely artificial. The fifteenth century was a period of labor shortage and high wages, and servants must have been difficult to get and harder to hold.

14. It should be noted that about twenty wills do survive from the City Court of Norwich, and have been used in this study.

15. Of the testators in Group 1, 34.5% were married.

16. This is an impressionistic, and not quantitative statement. Most of the parents appear to have been active and vigorous, judging from the wills of their offspring. The fact that so many—about three-quarters—were named as will executors is only one indication; another is that about half of them appeared to have been living and working their own tofts and messuages, and not dwelling in the houses of their children.

17. Of 197 testators in Age Group 1, only 5 had children.

18. It should be noted that this differs significantly from the data presented in a recent article by H. LeBras. In "Parents, grandparents, bisaïeux," *Population* 28, 1973, LeBras discusses the age of children at their parents' death, based on data from modern and "Ancien Régime" France. In "Ancien Régime" France, he found that most individuals had their fathers alive when they were 27, and their mothers at 32. More than half had both parents at 18; and at 21, only 13% had lost both. For the entire population, 31% had no parents, 28% had one parent, and 41% had both parents. For adults—those over 20 years—55% had no parents, and 86% had lost one. The median age of orphanage was 48 years. Although the author does not believe that modern and even early modern data can be compared accurately with medieval data, the discrepancies between the LeBras figures and those presented in this chapter are large enough to cast some doubt on the latter's validity. It must be stressed, however, that Group 1 testators comprise only 1.3% of the total sample, and therefore have little effect on the age tables in general.

19. There were only about fifty testators who met this godchild criterion, and their inclusion in the sample had little numerical significance, especially since about half of them also qualified for inclusion in Age Group 3 because they also had grandchildren or children of age.

20. There are some cases when the age of majority is actually given, and it is almost always 24 or 25 years. There are other cases where testators leave goods or land to their children when those children reach 24 or 25, although no mention is made about either of the above being the years of "coming of age."

21. See below, pp. 190–201.

22. P.C.C. testators have not been included in Table 6.2.2. This last statement is made on the basis of another age-wealth bivariate sample which has not been included in the text for reasons of economy. In this run, approximately 8% of the P.C.C. sample fell into Age Group 1 and Wealth Group A, a significant increase

over the proportions of the sample as a whole, and 35% fell into Age Group 3 and Wealth Group A, also an increase over the proportions for the sample as a whole.

23. This position is held by two historians of the will, A. J. Camp, *Wills and Their Whereabouts* (Canterbury: Phillimore, 1963), p. xi; and J. S. W. Gibson, *Wills and Where to Find Them* (Chicester: Phillimore, 1974), pp. xv–xvi.

It is worth noting again that the author is aware of the limitations of the wealth measure. Despite the legal imperatives discussed in the first chapter, we have no way of knowing exactly what proportion of a man's wealth was left to the church, either through bequest to the high altar, or total pious donations. The gift to the high altar may distort the wealth category, although in the fifteenth century it is not likely that anyone would have to scrimp on this bequest in order to provide more for his or her heirs. Attitudes change in a fifty-year period, and a subjective judgment of pious donations indicates a rise in secularism in the 1460's and 1470's, although this is mirrored in additional bequests, rather than those to the high altar. But even with these reservations noted, virtually all wills do have some donation to the high altar, and these donations appear to be in rough approximation of total wealth as portrayed in the wills. Perhaps more important, a wealth measure was devised because it was felt that some reasonably objective standard, even if it could not be absolutely substantiated, was better than no wealth standard at all. This justification may also be applied to the age measure, also imperfect, but again, the best data available. It was felt that admittedly crude measures were better than no measures at all.

24. This information comes to me from Dr. R. S. Schofield. For a survey of the comparative levels of wealth of the English counties in the later Middle Ages, see his "Geographical Distribution of Wealth in England, 1334–1649," *Ec.H.R.*, 2nd series, XVIII, 1965. By the early sixteenth century, Hertfordshire had risen significantly in the ranks of wealth, and Norfolk had declined, according to Schofield's figures.

25. *Ibid.* Although they are based on fourteenth century tax data, se R. A. Pelham, "Fourteenth Century England," in H. C. Darby, ed., *Historical Geography of England* (Cambridge: Cambridge Univ. Press, 1936); and R. F. Glasscock, "England, 1334," in H C. Darby, ed., *New Historical Geography of England* (Cambridge: Cambridge Univ. Press, 1973).

26. See above, pp. 21–22.

27. In his study of the bourgeoisie of Geneva, Louis Henry, *Anciennes familles genevoises* (Paris: Presses universitaires de France, 1956), found evidence of the practice of birth control. For birth control in pre-industrial England, see the works of E. A. Wrigley cited in the bibliography, especially "Family Limitation in Pre-Industrial England, *Ec.H.R.*, 2nd series, XIX, 1966.

28. See above, pp. 21–22.

29. See below, pp. 189–193, 197–201.

30. See below, pp. 189–193.

31. There were higher numbers of clerics in Norfolk and Suffolk than in Hertfordshire, as reported in the wills, but this factor is eliminated in Table 6.3.2.

32. See below, pp. 209–222.

33. J. Hajnal, "European Marriage Patterns in Perspective," in D. V. Glass

and D. E. C. Eversley, eds., *Population in History* (London: Edward Arnold, 1965).

34. For example, 18.3% of Group 1 testators came from the P.C.C. alone, as compared to 8.6% P.C.C. representation from the entire sample.

35. Less than 20% of the under-25's were women, and of these, only 10% were married. None of these had children. The fact that there were proportionally more under-25 women than men may indicate that the female age of first marriage was slightly lower.

36. Because the LeBras work, *op. cit.*, sheds doubt on the validity of Group 1, an alternative test for average age of first-marriage is necessary. Although argument by analogy is poor historical method, it was felt that if the will marriage ratios could be proved approximate with proportions married by age for data considered modern by Hajnal, then it could be used as further evidence for age of first-marriage after 25 years. T. H. Hollingsworth's data on the British peerage, from "A Demographic Study of the British Ducal Families," in Glass and Eversley, *op. cit.*, were selected. Although they are for the aristocracy, no alternative large-scale data for pre-industrial English population were available. Since the data are presented by proportions not married at five-year intervals, some adaptation was necessary. To get proportions married by age, the Hollingsworth figures were first subtracted from 1.00, and then multiplied by deaths at each age ($_n$dx). The $_n$dx values were taken from Ansley Coale and Paul Demeny, *Regional Model Life Tables and Stable Populations* (Princeton: Princeton University Press, 1973), Model West tables, female, $e_0 = 30$. The products of $_a$age (a) and $_n$dx (B) were added, and divided by the sums of B, or $\left[\dfrac{\Sigma (A) \quad (B)}{\Sigma (B)}\right]$. The will data were compared with the Hollingsworth cohorts from 1330–1479; 1480–1679; and 1680–1729. The will ratio for the entire sample was .78 for the group without clerics; the Hollingsworth figures were, respectively, .86, .86, and .73. Thus, the fifteenth century testamentary figures fall somewhere between the latter two Hollingsworth cohorts. Average ages of first-marriage for these two cohorts were 24.3 and 28.6. It would follow that the fifteen century will figures for age of first marriage would be between these two figures, or after age 25.

37. See below, pp. 195–196.

38. For the Beccles and Bungay replacement ratios, see below, pp. 200, 202.

39. Among others, see J. C. Russell, *British Medieval Population,* (Albuquerque: Univ. of New Mexico Press, 1948), pp. 371–396.

40. There is evidence from the individual wills that some of these clerical children were illegitimate, and more so than for the bulk of the population.

# CHAPTER VII

# *The Course of Population, 1430–1480*

## 7.1 Prospects for the Future: Children

Through the use of child-replacement ratios, and especially male replacement ratios, it is possible to discern long-term trends in the movement of population and different demographic responses and characteristics among the various groups and areas covered in the study. Three types of replacement ratios have been used in analyzing the data. First, the ratio of all male children to all testators has been taken. Despite the general and imprecise nature of this measure, it is essential for comparative purposes with groups containing female testators, since effective female replacement ratios cannot be constructed by use of the wills alone. The second was all male testators who could in theory marry—that is, all males less priests—by all male children. This is the replacement ratio referred to most frequently in the course of the chapter. Finally, a third measure, married male testators only to all their sons as reported in the wills was taken. This was an attempt to see if the will-making family units were replacing themselves.

An important qualification must be noted. The replacement ratio method is a complex and as yet not fully developed concept. The logic behind it holds that one group within a particular population within a given generation can be compared to a similar group in the corresponding population in the next generation. Ideally, this should be done at precisely the same point in time for each generation. If done this way, the replacement ratio for a growing population will measure above unity

187

(1.00), that of a stationary population at or about unity, and a declining population below 1.00. Unfortunately, the nature of the testamentary evidence permits only a generational *approximation* of age, and there is no way of knowing if the replacement ratio scheme does actually compare father and son at identical ages. This means that if a replacement ratio measures the generations at different times in their lives, it could conceivably be growing, even if it is below 1.00! The method used below, however, does assume that each generation married and had children at about the same age, that a ratio of above 1.00 represents demographic growth, and that one of about 1.00 represents demographic stability. But this cannot be proved; it can only be assumed.[1]

There is one other reservation to be noted. Grandchildren have been recorded, but the data are not presented in this chapter.[2] Even more than is the case when trying to deal with younger sons, the historian cannot be sure that the wills are reflecting an accurate portrayal of the numbers of grandsons. As the age data in Chapter 6 have shown, the number of adults who had children and then lived long enough to see their children have children was small indeed. The crude numbers of grandsons reported in the wills may in fact have been accurate, but there is no way of being certain. Grandsons could have been left out of the wills if things to bequeath ran out. Testators may have felt an immediate responsibility to provide only for their children and not future generations; and as it was probably assumed that the sons' sons, if not the daughters' sons, would inherit the bulk of the estate in due time at any rate, bequests to grandsons may simply have been viewed as superfluous. Therefore, the numbers of grandsons reported in the wills have been added to the raw numbers used for sons, but were considered to be too few and too unreliable to be dealt with individually.[3]

A few general impressions of the data, recorded in Tables 7.1.1 through 7.1.10 may be noted. Male replacement ratios and numbers of multiple sons are consistently higher for testators from the P.C.C. than for testators registering their wills in lower courts. This is the case with all three of the replacement ratio methods, presented in Tables 7.1.1 through 7.1.3. The P.C.C. ratios are highest because of the greater frequency of 2, 3, 4, 5 and 6-son families, but it will be noted that the numbers of P.C.C. families with no sons was also among the lowest in the sample. Part of the reason for more multiple-son families among the P.C.C. testators may have been their greater personal wealth, which enabled them to provide more adequately for their children. But more important—and also a function of greater wealth—male and especially female P.C.C. testators appear to have married at an earlier age than did

*Table 7.1.1.* Male Child Replacement Ratios:
Males to Entire Sample

| | R.R. | Mode | 0 | 1 | 2 | 3 | 4 | 5 | 6+ |
|---|---|---|---|---|---|---|---|---|---|
| | | | | | Distribution of Sons Per Family - in % | | | | |
| All 1430–80 | .68 | 0 | 57.9 | 24.8 | 11.6 | 4.0 | 1.2 | .4 | .1 |
| N 1430–80 | .69 | 0 | 58.0 | 23.8 | 12.3 | 4.0 | 1.5 | .2 | .2 |
| S 1430–80 | .65 | 0 | 57.5 | 26.0 | 11.6 | 3.6 | .9 | .3 | .1 |
| H 1430–80 | .69 | 0 | 58.6 | 25.0 | 9.1 | 4.9 | 1.2 | 1.0 | .2 |
| P.C.C. 30–80 | .76 | 0 | 57.6 | 21.8 | 11.8 | 5.8 | 2.0 | .7 | .3 |
| All 1430–40 | .49 | 0 | 68.2 | 20.3 | 7.3 | 2.9 | 1.1 | .2 | .0 |
| N 1430–40 | .45 | 0 | 71.0 | 18.6 | 6.9 | 1.9 | 1.4 | .2 | .0 |
| S 1430–40 | .49 | 0 | 68.1 | 19.9 | 8.0 | 3.1 | .7 | .2 | .0 |
| H 1430–40 | .60 | 0 | 60.6 | 26.3 | 8.0 | 4.0 | 1.2 | .0 | .0 |
| P.C.C. 30–40 | .52 | 0 | 68.4 | 18.9 | 6.8 | 4.4 | 1.0 | .5 | .0 |
| All 1441–50 | .61 | 0 | 62.1 | 22.9 | 9.4 | 3.9 | 1.2 | .2 | .1 |
| N 1441–50 | .64 | 0 | 61.5 | 22.1 | 10.5 | 4.3 | 1.2 | .1 | .2 |
| S 1441–50 | .58 | 0 | 61.5 | 25.3 | 9.4 | 2.9 | .7 | .2 | .1 |
| H 1441–50 | .63 | 0 | 63.6 | 20.8 | 8.5 | 5.1 | .8 | .8 | .4 |
| P.C.C. 41–50 | .67 | 0 | 62.0 | 20.4 | 9.9 | 4.2 | 3.5 | .0 | .0 |
| All 1451–60 | .65 | 0 | 58.9 | 24.9 | 10.7 | 3.9 | 1.2 | .2 | .1 |
| N 1451–60 | .66 | 0 | 60.6 | 22.5 | 10.1 | 5.0 | 1.2 | .3 | .3 |
| S 1451–60 | .62 | 0 | 58.6 | 26.4 | 10.8 | 3.0 | 1.1 | .1 | .0 |
| H 1451–60 | .67 | 0 | 58.2 | 26.5 | 8.6 | 3.4 | 1.9 | .7 | .4 |
| P.C.C. 51–60 | .77 | 0 | 56.1 | 21.1 | 14.0 | 7.0 | 1.8 | .0 | .0 |
| All 1461–70 | .69 | 0 | 56.4 | 25.9 | 12.0 | 4.0 | 1.1 | .3 | .1 |
| N 1461–70 | .70 | 0 | 55.0 | 27.0 | 12.7 | 3.4 | 1.5 | .2 | .0 |
| S 1461–70 | .66 | 0 | 58.0 | 25.5 | 11.4 | 3.9 | .8 | .3 | .1 |
| H 1461–70 | .79 | 0 | 52.0 | 26.2 | 14.5 | 5.9 | .9 | .5 | .0 |
| P.C.C. 61–70 | .77 | 0 | 56.0 | 23.4 | 11.4 | 7.4 | .9 | .3 | .6 |
| All 1471–80 | .78 | 0 | 52.8 | 26.0 | 14.5 | 4.5 | 1.4 | .6 | .2 |
| N 1471–80 | .83 | 0 | 51.4 | 24.6 | 16.7 | 5.0 | 1.8 | .3 | .2 |
| S 1471–80 | .74 | 0 | 53.0 | 27.7 | 14.0 | 3.9 | .9 | .5 | .1 |
| H 1471–80 | .76 | 0 | 57.9 | 24.8 | 7.8 | 5.8 | 1.2 | 2.3 | .3 |
| P.C.C. 71–80 | .96 | 0 | 49.5 | 23.9 | 16.2 | 4.7 | 3.4 | 2.0 | .3 |

*Table 7.1.2.* Male Child Replacement Ratios:
Males to Male Adults, Excepting Clerics

| | R.R. | Mode | Distribution of Sons Per Testator - in % | | | | | | |
|---|---|---|---|---|---|---|---|---|---|
| | | | 0 | 1 | 2 | 3 | 4 | 5 | 6+ |
| All 1430–80 | .76 | 0 | 53.1 | 27.5 | 12.9 | 4.5 | 1.4 | .4 | .1 |
| N 1430–80 | .82 | 0 | 50.3 | 27.9 | 14.8 | 4.7 | 1.8 | .3 | .2 |
| S 1430–80 | .71 | 0 | 54.1 | 28.2 | 12.5 | 3.8 | 0.9 | .3 | .1 |
| H 1430–80 | .69 | 0 | 58.9 | 25.1 | 8.8 | 4.9 | 1.3 | 1.0 | .3 |
| P.C.C. 30–80 | .85 | 0 | 52.8 | 24.8 | 12.1 | 6.8 | 2.5 | .8 | .3 |
| All 1430–40 | .62 | 0 | 59.9 | 25.3 | 9.4 | 3.8 | 1.4 | .3 | .0 |
| N 1430–40 | .62 | 0 | 60.0 | 24.9 | 10.1 | 2.8 | 1.6 | .4 | .0 |
| S 1430–40 | .65 | 0 | 58.3 | 25.8 | 10.6 | 3.9 | 1.1 | .4 | .0 |
| H 1430–40 | .58 | 0 | 61.9 | 25.7 | 8.4 | 4.5 | 1.5 | .0 | .0 |
| P.C.C 30–40 | .64 | 0 | 61.4 | 22.8 | 9.0 | 4.8 | 1.4 | .7 | .0 |
| All 1441–50 | .72 | 0 | 54.9 | 27.5 | 11.6 | 4.5 | 1.4 | .2 | .3 |
| N 1441–50 | .83 | 0 | 49.5 | 28.5 | 14.7 | 5.4 | 1.4 | .2 | .2 |
| S 1441–50 | .66 | 0 | 55.8 | 29.1 | 10.6 | 3.4 | .6 | .3 | .2 |
| H 1441–50 | .62 | 0 | 63.3 | 21.1 | 9.0 | 4.5 | 1.0 | .5 | .5 |
| P.C.C. 41–40 | .76 | 0 | 56.4 | 25.5 | 9.1 | 4.5 | 4.5 | .0 | .0 |
| All 1451–60 | .73 | 0 | 53.6 | 28.3 | 12.1 | 4.4 | 1.2 | .3 | .1 |
| N 1451–60 | .80 | 0 | 51.3 | 28.2 | 12.9 | 5.9 | 1.0 | .5 | .3 |
| S 1451–60 | .68 | 0 | 54.7 | 29.1 | 11.7 | 3.3 | 1.2 | .1 | .0 |
| H 1451–60 | .70 | 0 | 56.9 | 28.0 | 8.4 | 3.6 | 1.8 | .9 | .4 |
| P.C.C. 51–60 | .90 | 0 | 50.3 | 24.0 | 14.0 | 9.4 | 2.3 | .0 | .0 |
| All 1461–70 | .75 | 0 | 52.9 | 27.8 | 13.1 | 4.4 | 1.3 | .4 | .1 |
| N 1461–70 | .80 | 0 | 49.7 | 29.8 | 14.3 | 3.9 | 2.0 | .3 | .0 |
| S 1461–70 | .70 | 0 | 55.6 | 26.7 | 12.2 | 4.2 | .8 | .3 | .2 |
| H 1461–70 | .77 | 0 | 52.9 | 26.5 | 13.8 | 5.3 | 1.1 | .5 | .0 |
| P.C.C. 61–70 | .84 | 0 | 52.5 | 25.7 | 11.4 | 8.2 | 1.1 | .4 | .8 |
| All 1471–80 | .83 | 0 | 50.0 | 27.5 | 15.3 | 4.7 | 1.6 | .7 | .2 |
| N 1471–80 | .92 | 0 | 46.7 | 26.8 | 18.3 | 5.4 | 2.2 | .3 | .4 |
| S 1471–80 | .77 | 0 | 51.0 | 28.9 | 14.6 | 4.0 | .9 | .6 | .1 |
| H 1471–80 | .76 | 0 | 58.4 | 24.1 | 7.6 | 5.9 | 1.3 | 2.3 | .3 |
| P.C.C. 71–80 | 1.04 | 0 | 46.2 | 25.8 | 16.0 | 5.3 | 4.0 | 2.2 | .4 |

*Table 7.1.3.* Male Child Replacement Ratios:
Males to Married Male Testators

| | R.R. | Mode | Distribution of Sons Per Testator - % | | | | | | |
| | | | 0 | 1 | 2 | 3 | 4 | 5 | 6+ |
|---|---|---|---|---|---|---|---|---|---|
| All 1430–80 | .83 | 0 | 49.0 | 29.6 | 14.1 | 5.0 | 1.6 | .5 | .1 |
| N 1430–80 | .91 | 0 | 45.5 | 30.0 | 16.6 | 5.3 | 2.1 | .4 | .2 |
| S 1430–80 | .77 | 0 | 50.3 | 30.3 | 13.5 | 4.3 | 1.1 | .4 | .1 |
| H 1430–80 | .72 | 0 | 57.3 | 25.5 | 9.5 | 5.0 | 1.6 | .9 | .3 |
| P.C.C. 30–80 | .99 | 0 | 45.5 | 28.4 | 14.2 | 7.7 | 2.9 | 1.0 | .3 |
| All 1430–40 | .69 | 0 | 56.3 | 27.0 | 10.1 | 4.6 | 1.6 | .4 | .0 |
| N 1430–40 | .73 | 0 | 55.6 | 26.4 | 11.3 | 3.9 | 2.3 | .6 | .0 |
| S 1430–40 | .71 | 0 | 55.2 | 26.9 | 11.4 | 3.0 | 1.0 | .5 | .0 |
| H 1430–40 | .60 | 0 | 59.6 | 27.8 | 6.6 | 4.6 | 1.3 | .0 | .0 |
| P.C.C. 30–40 | .70 | 0 | 50.0 | 23.1 | 10.3 | 5.1 | 1.7 | .9 | .0 |
| All 1441–50 | .81 | 0 | 49.8 | 30.4 | 12.5 | 5.1 | 1.5 | .3 | .3 |
| N 1441–50 | .95 | 0 | 44.1 | 31.0 | 16.0 | 6.5 | 1.6 | .3 | .3 |
| S 1441–50 | .76 | 0 | 49.3 | 33.2 | 11.8 | 4.5 | .6 | .4 | .2 |
| H 1441–50 | .62 | 0 | 63.9 | 21.3 | 8.3 | 4.1 | 1.2 | .6 | .6 |
| P.C.C. 41–50 | .97 | 0 | 45.3 | 30.2 | 12.8 | 5.8 | 5.8 | .0 | .0 |
| All 1451–60 | .78 | 0 | 50.1 | 30.6 | 12.8 | 4.6 | 1.5 | .2 | .1 |
| N 1451–60 | .84 | 0 | 48.6 | 29.1 | 14.5 | 5.9 | 1.5 | .2 | .2 |
| S 1451–60 | .73 | 0 | 51.0 | 31.7 | 12.5 | 3.4 | 1.3 | .1 | .1 |
| H 1451–60 | .72 | 0 | 55.7 | 28.6 | 8.6 | 3.2 | 2.7 | .5 | .5 |
| P.C.C. 51–60 | 1.04 | 0 | 41.9 | 28.2 | 16.1 | 11.3 | 2.4 | .0 | .0 |
| All 1461–70 | .84 | 0 | 48.3 | 30.1 | 14.1 | 5.2 | 1.6 | .5 | .1 |
| N 1461–70 | .88 | 0 | 44.6 | 32.7 | 15.8 | 4.2 | 2.3 | .4 | .1 |
| S 1461–70 | .78 | 0 | 51.5 | 28.7 | 12.8 | 5.3 | 1.0 | .4 | .2 |
| H 1461–70 | .82 | 0 | 52.8 | 23.8 | 15.9 | 6.0 | 1.3 | .7 | .0 |
| P.C.C. 61–70 | .95 | 0 | 45.8 | 30.5 | 12.7 | 8.5 | 1.3 | .4 | .8 |
| All 1471–80 | .91 | 0 | 46.2 | 29.1 | 16.9 | 5.1 | 1.7 | .9 | .2 |
| N 1471–80 | 1.02 | 0 | 41.4 | 29.1 | 20.3 | 6.2 | 2.3 | .6 | .3 |
| S 1471–80 | .82 | 0 | 48.4 | 30.0 | 15.7 | 4.3 | 1.0 | .7 | .1 |
| H 1471–80 | .80 | 0 | 55.7 | 25.3 | 8.9 | 6.3 | 1.3 | 2.1 | .4 |
| P.C.C. 71–80 | 1.20 | 0 | 38.4 | 29.5 | 18.4 | 5.8 | 4.7 | 2.6 | .5 |

*Table 7.1.4.* Male Child Replacement Ratios:
Urban Males to All Urban Testators

| | R.R. | Mode | Distribution of Sons Per Testator - in % | | | | | | |
|---|---|---|---|---|---|---|---|---|---|
| | | | 0 | 1 | 2 | 3 | 4 | 5 | 6+ |
| All 1430–40 | .58 | 0 | 64.3 | 21.4 | 9.1 | 3.8 | .8 | .4 | .1 |
| London 30–80 | .71 | 0 | 58.6 | 23.0 | 11.3 | 4.5 | 1.9 | .5 | .2 |
| Norwich 30–80 | .59 | 0 | 65.5 | 20.6 | 8.4 | 4.5 | .6 | .3 | .1 |
| Ipswich 30–80 | .44 | 0 | 71.9 | 15.1 | 10.3 | 2.2 | .5 | .0 | .0 |
| St Alb. 30–80 | .63 | 0 | 62.3 | 22.6 | 8.6 | 4.4 | .5 | 1.1 | .5 |
| B.S.E. 30–80 | .44 | 0 | 69.8 | 20.1 | 7.5 | 2.3 | .2 | .2 | .0 |
| London 1430–40 | .54 | 0 | 67.2 | 18.9 | 7.4 | 5.7 | .8 | .0 | .0 |
| 1441–50 | .65 | 0 | 62.8 | 20.2 | 9.6 | 4.3 | 3.2 | .0 | .0 |
| 1451–60 | .66 | 0 | 59.2 | 22.5 | 13.4 | 3.5 | 1.4 | .0 | .0 |
| 1461–70 | .72 | 0 | 59.2 | 23.4 | 11.1 | 6.8 | .9 | .0 | .4 |
| 1471–80 | .91 | 0 | 50.0 | 26.8 | 15.2 | 2.0 | 3.5 | 2.0 | .5 |
| Norwich 30–40 | .42 | 0 | 70.6 | 21.2 | 5.9 | 1.2 | 1.2 | .0 | .0 |
| 1441–50 | .52 | 0 | 69.9 | 18.4 | 5.9 | 5.1 | .0 | .0 | .7 |
| 1451–60 | .63 | 0 | 64.2 | 17.4 | 9.2 | 9.2 | .0 | .0 | .0 |
| 1461–70 | .61 | 0 | 63.4 | 20. | 11.0 | 3.7 | 1.2 | .6 | .0 |
| 1471–80 | .56 | 0 | 62.4 | 24.4 | 8.6 | 2.6 | 1.0 | .0 | .0 |
| Ipswich 30–40 | .20 | 0 | (poor data) | | | | | | |
| 1441–50 | .66 | 0 | 65.8 | 13.2 | 10.5 | 10.5 | .0 | .0 | .0 |
| 1451–60 | .24 | 0 | 81.0 | 14.3 | 4.8 | .0 | .0 | .0 | .0 |
| 1461–70 | .48 | 0 | 70.8 | 15.4 | 10.8 | 1.5 | 1.5 | 1.5 | .0 |
| 1471–80 | .54 | 0 | 57.4 | 33.3 | 7.4 | 1.9 | .0 | .0 | .0 |
| St. Alb. 30–40 | .43 | 0 | 70.8 | 18.6 | 7.1 | 3.5 | .0 | .0 | .0 |
| 1441–50 | .55 | 0 | 64.8 | 25.0 | 6.0 | 4.0 | 1.0 | .2 | .0 |
| 1451–60 | .54 | 0 | 66.3 | 21.2 | 7.7 | 3.8 | 1.0 | .0 | .0 |
| 1461–70 | .74 | 0 | 56.4 | 23.6 | 12.7 | 5.5 | .9 | .9 | .0 |
| 1471–80 | .86 | 0 | 54.9 | 25.4 | 9.2 | 4.9 | 1.4 | 3.5 | .7 |
| B.S.E. 30–40 | .30 | 0 | 78.5 | 16.9 | 3.1 | 1.5 | .0 | .0 | .0 |
| 1441–50 | .46 | 0 | 67.1 | 22.1 | 8.6 | 2.1 | .0 | .0 | .0 |
| 1451–60 | .48 | 0 | 64.8 | 24.8 | 8.6 | 1.9 | .0 | .0 | .0 |
| 1461–70 | .33 | 0 | 77.0 | 14.8 | 5.9 | 2.2 | .0 | .0 | .0 |
| 1471–80 | .49 | 0 | 68.1 | 19.9 | 8.3 | 1.0 | 1.0 | .0 | .0 |
| Bungay 30–80 | .42 | 0 | 70.8 | 19.8 | 7.3 | 1.0 | 1.0 | .0 | .0 |
| Beccles 30–80 | .46 | 0 | 66.3 | 22.5 | 1.0 | 1.3 | .0 | .0 | .0 |
| Sudbury 30–80 | .68 | 0 | 55.9 | 26.5 | 11.8 | 5.9 | .1 | .0 | .0 |

*Table 7.1.5.* Male Child Replacement Ratios: Males to All Testators in Occupational and Special Groups

| | | | Distribution of Sons Per Testator - in % | | | | | | |
|---|---|---|---|---|---|---|---|---|---|
| | R.R. | Mode | 0 | 1 | 2 | 3 | 4 | 5 | 6+ |
| Rural Élite | | | | | | | | | |
| 1430–80 | 1.02 | 0 | 45.4 | 23.1 | 17.1 | 9.6 | 1.9 | 2.3 | .0 |
| 1430–40 | .89 | 0 | 54.3 | 19.6 | 13.0 | 10.9 | 2.2 | 2.2 | .0 |
| 1441–50 | 1.21 | 0 | 47.7 | 20.5 | 9.1 | 13.6 | 4.5 | 4.5 | .0 |
| 1451–50 | .92 | 0 | 51.1 | 19.1 | 19.1 | 8.5 | 2.1 | .0 | .0 |
| 1461–70 | 1.00 | 0 | 42.0 | 30.0 | 18.0 | 8.0 | 2.0 | .0 | .0 |
| 1471–80 | 1.23 | 0 | 32.8 | 27.9 | 4.9 | 3.3 | 1.6 | .0 | .0 |
| London Élite | | | | | | | | | |
| 1430–80 | .92 | 0 | 49.3 | 24.9 | 14.4 | 7.5 | 4.0 | .0 | .0 |
| 1430–40 | .75 | 0 | 56.3 | 21.9 | 15.6 | 3.1 | 3.1 | .0 | .0 |
| 1441–50 | .44 | 0 | 60.0 | 36.0 | 4.0 | .0 | .0 | .0 | .0 |
| 1451–60 | .95 | 0 | 51.3 | 23.1 | 7.7 | 15.4 | 2.6 | .0 | .0 |
| 1461–70 | 1.06 | 0 | 46.0 | 20.0 | 20.0 | 10.0 | 4.0 | .0 | .0 |
| 1471–80 | 1.12 | 0 | 40.5 | 26.2 | 21.4 | 4.8 | 7.1 | .0 | .0 |
| Select Urban Occ. 30–80 | .64 | 0 | 62.4 | 18.8 | 12.8 | 5.4 | .7 | .7 | .0 |
| Select Rural Occ. 30–80 | .54 | 0 | 65.8 | 19.0 | 11.4 | 2.5 | 1.3 | .0 | .0 |
| All Citizens 1430–80 | .85 | 0 | 50.7 | 27.2 | 13.0 | 5.7 | 2.6 | .4 | .2 |
| All Occ. 1430–80 | .79 | 0 | 54.7 | 24.4 | 12.6 | 5.6 | 1.9 | .7 | .2 |
| Female Test. 1430–80 | .63 | 0 | 59.6 | 24.4 | 10.9 | 3.9 | 1.0 | .2 | .1 |
| Testators w/servants 1430–80 | .80 | 0 | 55.5 | 19.8 | 17.0 | 6.3 | .8 | .3 | .3 |

testators registering their wills in lower courts, and therefore had longer periods of high fertility in which to give birth.[4]

The modal number of sons for all groups was always zero. Social mobility, if such a term may be used here, must have been very pronounced.[5] The number of families which failed to survive, in the male line for a mere three generations, would seem to approximate 75 percent of the will-making population; and in most of the replacement ratio measures taken, the proportions of testators who had no surviving sons was over 50 percent in the first generation—and this assumes a stationary population with no "wastage" of underage sons.[6] Families with one child of either sex, taken for the whole sample, constitute only half of the population, and families with both sons and daughters make up only about 19 percent of the population. It is probable that the modal figure of zero sons per family was predominant in most pre-industrial societies, but the low proportions described above may have been peculiar to fifteenth century England. Only in the late 1460's and 1470's did the dismal figures improve.

In East Anglia, the replacement ratios for sons were higher for Norfolk than for Suffolk. It is possible that this is a reflection of the predominance of consistory court wills in Norfolk, but the wealth and spouse data as presented in Chapter 6, however, shed considerable doubt on the "court" explanation for demographic discrepancies between counties and/or archdeaconries and there is no reason to believe that the situation for sons was any different. It is more probable that the numbers of recorded sons simply reflect local economic conditions and peculiarities, and, as discussed in Chapter 5, local epidemiological conditions. In all samples save the one which includes clerics, the Hertfordshire male replacement ratios are the lowest or next to lowest in the sample. This is in direct contrast to the high percentages of marriage among the Hertfordshire sample. There was a strong correlation between multiple sons and great per capita testator wealth, if not necessarily between single sons and wealth. This has been shown in Chapter 6, and can be seen by counties for the P.C.C. in Tables 7.1.1 through 7.1.3.

Urban male child replacement ratios were far lower than their rural counterparts. This was true for the wealthy London testators, but was most evident in the two provincial Suffolk towns, Bury St. Edmunds and Ipswich. The two Suffolk market towns, Beccles and Bungay, used for comparative purposes, showed equally dismal male replacement ratio figures, approximating the lows of Bury and Ipswich. Although little information as to the comparative average ages of initial urban and rural marriages can be gleaned from the wills for each county, it has been shown that urban marriage ratios and wealth levels were higher than those in the country, which makes the low male replacement ratios even more surprising. Of all the urban areas, only St. Albans had an approximately equal percentage of sons to that of the surrounding countryside. Except for the cities of London and St. Albans in the last two decades of the period, there were no major changes in these low replacement ratios through time—no swing upward, as there was to be for the rural areas, and in effect for the sample as a whole. Fifteenth century urban society appears to have been even more "fluid" than fifteenth century society as a whole. The urban areas acted as a demographic siphon on the neighboring rural areas. If they were to maintain their population levels, they must have relied heavily on massive immigration. Of the five urban areas discussed in the sample, London, Norwich, Ipswich, Bury St. Edmunds and St. Albans, it is probable that only London was as large in 1480 as it had been in 1430.[7] The decline was most pronounced in the Suffolk cases.

The failure of the urban populations to replace themselves is demonstrated by some of the occupational groups within the towns, as shown in Table 7.1.5. The London élite were among the wealthiest, oldest, most frequently married and remarried and earliest marrying of all the special occupational groups. They had the highest replacement ratios of any urban body, yet on average from 1430 to 1480 even they failed to reach a replacement level ratio of 1.00, something their rural counterparts, the gentry, esquires and knights did achieve. Only in the 1460's and 1470's did the London élite replacement ratios surpass unity, and even then over 40 percent of the wealthy merchants failed to produce a single male heir.

The other townsmen had lower male replacement ratios than did the wealthy and powerful London élite. A collection of testators claiming citizenship in their particular towns, presumably the wealthiest and most powerful inhabitants, could collectively produce a replacement ratio level of only 85 percent; more significantly, over 50 percent of them failed to leave a male heir. Urban craftsmen did far worse. They had a replacement ratio of 64 percent, over 62 percent mention no sons, and only 6.8 percent reported more than two sons. And all of these dismal figures are far higher than the replacement ratios for the mass of townsmen who did not list any occupation in their wills; and the townsmen were wealthier and had marriage ratios approximating those of their rural fellow Englishmen. The all important data on age of first-marriage for urban areas alone cannot be gleaned from the wills, but even with this crucial factor still a subject of speculation, it is obvious that geographic location and the local ecological conditions around a particular area were the most crucial factors in the comparative replacement ratios.

The countryside was the area of highest male replacement ratios. Not surprisingly, the group most successful in producing sons was the one which dominated the rural areas, the rural élite testators. Of all the bodies within the sample, urban or rural, prerogative court or consistory court, it was the gentry who most consistently replaced themselves and perhaps increased their numbers strictly by natural means, and not by immigration or new entrants into the class. As with the London élite, the rural élite were wealthier, married more frequently, and most important, married earlier than did members of other groups.[8] Yet in the fifteenth century there must surely have been a great flow of new candidates into the rural élite; only in the 1470's did less than 40 percent of the gentry die without male heirs. The key to their relative fertility was their larger number of multiple sons, as well as the fact that fewer of them died sonless.

As has been described in Chapter 1, there are distinct problems of underenumeration when using female replacement ratios, or male testator to female children replacement ratios, problems which did not have to be dealt with when using their all-male counterparts. Throughout the period 1430–1480, in all counties, and in most occupations without distinction between urban and rural, daughters were simply not included in the wills in what must have been their true proportions. There was a strong correlation between female progeny replacement ratios and testator wealth, one which was artificial rather than natural, the result of a quirk in the testamentary source which itself is a result of fifteenth century custom. There is no evidence nor any logical reason to postulate a shortage of up to 50 percent in the proportional relationship of males to females in fifteenth century England. Yet some sort of ratio concerning the numbers of female progeny within the sample can be useful in helping to determine both the individual peculiarities and characteristics of the society, and in plotting the long-term trends in population movements. The replacement ratios used show the proportions of the entire sample, and of male testators to their daughters, following the same three basic methods as described for the male ratios.

The data are shown in Tables 7.1.6 through 7.1.10. The most striking contrast between the male and female progeny ratios is the approximate parity among female replacement ratios between the urban and rural samples. This is in direct contrast with the male experience, as discussed above. While both the urban and rural ratios are grossly underenumerated, they are exactly the same—43 percent. This in turn is reflective of the general validity of the male replacement ratios.[9] We have seen that urban male replacement ratios were lower than rural male replacement ratios, and given the evidence of marriage and wealth, that these ratios were probably real, and not the result of an aberration in the source. Yet with female progeny, the urban-rural replacement ratios were equal. With female ratios as low as they were—generally below 50 percent—it is

*Table 7.1.6* Female Child Replacement Ratios:
Females to Entire Sample

|  | R.R. | Mode | % Test. No Daughters |
|---|---|---|---|
| All 1430–80 | .43 | 0 | 73.2 |
| N 1430–80 | .42 | 0 | 74.2 |
| S 1430–80 | .42 | 0 | 72.4 |
| H 1430–80 | .35 | 0 | 77.8 |
| P.C.C. 30–80 | .61 | 0 | 65.4 |
| All 1430–40 | .27 | 0 | 81.8 |
| N 1430–40 | .22 | 0 | 86.1 |
| S 1430–40 | .27 | 0 | 82.6 |
| H 1430–40 | .35 | 0 | 75.5 |
| P.C.C. 30–80 | .38 | 0 | 75.2 |
| All 1441–50 | .37 | 0 | 76.6 |
| N 1441–50 | .39 | 0 | 78.5 |
| S 1441–50 | .35 | 0 | 75.4 |
| H 1441–50 | .29 | 0 | 79.7 |
| P.C.C. 41–50 | .66 | 0 | 62.7 |
| All 1451–60 | .39 | 0 | 75.3 |
| N 1451–60 | .39 | 0 | 77.3 |
| S 1451–60 | .39 | 0 | 73.8 |
| H 1451–60 | .30 | 0 | 81.0 |
| P.C.C. 51–60 | .51 | 0 | 68.9 |
| All 1461–70 | .46 | 0 | 71.4 |
| N 1461-70 | .46 | 0 | 71.5 |
| S 1461–70 | .43 | 0 | 71.7 |
| H 1461–70 | .43 | 0 | 73.8 |
| P.C.C. 61–70 | .66 | 0 | 64.3 |
| All 1471–80 | .51 | 0 | 68.4 |
| N 1471–80 | .52 | 0 | 67.7 |
| S 1471–80 | .49 | 0 | 68.7 |
| H 1471–80 | .40 | 0 | 76.1 |
| P.C.C. 71–80 | .74 | 0 | 58.6 |

*Table 7.1.7.* Female Child Replacement Ratios: Females to
All Male Testators Excepting Clerics

|  | R.R. | Mode | % Test. No Daughters |
|---|---|---|---|
| All 1430–80 | .47 | 0 | 70.9 |
| N 1430–80 | .49 | 0 | 70.6 |
| S 1430–80 | .44 | 0 | 71.0 |
| H 1430–80 | .36 | 0 | 77.5 |
| P.C.C. 30–80 | .67 | 0 | 62.0 |
| All 1430–40 | .34 | 0 | 78.9 |
| N 1430–40 | .27 | 0 | 83.4 |
| S 1430–40 | .36 | 0 | 75.6 |
| H 1430–40 | .36 | 0 | 78.3 |
| P.C.C. 30–40 | .50 | 0 | 69.7 |
| All 1441–50 | .44 | 0 | 72.5 |
| N 1441–50 | .54 | 0 | 71.0 |
| S 1441–50 | .38 | 0 | 73.4 |
| H 1441–50 | .28 | 0 | 79.9 |
| P.C.C. 41–50 | .76 | 0 | 56.4 |
| All 1451–60 | .41 | 0 | 73.5 |
| N 1451–60 | .45 | 0 | 74.6 |
| S 1451–60 | .41 | 0 | 72.6 |
| H 1451–60 | .31 | 0 | 80.0 |
| P.C.C. 51–60 | .55 | 0 | 67.3 |
| All 1461–70 | .49 | 0 | 69.6 |
| N 1461–70 | .50 | 0 | 69.5 |
| S 1461–70 | .45 | 0 | 70.3 |
| H 1461–70 | .44 | 0 | 74.1 |
| P.C.C. 61–70 | .74 | 0 | 60.4 |
| All 1471–80 | .54 | 0 | 66.9 |
| N 1471–80 | .58 | 0 | 64.2 |
| S 1471–80 | .51 | 0 | 68.4 |
| H 1471–80 | .42 | 0 | 75.2 |
| P.C.C. 71–80 | .79 | 0 | 57.3 |

*Table 7.1.8.* Female Child Replacement Ratios: Females to
All Married Males

| | R.R. | Mode | % Test. No Daughters |
|---|---|---|---|
| All 1430–80 | .54 | 0 | 67.2 |
| N 1430–80 | .57 | 0 | 66.4 |
| S 1430–80 | .49 | 0 | 67.8 |
| H 1430–80 | .41 | 0 | 75.4 |
| P.C.C. 30–80 | .81 | 0 | 55.1 |
| All 1430–40 | .41 | 0 | 75.6 |
| N 1430–40 | .36 | 0 | 78.8 |
| S 1430–40 | .40 | 0 | 74.6 |
| H 1430–40 | .41 | 0 | 75.5 |
| P.C.C. 30–40 | .55 | 0 | 67.5 |
| All 1441–50 | .53 | 0 | 68.2 |
| N 1441–50 | .64 | 0 | 67.3 |
| S 1441–50 | .46 | 0 | 68.5 |
| H 1441–50 | .30 | 0 | 79.3 |
| P.C.C. 41–50 | 1.01 | 0 | 43.0 |
| All 1451–60 | .46 | 0 | 70.3 |
| N 1451–60 | .54 | 0 | 70.5 |
| S 1451–60 | .44 | 0 | 69.5 |
| H 1451–60 | .36 | 0 | 77.3 |
| P.C.C. 51–60 | .67 | 0 | 58.9 |
| All 1461–70 | .55 | 0 | 66.2 |
| N 1461–70 | .56 | 0 | 66.0 |
| S 1461–70 | .51 | 0 | 66.7 |
| H 1461–70 | .47 | 0 | 72.8 |
| P.C.C. 61–70 | .83 | 0 | 55.5 |
| All 1471–80 | .60 | 0 | 63.2 |
| N 1471–80 | .64 | 0 | 60.4 |
| S 1471–80 | .55 | 0 | 65.4 |
| H 1471–80 | .48 | 0 | 72.6 |
| P.C.C. 71–80 | .95 | 0 | 50.5 |

*Table 7.1.9.* Female Child Replacement Ratios: Females to
All Urban Testators

|  | R.R. | Mode | % Test. No Daughters |
|---|---|---|---|
| All 1430–80 | .43 | 0 | 73.1 |
| London 30–80 | .60 | 0 | 64.6 |
| Norwich 30–80 | .39 | 0 | 75.9 |
| Ipswich 30–80 | .33 | 0 | 77.3 |
| St. Albans 30–80 | .39 | 0 | 76.0 |
| Bury St. Edmunds 30–80 | .36 | 0 | 76.8 |
| London 1430–40 | .39 | 0 | 74.6 |
| 1441–50 | .64 | 0 | 62.8 |
| 1451–60 | .44 | 0 | 69.7 |
| 1461–70 | .66 | 0 | 63.8 |
| 1471–80 | .75 | 0 | 56.6 |
| Norwich 1430–40 | .24 | 0 | 81.2 |
| 1441–50 | .42 | 0 | 79.4 |
| 1451–60 | .38 | 0 | 72.5 |
| 1461–70 | .43 | 0 | 61.0 |
| 1471–80 | .40 | 0 | 74.1 |
| Ipswich 1430–40 | (poor data) |  |  |
| 1441–50 | (poor data) |  |  |
| 1451–60 | .25 | 0 | 81.0 |
| 1461–70 | .46 | 0 | 73.8 |
| 1471–80 | .32 | 0 | 77.8 |
| St. Albans 1430–40 | .33 | 0 | 82.3 |
| 1441–50 | .36 | 0 | 74.0 |
| 1451–60 | .26 | 0 | 79.8 |
| 1461–70 | .38 | 0 | 78.2 |
| 1471–80 | .52 | 0 | 67.6 |
| Bury St. Edmunds 30–40 | .31 | 0 | 76.9 |
| 1441–50 | .34 | 0 | 80.0 |
| 1451–60 | .32 | 0 | 80.0 |
| 1461–70 | .33 | 0 | 75.6 |
| 1471–80 | .43 | 0 | 74.1 |
| Bungay | .19 | 0 | 85.4 |
| Beccles | .33 | 0 | 77.5 |
| Sudbury | .39 | 0 | 67.6 |

*Table 7.1.10.* Female Child Replacement Ratios: Females to All Testators
in Occupational and Special Groups

|  | R.R. | Mode | % Test. No Daughters |
|---|---|---|---|
| Rural Élite |  |  |  |
| 1430– | .64 | 0 | 65.4 |
| 1430–40 | .40 | 0 | 71.7 |
| 1441–50 | .71 | 0 | 65.9 |
| 1451–60 | .53 | 0 | 68.1 |
| 1461–70 | .60 | 0 | 66.0 |
| 1471–80 | .90 | 0 | 54.1 |
| London Élite |  |  |  |
| 1430– | .86 | 0 | 55.2 |
| 1430–40 | .66 | 0 | 65.6 |
| 1441–50 | .96 | 0 | 52.0 |
| 1451–60 | .56 | 0 | 64.1 |
| 1461–70 | .96 | 0 | 56.0 |
| 1471–80 | 1.12 | 0 | 40.2 |
| Select Urban |  |  |  |
| Occ. 1430–80 | .30 | 0 | 82.6 |
| Select Rural |  |  |  |
| Occ. 1430–80 | .38 | 0 | 74.7 |
| All Citizens |  |  |  |
| 1430–80 | .73 | 0 | 57.8 |
| All Occ. 1430–80 | .59 | 0 | 65.9 |
| Female Testators |  |  |  |
| 1430–80 | .45 | 0 | 70.0 |
| Testators |  |  |  |
| w/servant |  |  |  |
| 1430–80 | .62 | 0 | 65.9 |

inconceivable that in underpopulated fifteenth century England they could drop much lower, even if the bulk of daughters had been provided for or dowered off in advance of the composition of the will.[10] Thirty to forty percent inclusion in wills is probably the minimal figure for daughters, whatever their true proportions in society, and this 30–40 percent was met in the towns as well as in the country. There are no biological reasons to believe that there were more daughters living in the towns than there were sons, at least not in the large proportions reflected in the data. In the towns, where conditions for a growing child of either sex must have been harsh, testators seem to have listed children of both sexes to their maximum "fifteenth century" degree; in the case of daughters, this may have been regulated by local peculiarities, but with sons, it appears to have been the full total alive at the time the wills were made. As we shall see in section 7.2, the numbers of daughters listed in the wills rises dramatically in times of crisis, when the quest for an heir of either sex who would survive the crisis was at its greatest. The case of the London élite in the 1440's is the classic example of this.[11] Since the numbers of daughters were underenumerated, there was much room to increase their proportions in the wills. But the numbers of sons in the wills did not rise at all in crisis periods; to the contrary, they usually declined, another barometer of the extent of mortality which gripped all members of the community. In fact, it is likely that the numbers of sons could not rise, because they were already at their maximum "will" levels.

There are exceptions to the general practice of underenumerating female progeny in the wills. One obvious instance which applies to all testators, regardless of wealth, occupation or social standing, was a family lacking a male heir; daughters were listed with far higher frequency and greater diligence when they had no brothers, a natural circumstance since daughters had customary rights to movables, as well as to land. Most of the other exceptional groups were wealthy ones. The London élite listed daughters more frequently than any other testator subgroup, and, in reality, probably had more daughters than did most of the other subgroups. In the 1470's, the numbers of daughters listed by them actually equalled the numbers of sons, the only instance where such a situation prevailed. It is likely that these London élite figures were accurate for all progeny, and in section 7.3, attempts will be made to assess conjugal family size from them.

The rural élite testators also had a far higher proportion of daughters in their wills than did the sample as a whole. They too must have had more daughters than did humbler folk. Yet unlike the London élite, it is not likely that the armigerous female progeny ever reflected their actual numbers, even in the 1470's. In direct contrast with the replacement ratios of their brothers, the female progeny figures never even reached unity. Although they were as wealthy or wealthier than the London merchants, the rural élite seem to have been a bit surer about the survival of their male heirs, and a bit more conservative in their ideas on inclusion of daughters in wills.

Citizens and all testators who mentioned occupations, regardless of location, listed more daughters than did testators of unspecified occupation. The former were also wealthier. It is not possible to say, as has been done for the London élite and the gentry, if these higher female replacement ratios represent a real increase in the numbers of daughters, or whether they represent mechanical increases brought on by middling wealth, conservation or custom. Perhaps townsmen were less conservative than peasants, and less inclined to follow older practices in regard to the inclusion of daughters in their testaments. But probably, with children of both sexes less likely to reach maturity in urban areas, the tendency was greater there to include all progeny of both sexes in the wills to increase the likelihood of naming at least one heir who would survive.

In all probate districts, P.C.C. testators had the highest numbers of daughters per family, and the replacement ratios of daughters closest to those of the sons. Even in the P.C.C., however, the total numbers of female progeny listed in the wills may never have reached completion. Of the counties, Norfolk consistently showed the highest ratios of daughters, just as it had the highest ratios of sons. Hertfordshire had the lowest numbers of daughters per testator, with Suffolk falling inbetween. In general, the counties stood in the same relationships to each other for female replacement ratios as they did for male replacement ratios. For all the major divisions in the sample the numbers of families without daughters was very high  rarely dipping under 70 percent. Only in the P.C.C. did the number of families listing daughters consistently rise above even 40 percent.

Wealth in general, and the quest for an heir of either sex in the towns were the key factors in the inclusion of daughters in fifteenth century wills. Perhaps wealth meant that a testator could marry earlier and provide more ably for his or her progeny; certainly, this was the case with the very wealthy, the London élite and the rural élite. In regard to male progeny, there is little correlation between wealth and sons in all but the cases of the very richest. But in the case of daughters, wealth at almost all levels meant more of the testamentary cake to distribute, and probably more daughters in the wills.

## 7.2 Movements of Population through Time

The most pronounced aspect of population movement in the period 1430–1480 was the concerted rise in both male and female replacement ratios in the late 1460's and throughout the 1470's, in all counties and special groups measured in the sample. Only the provincial urban centers failed to show increased replacement ratios, and even here there was an exception.[12] Part of the increase in the numbers of female progeny was mechanical—that is, a peculiarity in the nature of wills. But in light of the previous evidence given—the fact that the ratios of marriage remained approximately uniform and the average wealth per testator, which was somewhat linked to numbers of multiple sons per family, actually declined in the 1460's and 1470's—it seems likely that the rise in numbers of male progeny per testator was a real one. After a period of 150 or perhaps 200 years of first stagnation and then decline, replacement ratios and possibly overall population began a steady climb upward toward the end of our period.[13]

One of the most fascinating aspects of the replacement ratio increase was its encompassing nature. The upsurge began to appear for most areas sometime in the 1460's, and in the 1470's in Suffolk, where the population levels remained stable from 1440 to 1470.[14] The sheer numbers involved in the increase in male replacement ratios for the P.C.C. and Norfolk testators portend a forthcoming population upturn reflected not only in more surviving single-son families, but in more families with several sons. Even in the demographically troubled urban areas, there was an increase in male replacement ratios in two of the five centers, St. Albans and London. Only the East Anglian towns, Norwich, Ipswich and Bury St. Edmunds, showed something approaching continual demographic decline throughout the entire fifty-year period. The generalization established earlier of a continual drain on the rural populations of Norfolk and Suffolk holds true even in the decades of demographic upsurge. As the populations of both counties, with the possible exception of the delineated crisis-mortality regions, began to show signs of increases in the 1470's, the nonimmigrant populations of the towns continued to falter.

There were two principal factors in the rise of male replacement ratios in the 1470's. First, there was a rise in the number of testators listing multiple sons. It is possible that this was the result not of a natural rise in the numbers of sons born per family, but simply of a mechanical rise in the numbers of sons reported in the wills. It is hoped that the arguments presented in Chapter 6 concerning the relationship between wealth and multiple sons has effectively dispelled this doubt. In any case, the second and more significant factor in the population increase, and almost certain evidence that the increase in sons was natural and not mechanical, was the fall in numbers of testators having no sons. In all male replacement ratio measures, as shown in Tables 7.1.1 through 7.1.5, a sharp fall can be seen in those families which failed to produce a single male heir. This fall was general, if not always continual, from about 1440, but did not become pronounced until the 1470's. Although the modal figure for sons per testator remained zero in all measurements, the aggregate number of families failing to produce a male heir fell to under 50 percent for the first time in the last decade of the period. In the P.C.C., the number of families without male heirs fell below 40 percent.

The difference by county is significant. Hertfordshire, the poorest of the three counties, but the one with the highest marriage ratios, reflected the lowest male replacement ratios. Suffolk showed relatively low replacement ratios, even during the increases of the 1470's. Norfolk, on the other hand, exhibited higher replacement ratios throughout most of the fifty-year period, reflecting figures close to unity on average, and over unity in the last decade. As the individual testators from Norfolk do not appear to have married earlier, or been richer than those from Suffolk, the discrepancy in replacement ratios becomes something of a puzzle. To see if the answer to the problem lay in the predominance of consistory court wills in Norfolk and archdeaconry court wills in Suffolk, wills from the N.C.C. only were analyzed for testators from both counties. The results show that the replacement ratios from just the N.C.C. reflected the same proportions for both counties as had the replacement ratios from both counties using all the courts. The answer to Norfolk's high replacement ratios did not lie in the predominance of consistory court wills.[15] Rather, the low Suffolk figures were the result of the chronic and consistently low survival ratios of children in the two Suffolk towns, Bury St. Edmunds and Ipswich, and the large number of high crisis-mortality regions in the county. Thus, the statement made in Chapter 4 in regard to the decline of population in Suffolk in the 1470's can probably be limited to particular areas. Conversely, an answer to the high Norfolk replacement ratios may be the lack of crisis-mortality regions. It cannot be said with complete certainty that the endemic regions delineated for Norfolk would stand finally and unaltered as they do now if the wills from the Norwich archdeaconry court were available. Also, two Norfolk towns, King's Lynn and Great Yarmouth, which may have acted as "demographic siphons," could not be included in the sample. But continual endemic disease does appear to have been less frequent and less common in Norfolk than in Suffolk, and this may have been the major factor in the differing levels of replacement ratios in two neighboring counties with similar levels of testator wealth and frequency of marriage.

While the replacement ratios for the 1470's are on the whole higher than at any time in the fifty-year period studied, they are not large enough to give firm evidence that population was growing at significant levels, or even growing at all. If one allowed for 10 percent underenumeration in the wills, the ratios in most of the samples were not much greater than unity, and only in the P.C.C. and among the rural élite do we have figures which hint of consistent and continual demographic growth from the 1450's onward. By all accounts and for almost all calculations in the sample, the 1430's and 1440's were decades of population decline, as had been the decades before them for four or five generations. For the region covered in the sample as a whole, population continued in its decline for the first twenty and perhaps thirty years of the period under study; and it may be that in the 1440's, 1450's, and even the 1460's the decline was slowing down, but not stopping. At best, much of the 1460's were a time of stagnation, and not demographic growth. It is only in the 1470's that we have the first indications via the vector of male replacement ratios, of demographic development; and even in this decade, they are hardly overwhelming. At worst, the 1470's themselves may reflect little more than stagnation, and it is feasible that the long decline in population, probably extending back into the late thirteenth or early fourteenth century, was halted in East Anglia only in this decade.

The data for the special groups within the sample reflected some long-term trends. The rural élite testators were most successful in producing sons, and this success is increasingly evident through time. Only in the 1430's and 1450's were their replacement ratios below unity. Significantly, the low figure for the 1450's came after a remarkably fecund period in the 1440's. The knights and squires showed signs of considerable increases in their numbers in the 1440's and 1470's, and in the 1470's the number of rural élite families failing to leave behind a male heir at the time the will was made had fallen below one-third. It is possible that the children of the 1440's had become the testators of the 1470's.[16]

The replacement ratios of the London élite showed stagnation when viewed in mass, with about half of the wealthy merchants failing to produce a male heir who survived beyond his early years. A closer examination shows that this situation of seeming stagnation can be divided into distinct periods. The 1430's and especially the 1440's proved particularly dismal for the London élite, with a male replacement ratio of less than 50 percent in the latter decade. Significantly, the numbers of female progeny per London élite testator in the 1440's rose almost to unity. A logical medical explanation for this curious phenomena cannot be offered; it was a decade of extensive epidemic disease in the city of London, and perhaps the epidemics proved most lethal to male children. From 1450 onward, and the 1470's in particular, there was a sharp increase in the male replacement ratios of this group, and the London élite, as well as the rural élite, probably increased their numbers by means of birth alone in the last decade of the period 1430–1480.

None of the other urban or occupational subgroups surveyed—not widows, nor urban or rural craftsmen, nor families with servants, nor even the testators claiming citizenship in one of the urban centers— exhibited male replacement ratios approaching one male child per one male testator. The bulk of the male child increase came in the rural areas, especially in Norfolk. We are confronted once again with the realization that the urban centers covered in the study with the possible exception of London must have declined in population during the middle decades of the fifteenth century, and only continual immigration could have confined the proportion of decline within moderate, gradual levels.[17] London alone must have been able to offer the necessary incentive and economic opportunity in an era of relatively easily obtained land to have continued to attract enough immigrants to maintain its population. With a few exceptions, such as Bristol and Exeter, the paradigm of declining urban population formulated for eastern England held true for all provincial urban centers in fifteenth century England.[18]

Like their male counterparts, female progeny replacement ratios showed an upward secular trend for the period 1430–1480. Because of the chronic underenumeration of female progeny, the rise in the female child ratios was even more pronounced than those for males. For reasons similar to those given for their male counterparts—the steady ratios of marriage per testator, and the decline in wealth levels, with wealth being very closely related to female replacement ratios—it is apparent that the bulk of the replacement ratio increase was real and not due to an aberration in the source. Yet simply because the female replacement ratios, especially in the earlier decades of the fifty-year period, were so low, it is obvious that a certain part of the increase was due to mechanical causes, that is, the greater inclusion of females within the context of the last testament. And once again, assuming that there were no unknown biological reasons for male children to exist in 25 to 50 percent greater frequency in the fifteenth century than female children, it is evident that even in the 1470's, female progeny continued to be at least partially underenumerated.

It is in the P.C.C. that the few seemingly complete recordings of female sibling progeny can be found. In the 1440's, the 1470's, and to a lesser extent the 1460's, the P.C.C. testators probably listed something approaching the totality of their female children. The 1440's figures—over unity for one measure—remain a bit of a puzzle, even though the meteoric rise in the female child replacement ratio must be directly related to the correspondingly mysterious drop in the male child replacement ratios for the P.C.C. Female children came into their own in the wills of the London élite during the 1470's, when they equalled the ratios for males, and in the 1460's when their numbers were almost as high as their male counterparts. A similar situation existed for the rural élite daughters during the latter years of the period 1430–1480.

Despite very significant increases through time, even in the 1470's, testators from none of the three counties surveyed showed listings of daughters as accurate as those shown by the P.C.C. testators. Increases in the period were most pronounced among testators from Norfolk, as were those in the male replacement ratios. This is further evidence that it was in Norfolk, especially rural Norfolk, that replacement ratios expanded most significantly in the last two decades of the period under study. But the Suffolk figures also showed a steady rise in the numbers of daughters listed; and even Hertfordshire, with the lowest female child replacement ratios of the three counties, had an upward secular trend.

It can thus be stated with some confidence that if the population of eastern England had not begun to rise, it had at least stopped declining in the last years of the period 1430–1480. Further testamentary evidence shows a sharp upward rise in male and female replacement ratio levels in the 1480's, a rise which was far greater than that of the 1470's.[19] But with the trend of fifteenth century population deciphered, at least in part, a fundamental question still remains: what was the major factor behind the population increase—a rise in fertility or a decrease in mortality? Many historical demographers have argued that a decline in mortality was almost always the cause of an increase in pre-industrial population.[20] And when and if a satisfactory explanation for the causes of the replacement ratio increase of the 1470's can be offered, the reason why population was so slow in rising throughout the bulk of the fifteenth century must be given. As has been the practice throughout the thesis, definitive answers cannot and will not be advanced on the basis of the testamentary evidence alone. Such things as the age of marriage through time, a crucial factor in the control of birth, are at present beyond the scope of the will data alone. Until, if ever, such questions can be answered, only informed guesses can be offered.

We have seen that there was no overall rise in percentages of marriage, at least from 1440 to 1480, although the ratios of remarriage did rise in the latter decades in certain segments of the population. It is not likely then that the higher male and female replacement ratios of the 1470's were the result of greater frequency of marriage. As has been repeatedly stressed, the crucial factor of age of marriage by decade cannot be examined. But as was demonstrated in Chapters 4 and 5, the frequency of epidemic disease and the figures of raw mortality were at least as high in the 1460's and 1470's as they had been at any previous time in the five decades. Thus a decrease in overall crude, adult mortality was also probably not responsible for the increase. We are left with three major possible causes: a rise in individual fertility, induced perhaps by an earlier age of marriage; a decrease in infant mortality; and/or a change in the nature and aetiological character of epidemic disease in the 1460's and 1470's. The possibilities of an increase in fertility have been discussed throughout this chapter. Given the evidence of fewer families with no children and more families with multiple children, it seems likely that an increase in individual testator fecundity was at least in part an effective agent in the population increase.

The very nature of the will evidence—including the fact that it measures adult, and essentially adult male mortality, and the fact that the replacement ratio increases which have been referred to were increases in numbers of children (although many of these children were adult when their parents drew up their last wills)—makes it necessary to examine the possibility of a change in the aetiological character of the diseases of the 1460's and especially the 1470's. Perhaps the diseases most prevalent in the early decades of the fifteenth century were especially lethal to children, and this situation changed during the course of the century. An aetiological change in the nature of infectious disease could have caused a decrease in infant mortality, a result which would have sent the replacement ratios rising as they did.[21] Unfortunately, there is no way wills or any other sources can measure this crucial factor on a large scale for fifteenth century England. Thus, as was the case with an earlier age of marriage, the possibility of a decrease in infant mortality as a major cause in the population upsurge of the late 1460's and 1470's must remain a major imponderable. But the mutability of infectious diseases over time has been a major theme of this thesis, and, as we have seen, after two decades of relative epidemiological calm, infectious disease flared up again in the mid-1460's and 1470's. Further, the names of the diseases, pockeys, styche, flyx, and—a bit after our period—sweat, were decidedly different from the pestilences of the earlier decades, though pestilences too remained in the 1460's and 1470's. It is possible that replacement ratio increases of the 1460's and 1470's were the result of changes in both mortality and fertility.

In an attempt to answer these questions, the responses of population will be examined in detail during and immediately after certain select quarters of protracted mortality caused by epidemic disease. Ratios of marriage and remarriage, and male and female progeny replacement ratios will be examined in this section for the autumn quarters of the epidemic years of 1439, 1452 and 1465,[22] as well as the fall quarters of 1441 and 1455. As can be seen from the graphs accompanying Chapter 4, the latter two quarters were periods of "average" autumnal mortality; and are included in the survey for comparative purposes. Because of the significance of crisis mortality in the 1470's, the entire decade by quarter will be examined in detail for spouse, and male and female replacement ratios in section 7.3.

The demographic data for the autumn quarters of 1439, 1441, 1452, 1455 and 1465 are presented in Tables 7.2.1 to 7.2.3. Samples were taken for all testators, male testators less clerics, and married male testators, for male and female children. For spouses, samples for all testators and male testators less clerics have been taken. As has been shown, mortality for the autumns of 1439, 1452 and 1465 were very high—up to five times higher than the previous quarters' records. By definition of selection, mortality for the autumn quarters of 1441 and 1455 was average for the fall.

During and immediately after the last severe epidemic of the terrible 1430's, marriage and remarriage levels were significantly higher than the decennial and five-year averages before the epidemic quarter had been.

*Table 7.2.1.* Special Quarterly Ratios: Spouse*

| | Marriage Per Test. | Mode | % Test. Not Married | Remarriage |
|---|---|---|---|---|
| Spouse to Entire Sample | | | | |
| 1439 | .69 | 1.0 | 36.9 | 4.8 |
| 1441 | .48 | .0 | 52.2 | .0 |
| 1452 | .66 | 1.0 | 36.3 | 2.0 |
| 1455 | .87 | 1.0 | 13.5 | .0 |
| 1465 | .66 | 1.0 | 34.8 | 1.0 |
| Spouse to All Males Less Clerics | | | | |
| 1439 | .77 | 1.0 | 64.3 | 5.7 |
| 1441 | .60 | 1.0 | 40.0 | .0 |
| 1452 | .75 | 1.0 | 27.2 | 2.5 |
| 1455 | .91 | 1.0 | 9.4 | .0 |
| 1465 | .69 | 1.0 | 31.9 | .6 |

*All years are autumn quarters in Tables 7.2.1, 7.2.2 and 7.2.3.

*Table 7.2.2.* Special Quarterly Ratios: Male Children

| | R.R. | Mode | Distribution of Sons per Testator - in % | | | | | | |
| | | | 0 | 1 | 2 | 3 | 4 | 5 | 6+ |
|---|---|---|---|---|---|---|---|---|---|
| **Males to Entire Sample** | | | | | | | | | |
| 1439 | .50 | 0 | 65.5 | 22.6 | 9.5 | 1.2 | 1.2 | .0 | .0 |
| 1441 | .52 | 0 | 69.6 | 15.2 | 8.7 | 1.5 | .0 | .0 | .0 |
| 1452 | .61 | 0 | 60.8 | 26.5 | 6.9 | 4.9 | .0 | .0 | .0 |
| 1455 | .68 | 0 | 56.8 | 21.6 | 18.9 | 2.7 | .0 | .0 | .0 |
| 1465 | .61 | 0 | 66.2 | 16.9 | 11.4 | 3.5 | 1.0 | .5 | .5 |
| **Males to All Males Except Clerics** | | | | | | | | | |
| 1439 | .59 | 0 | 60.0 | 25.7 | 11.4 | 1.4 | 1.4 | .0 | .0 |
| 1441 | .70 | 0 | 56.7 | 23.3 | 13.3 | 6.7 | .0 | .0 | .0 |
| 1452 | .73 | 0 | 54.3 | 29.6 | 8.6 | 6.2 | 1.2 | .0 | .0 |
| 1455 | .69 | 0 | 59.4 | 15.6 | 21.9 | 3.1 | .0 | .0 | .0 |
| 1465 | .61 | 0 | 68.1 | 15.3 | 10.4 | 3.7 | 1.2 | .6 | .6 |
| **Males to Married Male Testators** | | | | | | | | | |
| 1439 | .64 | 0 | 56.0 | 30.0 | 10.0 | 2.0 | 2.0 | .0 | .0 |
| 1441 | .78 | 0 | 55.6 | 22.2 | 11.1 | 11.1 | .0 | .0 | .0 |
| 1452 | .85 | 0 | 43.3 | 36.7 | 11.7 | 8.3 | .0 | .0 | .0 |
| 1455 | .76 | 0 | 55.2 | 17.2 | 24.1 | 3.4 | .0 | .0 | .0 |
| 1465 | .80 | 0 | 59.5 | 18.9 | 12.6 | 5.4 | 1.8 | .9 | .9 |

*Table 7.2.3.* Special Quarterly Ratios: Female Children

| | R.R. | Mode | % Test. No Daughters |
|---|---|---|---|
| **Females to Entire Sample** | | | |
| 1439 | .35 | 0 | 79.8 |
| 1441 | .22 | 0 | 84.8 |
| 1452 | .40 | 0 | 69.6 |
| 1455 | .30 | 0 | 78.4 |
| 1465 | .44 | 0 | 75.1 |
| **Females to All Males except Clerics** | | | |
| 1439 | .40 | 0 | 77.1 |
| 1441 | .30 | 0 | 80.0 |
| 1452 | .46 | 0 | 65.4 |
| 1455 | .31 | 0 | 78.1 |
| 1465 | .46 | 0 | 74.2 |
| **Females to Married Male Testators** | | | |
| 1439 | .46 | 0 | 78.0 |
| 1441 | .50 | 0 | 66.7 |
| 1432 | .55 | 0 | 56.7 |
| 1455 | .34 | 0 | 75.9 |
| 1465 | .57 | 0 | 69.4 |

Only two years later, in 1441, as perhaps should be expected, the marriage and remarriage ratios had dropped significantly. In the ratio for the entire sample, marriage per testator actually fell below 50 percent. As the marriage ratios as defined in section 6.3 include recently deceased spouses, the remarriage ratios are the most accurate barometer of the immediate nuptial response to severe demographic dislocation. In a sample of well over 100 testators, there was no remarriage at all reported in the autumn of 1441![23] Barring death, marriage in the fifteenth century was essentially a one-time affair, and it is not surprising that after a period of protracted mortality and higher than usual marriage and remarriage ratios, nuptial ratios would drop significantly—at least until the next period of concerted mortality.

The next period of concerted mortality came in the early 1450's. Mortality was high throughout the early 1450's, and was as sharp and well defined, if not always as severe, as it had been in the pestilential quarters of the 1430's. Two years after the quarter of peak mortality, in 1452, mortality was still a bit higher than normal in certain areas, and it was decided to use the fall quarter of 1455 rather than that of 1454. For autumn, 1452, in the midst of a period of extended mortality, marriage ratios were about the same as they had been and would be on average for the decade as a whole. But three years later, in autumn, 1455, they were high; and all of the increase by 1455, as in 1441, was first-marriage and not remarriage. The 1455 figures were among the highest for any quarter for the entire fifty-year period, with 87 percent of total population, including clerics, and 91 percent of the male population less clerics claiming to be married. For the rest of the decade, the figures were far lower. Thus, while it took longer for a response, marriage ratios rose significantly after the epidemic of 1452, as they had immediately after the epidemics of the late 1430's. The situation in the autumn, 1465, was almost identical to that of 1452. They began to decline from the epidemic of pox in the spring quarter, 1462, and were still below the decennial norm by the 1460's highest overall quarter of mortality, autumn, 1465. By 1466, they were rising again, only to decline from 1467, with the beginning of another series of epidemics.[24]

Marriage, the characteristic social precondition for childbirth in fifteenth century society, was quite responsive to epidemic disease. During the most protracted periods of epidemic, it fell as mortality increased. But almost immediately upon the return of normality, the ratios rose, until they had first surpassed and then settled back to their pre-epidemic levels. Thus the most important medium of childbirth was in the long term relatively unaffected by epidemic disease from 1440 to 1465. From looking at marriage and remarriage ratios for select crisis- and noncrisismortality quarters before 1470, we can get little insight into why replacement ratios increased as they generally did in the last decade of the period 1430 to 1480.

Child replacement ratios also proved to be responsive to quarters of crisis mortality. Male replacement ratios were below decennial averages for both 1439 and 1441, and female replacement ratios were up for 1439, typical signs of crisis mortality as seen from the testamentary evidence. Although the data for autumn, 1452, are inconclusive, male replacement ratios were below decennial levels in autumn, 1465, and about equal to the ten-year average for the fall, 1435, a normal quarter. But it cannot be said that the replacement ratios for children were dramatically lower during quarters of high mortality before 1470 than they were during normal quarters. From the selective quarterly testamentary evidence, it does not appear that infectious disease until 1470 was more lethal among children than it was among adults. Both parent and progeny seem—and no stronger word can be used on the basis of the testamentary data alone—to have been afflicted by epidemic disease in equal proportions. Despite the rapid and resilient response by the population after a crisis-mortality quarter, infectious diseases occurred and recurred frequently enough to curtail population growth. Yet in the 1470's, when epidemic disease was as frequent and virulent as it had been at any other time in the fifty-year period, 1430–1480, child replacement ratios are generally well above their previous forty-year levels. In many areas in East Anglia, population was growing. We must turn to a seasonal analysis of the 1470's to see why population responded as it did.

## 7.3 The 1470's: A Decade of Contradictions

It has been stated that population began to rise, or at least stopped declining, in the 1470's. We have seen that both male and female replacement ratios in the 1470's were on the whole above their levels for the previous forty years. At the same time, it has been shown that the decade was one of several severe epidemics. There were national epidemics in 1471, 1473 and 1479–1480, lesser epidemics in 1475 and 1476–1477, and perhaps in 1474 and 1478.[25] Crude mortality was extremely pronounced, as high or higher than it had been at any time in the period, 1430–1470. The demographic evidence from quarters of excessive mortality before 1470 indicate that children do not appear to have been any more susceptible to infectious diseases than were their parents. Can the new demographic equation of the 1470's be balanced by factors of fertility alone?

In an attempt to answer this, the major factors of fertility which can be gleaned from the wills—marriage and male and female child replacement ratios—were analyzed by quarter for the entire decade. The data are presented in Tables 7.3.1 to 7.3.3, and are for the relationships of the entire sample, women and clerics included, to spouse, males, and females. The emphasis of the analysis will be on the immediate response of population to severe, short-term dislocation. Decennial mortality has already been covered in Chapter 4. Briefly, it was extremely pronounced in the autumn of 1471, the autumn of 1473, the winter and spring of 1476– 1477, and the autumn and winter of 1479 and 1479–1480, or about every other year, a death pattern unique in the fifty-year period. All but the 1475 epidemic resulted in sample-wide mortality; the flux of 1473 did not affect Hertfordshire, judging from the testamentary evidence. Average mortality subsequent to that of the periods of extreme dislocation, such as the spring quarters (and it was spring mortality which was generally most severe in nonepidemic years) following an autumn epidemic, was usually quite low. Mortality in the 1470's was very high, higher by far than in any other decade, even the 1430's.[26]

As expected, remarriage ratios reacted to crisis mortality by rising soon after the peak death periods; however, they rose only after two of the four periods of extremely high death tolls. Although adult mortality was very heavy during the pestilence of 1471, the marriage ratios themselves were virtually unaffected, remaining stable at around 70 percent of the total will-making population, including clerics, from late 1470 through 1473. The levels of the second half of the 1460's were maintained during the first three years of the 1470's. By definition, the marriage ratios employed in this study measure dead spouses as well as live ones, and therefore a significant change in the marriage ratio *per se* cannot be expected. A change in the remarriage ratio and in the percentage of widows and widowers can be expected, however, and while the latter does increase after autumn, 1471, the remarriage ratio does not perceptibly alter until the winter and spring, 1473, and autumn, 1473. In fact, for the summer and autumn quarters of 1472, just when a large remarriage ratio might be expected, two samples of over 100 testators showed absolutely no record of remarriage.

After the next epidemic, that of 1473, however, the marriage and remarriage ratios did rise substantially. The numbers of widows and widowers also rose. Marriage ratios fell during the summer, autumn and winter quarters of 1473–1474, close to their lowest levels of the sample; and remarriage during the fall, the quarter of most severe epidemic virulence, fell to .4 of 1 percent of the will-making sample. From the spring, 1474, the marriage and remarriage ratios continued their general increase until the autumn, 1477—well after the peak death tolls during

*Table 7.3.1.* Quarterly Data, 1470–1480: Spouse Ratios to Entire Sample

|  |  | Marriage Per Test. | Mode | % Test. Not Married | Remarriage |
|---|---|---|---|---|---|
| 1470 | 1 | .66 | 1.0 | 38.6 | .8 |
|  | 2 | .64 | 1.0 | 36.5 | .9 |
|  | 3 | .82 | 1.0 | 22.2 | 4.2 |
|  | 4 | .72 | 1.0 | 32.2 | 4.3 |
| 1471 | 1 | .70 | 1.0 | 31.0 | 1.1 |
|  | 2 | .71 | 1.0 | 32.6 | 2.9 |
|  | 3 | .70 | 1.0 | 30.6 | 1.0 |
|  | 4 | .74 | 1.0 | 27.0 | 1.0 |
| 1472 | 1 | .70 | 1.0 | 30.8 | .7 |
|  | 2 | .73 | 1.0 | 28.8 | 1.4 |
|  | 3 | .79 | 1.0 | 21.0 | .0 |
|  | 4 | .72 | 1.0 | 27.8 | .0 |
| 1473 | 1 | .69 | 1.0 | 33.3 | 2.7 |
|  | 2 | .71 | 1.0 | 33.6 | 4.1 |
|  | 3 | .63 | 1.0 | 39.1 | 1.8 |
|  | 4 | .68 | 1.0 | 32.7 | .4 |
| 1474 | 1 | .67 | 1.0 | 35.4 | 2.1 |
|  | 2 | .75 | 1.0 | 26.9 | 2.0 |
|  | 3 | .77 | 1.0 | 27.0 | 2.4 |
|  | 4 | .81 | 1.0 | 20.3 | 5.7 |
| 1475 | 1 | .84 | 1.0 | 20.8 | 5.2 |
|  | 2 | .75 | 1.0 | 28.4 | 3.7 |
|  | 3 | .72 | 1.0 | 30.6 | 2.8 |
|  | 4 | .79 | 1.0 | 31.7 | 5.0 |
| 1476 | 1 | .76 | 1.0 | 31.7 | 6.1 |
|  | 2 | .82 | 1.0 | 24.6 | 5.6 |
|  | 3 | .83 | 1.0 | 26.6 | 6.3 |
|  | 4 | .66 | 1.0 | 35.8 | 1.9 |
| 1477 | 1 | .89 | 1.0 | 14.6 | 2.7 |
|  | 2 | .75 | 1.0 | 28.8 | 3.7 |
|  | 3 | .77 | 1.0 | 29.1 | 5.8 |
|  | 4 | .79 | 1.0 | 25.9 | 3.6 |
| 1478 | 1 | .68 | 1.0 | 35.5 | 3.9 |
|  | 2 | .72 | 1.0 | 34.4 | 5.2 |
|  | 3 | .75 | 1.0 | 29.2 | 4.2 |
|  | 4 | .84 | 1.0 | 20.0 | 4.4 |
| 1479 | 1 | .76 | 1.0 | 29.6 | 5.6 |
|  | 2 | .77 | 1.0 | 25.3 | 2.4 |
|  | 3 | .81 | 1.0 | 24.4 | 3.9 |
|  | 4 | .72 | 1.0 | 30.1 | 1.7 |
| 1480 | 1 | .66 | 1.0 | 35.7 | .8 |
|  | 2 | .78 | 1.0 | 23.8 | 1.3 |
|  | 3 | .80 | 1.0 | 22.4 | 2.0 |
|  | 4 | .77 | 1.0 | 25.0 | 1.5 |

winter and spring, 1476–1477. Thus the crisis mortality of 1476–1477, like that of 1471, had little effect on marriage and remarriage ratios. Remarriage, the most accurate measurement of the immediate effect on population of successive periods of crisis mortality, increased in 1474 and through 1476 and 1477, into the early months of 1479 in higher levels than it had in the earlier years of the decade. This expansion came to a sudden halt during the great plague epidemic of 1479–1480. Marriage and remarriage ratios fell sharply in the autumn and winter quarters of these years, with remarriage ratios at .8 of 1 percent during the winter, 1479–1480. But the marriage ratios again proved their resilience to relatively brief periods of excessive mortality, and by spring quarter, 1480, showed signs of recovery.

Thus in two of four cases, testators appear to have quickly remarried after periods of decline caused by crisis mortality. It should be noted that the two cases, the epidemics of 1473 and 1479–1480, were the most severe epidemics in the period, 1430–1480. As we have seen in Chapter 6, epidemic disease and the crisis mortality that it caused had little effect on the long-term marriage ratios over a fifty-year period, and seemed to cause relatively few dislocations even on a decennial basis. The overall marriage ratios of the 1470's were close to those of the other four decades. Within the individual quarters of the decade of the 1470's, marriage ratios show that first-marriages were highest, albeit slightly, in the middle years of the decade, at precisely the time when remarriage was at its decennial peak. This in turn may explain the relatively low remarriage ratios immediately after the high mortality quarters of 1471 and 1476–1477. There can be little doubt, both from the widow-widower data[27] and the figures for testators who were not married, that epidemic disease had an immediate quarterly and perhaps yearly effect on the marriage ratios. The percentage of testators who did not list a spouse right after a major epidemic was always high—30 percent or more during the winter quarters of 1472, 1474 and 1479, and close to 30 percent in the summer, 1477, the quarters after the seasons of highest decennial mortality. Thus, having been reduced during the epidemic of 1473 and, to a much lesser extent, that of 1471, marriage ratios recovered strongly during the middle years of the decade, declined again during the epidemic of 1479–1480, and seemed to be well on their way to recovering their previous levels once more by mid-1480. The French Pox of 1475 appears to have had no effect whatsoever on the marriage results. This pattern of rapid nuptial recovery is similar to that of the sample as a whole from 1430 to 1470, and to that of the crisis-mortality quarters analyzed in section 7.2. The demographic upsurge of the 1470's cannot be explained in terms of

*Table 7.3.2.* Quarterly Data, 1470–1480: Male Child Replacement
Ratios to Entire Sample

| | | | | Distribution of Sons per Family - in % | | | | | |
| | R.R. | Mode | 0 | 1 | 2 | 3 | 4 | 5 | 6+ |
|---|---|---|---|---|---|---|---|---|---|
| 470 1 | .70 | 0 | 59.8 | 20.5 | 11.8 | 6.3 | .8 | .8 | .0 |
| 2 | .68 | 0 | 53.9 | 28.7 | 13.0 | 4.3 | .0 | .0 | .0 |
| 3 | .86 | 0 | 51.4 | 23.6 | 12.5 | 11.1 | 1.4 | .0 | .0 |
| 4 | .83 | 0 | 49.6 | 30.4 | 11.3 | 5.2 | 3.5 | .0 | .0 |
| 471 1 | .58 | 0 | 64.4 | 18.4 | 14.9 | 2.3 | 1.0 | .0 | .0 |
| 2 | .86 | 0 | 51.1 | 25.9 | 15.6 | 5.9 | .7 | .7 | .0 |
| 3 | .70 | 0 | 56.1 | 23.5 | 14.3 | 6.1 | .0 | .0 | .0 |
| 4 | .69 | 0 | 53.4 | 28.9 | 14.7 | 1.5 | 1.0 | .5 | .0 |
| 472 1 | .53 | 0 | 64.4 | 24.7 | 5.5 | 4.1 | 1.4 | .0 | .0 |
| 2 | .69 | 0 | 55.7 | 25.0 | 15.6 | 2.8 | .0 | .9 | .0 |
| 3 | .77 | 0 | 53.2 | 24.2 | 17.7 | 1.6 | 3.2 | .0 | .0 |
| 4 | .74 | 0 | 56.9 | 26.4 | 9.7 | 4.2 | 1.4 | 1.4 | .0 |
| 473 1 | .83 | 0 | 52.0 | 22.7 | 20.0 | 2.7 | 1.3 | 1.3 | .0 |
| 2 | .80 | 0 | 50.0 | 25.4 | 19.7 | 4.9 | .0 | .0 | .0 |
| 3 | .82 | 0 | 47.3 | 33.6 | 11.8 | 4.5 | 2.7 | .0 | .0 |
| 4 | .81 | 0 | 51.2 | 27.2 | 14.6 | 4.7 | 1.6 | .8 | .0 |
| 474 1 | .94 | 0 | 43.9 | 28.6 | 20.1 | 4.8 | 2.6 | .0 | .0 |
| 2 | 1.06 | 0 | 44.2 | 25.9 | 17.3 | 7.1 | 2.5 | 1.0 | .0 |
| 3 | .64 | 0 | 61.1 | 20.6 | 13.5 | 3.2 | 1.6 | .0 | .0 |
| 4 | .88 | 0 | 51.0 | 21.6 | 17.6 | 7.8 | 2.0 | .0 | .0 |
| 475 1 | .74 | 0 | 51.9 | 27.3 | 15.6 | 5.2 | .0 | .0 | .0 |
| 2 | .75 | 0 | 55.6 | 22.2 | 16.0 | 3.7 | 2.5 | .0 | .0 |
| 3 | .81 | 0 | 55.6 | 19.4 | 16.7 | 5.6 | 2.8 | .0 | .0 |
| 4 | 1.00 | 0 | 48.8 | 27.5 | 15.0 | 3.8 | 2.5 | 1.3 | 1.3 |
| 1476 1 | .68 | 0 | 54.9 | 30.5 | 8.5 | 4.9 | .0 | 1.2 | .0 |
| 2 | .94 | 0 | 50.8 | 22.2 | 16.7 | 4.8 | 4.0 | 1.6 | .0 |
| 3 | .82 | 0 | 48.1 | 27.8 | 19.0 | 3.8 | 1.3 | .0 | .0 |
| 4 | .79 | 0 | 53.8 | 24.5 | 14.2 | 5.7 | .9 | .9 | .0 |
| 1477 1 | .88 | 0 | 48.9 | 27.0 | 16.1 | 4.4 | 2.2 | 1.5 | .0 |
| 2 | .75 | 0 | 53.4 | 25.7 | 14.7 | 4.7 | 1.2 | .0 | .0 |
| 3 | .78 | 0 | 48.8 | 31.4 | 14.0 | 4.7 | 1.2 | .0 | .0 |
| 4 | .76 | 0 | 50.0 | 29.5 | 15.2 | 5.4 | .0 | .0 | .0 |
| 1478 1 | .80 | 0 | 55.3 | 22.4 | 15.8 | 2.6 | 1.3 | 2.6 | .0 |
| 2 | .81 | 0 | 53.1 | 25.0 | 13.5 | 5.2 | 2.1 | 1.0 | .0 |
| 3 | .88 | 0 | 54.2 | 25.0 | 12.5 | 4.2 | 2.1 | .0 | 2.1 |
| 4 | 1.00 | 0 | 40.0 | 37.8 | 11.1 | 8.9 | 8.9 | 2.2 | .0 |
| 1479 1 | .82 | 0 | 51.9 | 22.2 | 20.4 | 3.7 | 1.9 | .0 | .0 |
| 2 | .72 | 0 | 54.2 | 28.9 | 10.8 | 3.6 | 1.2 | 1.2 | .0 |
| 3 | .74 | 0 | 61.5 | 16.7 | 14.1 | 3.8 | 1.3 | 2.6 | .0 |
| 4 | .70 | 0 | 57.6 | 25.0 | 10.6 | 5.1 | .8 | .4 | .4 |
| 1480 1 | .70 | 0 | 55.8 | 26.4 | 14.0 | 1.6 | 1.6 | .0 | .8 |
| 2 | .70 | 0 | 60.0 | 22.5 | 8.8 | 6.3 | 1.3 | 1.3 | .0 |
| 3 | .80 | 0 | 57.1 | 28.6 | 6.1 | 2.0 | 2.0 | 2.0 | 2.0 |
| 4 | .83 | 0 | 42.6 | 36.8 | 16.2 | 4.4 | .0 | .0 | .0 |

*Table 7.3.3.* Quarterly Data, 1470–1480: Female Child
Replacement Ratios to Entire Sample

|       |   | R.R. | Mode | % Test. No Daughters |
|-------|---|------|------|----------------------|
| 1470  | 1 | .31  | 0    | 78.7                 |
|       | 2 | .23  | 0    | 84.3                 |
|       | 3 | .74  | 0    | 55.6                 |
|       | 4 | .38  | 0    | 70.4                 |
| 1471  | 1 | .44  | 0    | 73.6                 |
|       | 2 | .43  | 0    | 73.3                 |
|       | 3 | .47  | 0    | 73.5                 |
|       | 4 | .46  | 0    | 71.6                 |
| 1472  | 1 | .50  | 0    | 71.9                 |
|       | 2 | .36  | 0    | 78.3                 |
|       | 3 | .31  | 0    | 79.0                 |
|       | 4 | .33  | 0    | 73.6                 |
| 1473  | 1 | .44  | 0    | 66.7                 |
|       | 2 | .54  | 0    | 64.8                 |
|       | 3 | .63  | 0    | 65.5                 |
|       | 4 | .51  | 0    | 64.2                 |
| 1474  | 1 | .56  | 0    | 64.0                 |
|       | 2 | .70  | 0    | 56.3                 |
|       | 3 | .50  | 0    | 67.5                 |
|       | 4 | .50  | 0    | 68.6                 |
| 1475  | 1 | .59  | 0    | 68.6                 |
|       | 2 | .56  | 0    | 63.0                 |
|       | 3 | .84  | 0    | 55.6                 |
|       | 4 | .65  | 0    | 63.8                 |
| 1476  | 1 | .53  | 0    | 69.5                 |
|       | 2 | .25  | 0    | 78.6                 |
|       | 3 | .65  | 0    | 62.0                 |
|       | 4 | .52  | 0    | 69.5                 |
| 1477  | 1 | .71  | 0    | 59.1                 |
|       | 2 | .44  | 0    | 69.6                 |
|       | 3 | .64  | 0    | 64.0                 |
|       | 4 | .36  | 0    | 74.1                 |
| 1478  | 1 | .40  | 0    | 73.7                 |
|       | 2 | .54  | 0    | 68.8                 |
|       | 3 | .63  | 0    | 62.5                 |
|       | 4 | .47  | 0    | 73.3                 |
| 1479  | 1 | .65  | 0    | 61.1                 |
|       | 2 | .55  | 0    | 66.3                 |
|       | 3 | .47  | 0    | 73.1                 |
|       | 4 | .47  | 0    | 70.5                 |
| 1480  | 1 | .51  | 0    | 72.9                 |
|       | 2 | .49  | 0    | 67.5                 |
|       | 3 | .67  | 0    | 67.3                 |
|       | 4 | .38  | 0    | 70.6                 |

the emergence of new patterns of marriage, caused by epidemic disease or anything else.

Child replacement ratios by quarter for the 1470's followed patterns similar to those of the marriage ratios, but proved to be even more responsive and more sensitive on a short-term basis to the immediate dislocations caused by crisis mortality. The data shown in Tables 7.3.2 and 7.3.3 were taken for the entire sample including clerics and females, and therefore are to be compared with the data from Tables 7.1.1 and 7.1.6, rather than those of 7.1.2, 7.1.3, 7.1.7 or 7.1.8. The reader is reminded that the figures reflect numbers of children as seen from the wills—that is, as recorded by their parents, and not from independent fertility data. Also, it is not possible to say precisely how an epidemic affected the numbers of children. Perhaps it did so directly, through high mortality; or perhaps indirectly through reducing conceptions for a variety of physical reasons or because of the psychological trauma of not wishing to conceive during a period of great emotional and physical stress.[28] These factors are in turn partially balanced by the possibility of more diligent recording of female progeny during periods of crisis mortality, all of which must be kept in mind before turning to the data.

Male replacement ratios were down significantly during and immediately after the pestilence of autumn, 1471; at one point, the number of sonless families rose to over 64 percent of the will-registering population, an increase of about 12 percent over the comparable decennial average, and the lowest replacement ratio for the ten-year period. Yet within a year, male replacement ratio levels were well over 80 percent in a sample which included clerics and unmarried testators. At one point, the ratios hovered at or around unity for the entire sample for six months. Female replacement ratios, underenumerated as usual, rose during the period of low male ratios, and then fell again as the numbers of sons increased, a pattern reminiscent of the replacement ratios of the London élite for the 1440's.

The high male replacement ratios continued with few exceptions into 1477, surpassing unity twice. At first glance, it appears that the epidemic of 1473 had little effect on the male ratios. On closer examination, however, it can be seen that the replacement ratios immediately following the quarter of greatest mortality, autumn, 1473, were extremely high, being in fact the highest "back-to-back" ratios in the entire sample, and in any case a significant increase over the figures for the months of 1473. The 1473 data only appear to be large when compared with the figures of 1471 and 1472. The same can be said about the female progeny replacement ratios. Further, it will be recalled from Chapter 5 that the scope of the 1473 epidemic of flux was largely limited to Norfolk. When Norfolk is singled out for individual analysis, the differences between the low 1473 figures and the high 1474 figures are more pronounced.[29]

The crisis mortality of winter, 1476–1477, and spring, 1477, the quarters which showed the lowest levels of excessive mortality of the four 1470's crisis-mortality periods, seems to have had little effect on the male and female replacement ratios. Although there was a slight slump in spring, 1477, both male and female ratios reached their highest levels for several quarters in the winter of 1476–1477. But in the autumn and winter, 1479–1480, the period of highest overall mortality in the fifty years surveyed, the decline in child replacement ratios was quite pronounced, almost matching proportionally those following the epidemic of 1471. And again, depressing effects on the replacement ratios do not seem to have been long-lasting; for by the summer quarter, 1480, there were already signs of improvement.

Thus, like their parents, the children in the wills proved responsive on a short-term basis to epidemic disease. Population losses were quickly recouped after a period of crisis-level mortality. The middle years of the 1470's were a time of recovery from the epidemics of the late 1460's and early 1470's, and, in effect, preparation for the onslaughts to come. But the rapid demographic recovery after a period of severe epidemic does not mean that infectious diseases were not the major factor in controlling population in the 1470's; to the contrary, the evidence would seem to indicate that they were the primary element in controlling population growth. It was the continual recurrence of infectious disease, primarily in epidemic form, which kept population levels low. At the risk of oversimplification, it should be said that while population seems to have been capable of quickly recouping all or most of its precrisis-mortality levels, the arrival of a new epidemic once again reduced the level of population to the point where it had been at the end of the last demographic catastrophe. The upsurge in replacement ratios which took place in the 1470's was the result of a few bountiful years crowded together in the middle of the decade, and not the result of unimpeded and continual demographic recovery, as the decennial data lead us to believe.

It was suggested earlier that the replacement ratio and perhaps population increase in the 1470's was due either to a change in the aetiological character of infectious diseases, a diminution in the levels of infant mortality, or a rise in fertility. As with the previous quarters of crisis mortality examined, the replacement ratios for crisis-mortality quarters in the 1470's showed a decline proportional to the rises in levels of mortality among adults, as indicated in the wills. Based on the testamentary evidence, there is no justification for claiming that the replacement ratio increase of the 1470's was due to a change in the nature of infectious diseases, which in turn proved less lethal to children than they had in the period, 1430–1460. As stated above, there is no way to measure changes in infant mortality. But it is possible, almost by default, that the increase was the result of greater fertility. In the 1470's the levels of fertility appear to have outstripped the claims of mortality. Although we lack sufficient data to comment on trends in the age of marriage, we do know from the testamentary data that the percentage of the population which was married did not change significantly from 1430 to 1480. Higher replacement ratios in the 1470's were not the result of more married testators, but more children within the individual families. There were more families with more children, and fewer families with no children.

Some additional figures can be given to illustrate the increase in family size in the 1470's.[30] For the entire sample, including unmarried testators, from 1430 to 1480, 54 percent of the population had no children; only 18 percent of the total population had at least one child of both sexes. In the 1470's, the number of childless families dropped dramatically. The decennial averages for the 1470's show that 59 percent of the population, as opposed to 46 percent for the entire sample from 1430 to 1480 and 42 percent of the population for the entire sample from 1430 to 1470, had at least one child of either sex, increases of 13 and 17 percent. Further, the figure for the 1470's marks an increase of over 20 percent in total numbers of families with children from the figures of the 1440's. By the 1470's over 25 percent of all testators, including clerics and the unmarried, had both male and female children. Part of the enlarged figures for the 1470's came from an increased mechanical inclusion of daughters in the wills; but the bulk of it simply reflects the natural rise in numbers of children in the last decade of the survey.

Proposing estimates about family size based only on the data from the testamentary evidence is a dangerous affair. Mechanical omissions, especially of daughters, make any sort of speculation about household denominators a risky business, even for the 1470's, the only decade in which it can be done with some statistical justification. Further, for the 1470's, the data are relatively reliable for only the two wealthiest groups of the sample, the London and rural élite. Conjugal family size, with conjugal family being defined as father and mother, and sons and daughters who were not married and not of age at the time the will was made, but excluding grandparents and grandchildren, was well over 4 per family unit in the 1470's for both of these groups. Subtracting married progeny and progeny of age, the figures as deduced from the wills are about 4.4 for the rural élite, and about 4.1 for the London élite. Conjugal family size for the sample as a whole in the 1470's, based primarily on the data from Tables 7.1.3 and 7.1.8, was just over 4 per family. Household size, with household being defined to include all testators but clerics (that is, including unmarried nonclerical testators) was about 3.1. Modest as these figures for the 1470's may appear, they represent a considerable increase over those of the previous four decades.[31]

# Notes

1. For descriptions of the replacement ratio method, see E. A. Wrigley, *Population and History* (New York: McGraw-Hill, 1969), pp. 20–21; T. H. Hollingsworth, *Historical Demography* (Ithaca, N. Y.: Cornell Univ. Press, 1969), pp. 375–388; and S. L. Thrupp, "Problem of Replacement Rates in Late Medieval English Population," *Ec.H.R.*, 2nd series, XVIII, 1965. As the text indicates, the replacement ratio method is by no means a definitive one. Much of its theory remains to be worked out, and it can only be hoped that this is being done by mathematical demographers. It would be ideal to use more direct and more proven methods to establish trends in fertility, but given the realities and limitations of the testamentary and other fifteenth century data, this is not possible.

2. For an example of the use of grandchildren, see above, p. 161.

3. Less than 5% of the total number of male progeny were grandsons.

4. See above, pp. 175–183.

5. For two studies on the shadowy subject of social mobility in late medieval England, see Thrupp, *The Merchant Class of Medieval London* (Chicago: Univ. of Chicago Press, 1948), pp. 191–233; and K. B. MacFarlane, *The Nobility of Later Medieval England* (Oxford: Oxford Univ. Press, 1973), pp. 142–176.

6. Wrigley, *op. cit.;* Hollingsworth, *op. cit.* Also, see Wrigley, "Fertility Strategy for the Individual and the Group," in Charles Tilly, ed., *Historical Studies of Changing Fertility* (forthcoming).

7. For further reference, see M. M. Postan, "Fifteenth Century," *Ec.H.R.*, IX, 1939; and his "Some Agrarian Evidence of Declining Population in the Later Middle Ages," *Ec.H.R.*, 2nd series, II, 1950.

8. For a discussion of the demographic characteristics of the late medieval nobility, a group, included within but more narrowly defined than the rural élite, see MacFarlane, *op. cit.;* Hollingsworth, "A Study of the British Ducal Families," *Population Studies*, XI, 1957; and his *Demography of the British Peerage*, supplement to *Population Studies*, XVIII, 1965; and J. T. Rosenthal, "Medieval Longevity and the Secular Peerage, 1350–1500," *Population Studies*, XXVII, 1973.

9. The possibility exists that younger or even eldest sons were provided for in advance of the wills and hence excluded from them. There is, however, little evidence to support this view. For comment on the remark of Gwyn Williams, *Medieval London: From Commune to Capital* (London: Athlone Press, 1963), pp. 315–317, see above, Chap. 4, footnote 70.

10. Underpopulation is a relative term, having to do with a variety of social,

economic and technological conditions. Nevertheless, despite the debate in regard to the standard of living in late medieval England, it is the consensus of most scholars that fifteenth century England was sparsely populated. For two opposing views on the topic, see: Postan, "Fifteenth Century" and "Some Agrarian Evidence"; and A. R. Bridbury, *Economic Growth: England in the Later Middle Ages* (London: G. Unwin, 1962).

11. See above, pp. 206–208.

12. The exception was St. Albans. For discussion, see above, p. 195.

13. For varying viewpoints on which, how and why the English population stopped growing, see J. Z. Titow, *English Rural Society* (London: George Allen and Unwin, 1969), pp. 65–96; Postan, "Medieval Agrarian Society in its Prime: England," in Postan, ed., *Cambridge Economic History of Europe*, I, 2nd ed. (Cambridge: Cambridge Univ. Press, 1966); J. C. Russell, "Pre-Plague Population of England," *Journal of British Studies*, V, 1966; Barbara Harvey, "The Population Trends in England, 1330–1348," *Transactions of the Royal Historical Society (T.R.H.S.)*, 5th series, XVI, 1966; and D. G. Watts, "A Model for the Early Fourteenth Century," *Ec.H.R.*, 2nd series, XX, 1967.

14. It was postulated in Chapter 4 on the basis of literary and mortality evidence that the population of Suffolk may have been declining in the mid-1470's. For a discussion of this in light of the replacement ratios, see above, pp. 205–206.

15. For example, for the replacement ratios of all male testators to all male progeny, the Norfolk ratio for the 1470's was .91, and the Suffolk ratio .75. For all married males to all male progeny, the ratios were 1.02 for Norfolk, and .83 for Suffolk.

16. It is interesting to compare these figures with those reached by MacFarlane, *op. cit.*, pp. 169–176.

17. By 1525, the situation of the East Anglian cities appears to have improved. The tax assessment of 1523/24 and 1524/25, based on wealth rather than on sheer size and omitting some important cities, lists Norwich as the second most heavily taxed urban area; Ipswich, seventh; King's Lynn, eighth; Bury St. Edmunds, thirteenth; Lavenham, fourteenth; Yarmouth, twenty-first; and Hadleigh, twenty-fifth. For a discussion of the tax assessment and early sixteenth century population, see W. G. Hoskins, "English Provincial Towns in the Early Sixteenth Century," *T.R.H.S.*, 5th series, VI, 1956; J. Cornwall, "English Population in the Early Sixteenth Century," *Ec.H.R.*, 2nd series, XXIII, 1970; and his "English Country Towns in the Fifteen Twenties," *Ec.H.R.*, 2nd series, XV, 1962.

18. See Chapter 5, footnote 41, for references to studies of these and other late medieval provincial towns. Also, see above, footnote 17.

19. For example, for wills from Norfolk and Suffolk taken exclusively from the Norwich Consistory Court (N.C.C.), a married male testator to all male progeny replacement ratio for 1480–1485 is 1.22. The author hopes to present data from the 1480's in the near future.

20. This is especially applicable to historical demographers writing on the population rise in many European countries during the early modern period. See

the articles in D.V. Glass and D. E. C. Eversley, eds. *Population in History* (London: Edward Arnold, 1965), especially K. F. Helleiner, "The Vital Revolution Reconsidered," pp. 79–86.

21. Smallpox, for instance, is especially lethal to very young children. For a discussion of infant mortality, among other things, see Wrigley, "Mortality in Pre-Industrial England: The Example of Colyton, Devon, over Three Centuries," *Daedalus*, 97, 1968.

22. These quarters were chosen because they were felt to be the quarters of most virulent epidemics in the period 1439–1465, with the possible exception of spring, 1462. The data from 1430 to 1439 could not be used because it is incomplete for most of the court jurisdictions.

23. The total absence of any remarriage whatsoever leads to some suspicion in regard to the data. Nonetheless, when doublechecked, the same results were obtained. Similar evidence was found for 1455, as shown above, p. 210.

24. To save space, the data from 1466 were not included in Tables 7.2.1 to 7.2.3. They followed patterns approximate to those of 1455, but were immediately affected by the epidemic of pestilence in the following year.

25. There is some doubt about the mortality of 1476–1477 being the result of an epidemic. See above, pp. 102–103.

26. This is based not only on the figures of crude mortality, as presented in the graphs in Chapter 4, but also on the shapes and relative sizes of each of the crisis-mortality peaks. See above, pp. 86–94.

27. The widow-widower data have not been published because of the method used to establish the spouse ratios. Some widows and widowers would be included in the married category. With this reservation in mind, however, it can be noted that the widow-widower data, albeit incomplete, exceeded 10% only in the winter of 1472, the autumn of 1473, and the autumn and winter of 1479 and 1479–1480.

28. For a discussion of some of the psychological factors involved in childbirth, see Louis Chevalier, "Towards a History of Population," in Glass and Eversley, eds., *op. cit.,* and S. L. Thrupp, "Problem of Replacement Rates."

29. For example, the Norfolk figures of 1473 are approximate to those of the sample as a whole, being in the low .80's. But in the first three quarters of 1474, the replacement ratios were all over unity and in winter, 1474, it was 1.00 for a sample which included clerics and unmarried testators.

30. A partial listing of the data appears in Table 6.1.1. The rest are enumerated in the text, when appropriate.

31. The incomplete data regarding family size was about 2.6.

# CHAPTER VIII

# Conclusions: Fifteenth Century England

This study has tried to employ new methods and techniques in the study of late medieval England. Large numbers of testamentary data have been used to analyze some demographic aspects of fifteenth century life in broader and more scientific terms than have generally been attempted before. Although some scholars such as M. M. Postan have forwarded important theories about fifteenth century demography, they have based their ideas on local, little, or no quantitative evidence.[1] Only J. C. Russell has presented large-scale statistical evidence for the later Middle Ages, and much of his work is based upon life-tables constructed from modern data.[2] While the data presented above are derived from eastern England, some generalization may be helpful in putting the evidence in broader perspective.

What were the demographic facts of life and death in fifteenth century England? The most important factor of mortality was epidemic disease, especially plague; and the most important feature of plague was not the virulence of any given epidemic, but rather the frequency of continual epidemics. From 1430 to 1470 and perhaps 1480, infectious disease was the primary factor in controlling population growth. Medical authorities were aware of its significance, but did not understand its origins or causes, and were essentially helpless in allaying its depredations. Epidemic and endemic disease and the incidence of regions of crisis mortality were probably of major importance in all pre-industrial societies, but few periods in history appear to have been subjected to as virulent and, most important, as frequent outbreaks of infectious disease as was fifteenth

225

century England. This factor of recurring epidemics, along with the continual presence of endemic disease in the community served to depress the population of at least eastern England from 1430 until the late 1460's. Of the other variables most commonly thought to have directly affected demographic growth in pre-industrial Europe, famine does not seem to have been a major problem in fifteenth century England, in part because infectious disease itself kept population at relatively low levels from at least the time of the Black Death. Climatic changes, however, may have played a role. Although much work on the history of climate remains to be done, the later Middle Ages in Europe is believed to have been an era of colder temperatures.[3] In the decades of worst virulence and highest frequency of epidemic disease in the period under study, the 1430's and 1470's, the narrative sources speak of unusually cold and wet weather. But infectious disease was the major causative element in the low fifteenth century population figures, and its frequency—at least twenty-seven of the fifty years covered in parts of England—was the major reason.

To answer a question posed in the introduction, East Anglia followed the biological pattern of demographic development more closely than the Malthusian pattern. With the possible exception of the 1470's, mortality and not fertility was the demographic pacesetter. And while Saltmarsh *may* have overestimated the general socio-economic effects of plague, Bean clearly underestimated them.

Epidemic disease, including plague, was not restricted solely to urban areas in the fifteenth century. Urban mortality was high, but on the average was no higher than rural mortality, and only London appears to have had as pronounced ratios of mortality as did those select rural areas which have been designated as regions of crisis mortality. Fertility, at least as shown by replacement ratios, was lower in the urban centers than it was in the countryside, but there is no evidence to indicate that this was the result of higher child mortality in the towns. Various factors of fertility, things which cannot be measured directly by the testamentary sources, such as levels of infant mortality and the very demographic constitution of the towns themselves, must have also played a large role in the comparative numbers of rural and urban offspring. In any case, massive migration into towns was necessary in order to maintain urban population. As it was, all the urban areas in the sample except London probably declined in numbers from 1430 to 1480. By contrast, much of rural East Anglia, especially Norfolk, seems to have maintained its numbers throughout most of the period, and even increased toward its end. One thing is certain: there can be no set rules about the preponderance of epidemic and endemic disease in the cities in the fifteenth century. Norwich actually appears to have suffered from disease less frequently than most rural areas. The presence of infectious disease appears to have depended primarily on local ecological conditions. While population density must have been an important factor in the transmission of infectious disease, only London had a population density large enough to make it a continual haven for viruses, bacilli and protozoa of all sorts.

In addition to the recurring presence of infectious disease, the major demographic peculiarity of fifteenth century England concerns fertility, or, in this case, a lack of it. There are few periods in western history where population declined or remained stagnant for as long as it did in fifteenth century England. Judging from the testamentary evidence, this was due not only to protracted high mortality, but also to low levels of fertility, a condition which does not seem to have changed until the 1470's. The replacement ratios given by Laslett and Goubert for the seventeenth century are dismal, but they are far better than those of the fifteenth century.[4] Stone laments the low replacement ratios of the English nobility in the late sixteenth and early seventeenth centuries—purportedly a period of demographic growth—but his figure of 29 percent sonless families is far lower than even the best fifteenth century will figures, and better even than Thrupp's figures for late medieval London merchants.[5] Replacement ratios in fifteenth century England appear to have been lower than they were in almost all periods and cultures in pre-industrial Europe. In terms of sheer population size, fifteenth century England was probably similar to twelfth century England; but there was a major difference. The population of twelfth century England was rising, while that of fifteenth century England was declining, or stagnant. In the twelfth century, there was very little, if any, plague. In the fifteenth century, plague recurred constantly.

In at least one demographic aspect, marriage, fifteenth century England was quite similar to early modern Europe. Marriage for both men and women appears to have taken place after age twenty-five, with the bulk of the pre-twenty-five marrieds coming from the merchant and rural élite testators. There was only a slight connection between first-marriages and wealth, as would be expected in a century of comparatively easily obtainable land. An overwhelming number of those who could marry did; in the case of the greater London merchants, this was well over 90 percent of the total population. Remarriage, however, was dependent on personal wealth. Among the wealthy, it probably took place quickly after the death of the first spouse, in pursuit of an elusive heir. Marriage and fertility were very responsive to the immediate short-term onslaughts of epidemic disease. After a severe epidemic period, marriage and replacement ratios recovered strongly—until the next epidemic. There was only a slight relationship between personal wealth and number of sons, except in the most extreme situations.

Speculative abstract attempts to view population trends can be made. A pattern of mid-fifteenth century population trends begins in the 1420's and 1430's with a period of extensive epidemic disease and continual and continued demographic decline. Theoretically with the relative abatement of epidemic disease on a national and regional scale, population would be expected to grow considerably in the 1440's, 1450's and early 1460's, as the result of earlier first-time marriage and more remarriage, and a considerable drop in mortality. With the return of epidemic disease on a national scale in the 1470's, population growth would have ceased, only to begin again in the relatively epidemic-free 1480's and 1490's.

With the exception of the enigmatic 1470's, most of this pattern holds true when considered in light of the testamentary evidence. The 1430's were a period of considerable demographic decline. Despite flaws in the testamentary evidence for this decade, the wills show that mortality was severe and protracted, marriage ratios were comparatively low, and fertility as represented by child replacement ratios was abnormally low by any standards. The 1440's and 1450's marked at least a slowing down of the demographic decline. Mortality was severe for certain quarters and even for periods of several quarters in succession in the early and late 1450's, though on a far lesser scale than was the case in the 1430's. Marriage and remarriage ratios were way up, although there is little evidence in regard to the comparative ages of first marriage. Child replacement ratios also were up, and in a few select subgroups in the sample, passed the unity mark. In the 1460's, there are considerable signs of demographic expansion, with increases in all the fertility and marriage measures. But the 1470's do not follow the proposed model path. Although mortality was as high as it was in the 1430's, child replacement ratios reached their highest levels in the fifty-year period studied. Instead of declining in the 1470's, population showed signs of increasing as it never had in the previous three decades of less frequent and less virulent epidemic disease.

We have seen that the replacement ratios' increase of the 1470's was not the result of decreased mortality or the increased ratios of marriage. It is conceivable that people married earlier in the 1470's than they had in the previous decades, and that infant mortality declined; unfortunately, the testamentary sources give little information on this. However, it would logically follow that people would have married earlier and infant mortality would have declined in the disease-free 1440's and 1450's rather than in the disease-ridden 1470's, but population did not rise then. Another answer to possible demographic growth in the 1470's may lie in a change in the aetiological character of the more common and more lethal epidemics, a change which made them less deadly to children, the group whose numbers increase so significantly in the 1470's. But it is not likely that a change in the nature of the most common infectious diseases of the century—a distinct possibility in itself—was the major factor in the replacement ratio increase. It is probable that the increase was due to a rise in fertility within individual testamentary families. In the wills, this is reflected by more families listing multiple numbers of children and decreased numbers of families which died without legitimate issue.

But if fertility improvement was the crucial factor in the replacement ratio rise, what caused it and why did it not occur sooner, after the decade of the 1430's? The fifteenth century was a period of relatively easily obtained land and comparatively abundant foodstuffs, at least in regard to bulk, if not quality. Those elements conducive to population growth existed throughout the century, and would be expected to contribute to a population increase from 1440 onward. The failure of population to respond immediately after the 1430's may have been due to psychological factors. Wrigley has found similar population lags in the seventeenth century—periods when population levels simply failed to respond to apparently ideal conditions of growth.[6] Chevalier has stressed a cultural reluctance to reproduce in periods of crisis,[7] although it would seem that the bulk of the population would be inured to the stress of pestilence by the fourth decade of the fifteenth century. It is possible that levels of nutrition improved in the 1470's, and directly affected personal fertility. Whatever the explanation, replacement ratios and perhaps overall population appear to have begun increasing, at least in eastern England in the 1470's, and continued to grow in the 1480's and 1490's.

None of these explanations can be tested by the data presented above. But large collections of records from which further demographic studies of late medieval England can be made do exist. There is adequate testamentary evidence to extend a study of this sort into at least the 1520's. Since it has been postulated that population began to increase in the 1470's and 1480's, work along these lines would be especially valuable. Excellent testamentary data also survive for London, Kent and Essex from 1430 to 1480. If wills from these areas were aggregated and analyzed, many of the theories and gaps presented in the thesis could be tested and filled in. For some areas and jurisdictions, notably London and the P.C.C., it is possible to extend a testamentary-demographic study into the fourteenth century.

There are other records from which demographic studies can be conducted on both a local and regional level. The tax data from 1377–1381 and 1523–1525 have been worked before, but can be further developed.

The same is true of the I.P.M.'s. Manorial documents also present population data, although they diminish in numbers and quality during the fifteenth century. The demographic evidence can be combined with other quantitative data, such as series of prices and wages on a local and perhaps even regional level.[8] Data for the quantitative study of late medieval England to exist, are accessible to the historian, and should be exploited.

## Notes

1. M. M. Postan, "The Fifteenth Century," *Ec.H.R.*, IX, 1939; and his "Some Agrarian Evidence of Declining Population in the Later Middle Ages," *Ec.H.R.*, 2nd series, II, 1950. For examples of local demographic studies in the fifteenth century, see W. G. Hoskins, "The Population of an English Village, 1086–1801," *Leicestershire Archeological and Historical Society*, 33, 1957; and S. L. Thrupp, "Problem of Replacement Ratios in Late Medieval English Population," *Ec.H.R.*, 2nd series, XVIII, 1965. Thrupp's *The Merchant Class of Medieval London* (Chicago: Univ. of Chicago Press, 1948), contains perhaps the best demographic analysis of any fifteenth century group on a greater than local level.

2. J. C. Russell, *British Medieval Population* (Albuquerque: Univ. of New Mexico Press, 1948).

3. See E. Leroy Ladurie, *Times of Feast and Times of Famine* (Garden City, N.Y.: Doubleday, 1971), although his chronology is somewhat different from the usual interpretations. See also J.Z. Titow, "Evidence of Weather in the Account Rolls of the Bishopric of Winchester, 1209–1330," *Ec.H.R.*, 2nd series, XII, 1960.

4. Peter Laslett, *The World We Have Lost* (New York: Scribner's, 1965), pp. 100–106; Pierre Goubert, *Beauvais et le Beauvaisis de 1600 à 1730* (Paris: S.E.V.P.E.N., 1960), chap. 3.

5. Lawrence Stone, *The Crisis of the Aristocracy* (Oxford: Oxford University Press Paperback, 1967), pp. 76–88; Thrupp, *Merchant Class*, pp. 191–206.

6. E. A. Wrigley, *Population and History* (New York: McGraw-Hill, 1969), chap. 4.

7. Louis Chevalier, "Toward a History of Population," in D.V. Glass and D.E.C. Eversley, eds., *Population and History* (London: Edward Arnold, 1965).

8. The role of price levels and their effect on population growth and decline have barely been touched upon in this thesis. They are a very complicated topic, and merit a thesis in their own right. It is possible that agricultural prices were low enough in mid-fifteenth century East Anglia to fail to provide incentive for peasant producers to expand their cultivation, even when the opportunity presented itself, and hence discouraged earlier age of first-marriage and larger families. Until adequate price data can be presented for a variety of goods on a local level for more than a few selected years, this idea cannot be pursued on an empirical level.

# APPENDIX A

# *Parish and Deanery Jurisdictions*

The individual parishes in the N.C.C. are too numerous to be listed.
Many are listed elsewhere, as the Sudbury parishes are in Tymms' index
to the West Suffolk wills (see bibliography). Thumbnail sketches of most
of the East Anglian parishes can be found in various gazetteers of England, such as Frank Smith, *A Genealogical Gazetteer of England* (Baltimore:
Genealogical Publishing Co., 1968), and Oliver Mason, *The Gazetteer of
England,* 2 vols. (Newton Abbot: David Charles, 1972). C.J.W. Messent's
*Parish Churches of Norfolk and Norwich* (Norwich: W. H. Hunt, 1936) is an
excellent study of virtually all parish churches in Norfolk, including those
gone to ruin. Maurice Beresford's *Deserted Medieval Villages* (London:
Lutterworth, 1968) provides a list of abandoned medieval parishes.
Therefore, only the N.C.C. deaneries are listed. Unlike the parishes of the
N.C.C., those in the archdeaconry of St. Albans are scattered throughout
the counties of Hertfordshire and Buckinghamshire. For this reason, and
because there are many fewer parishes in the archdeaconry, they are
given below.

*Archdeaconry of St. Albans*

Parishes in Hertfordshire

| | |
|---|---|
| Barnet Chipping | Rickmansworth |
| Barnet East | Ridge |
| Bushey | Saratt |
| Codicote | Sandridge |
| Elstree | Shephall |
| Hexton | St. Albans |
| Langeley Abbot | St. Albans St. Michael |
| Newnham | St. Albans St. Peter |
| Northaw | St. Albans St. Stephan |
| Norton | Walden St. Paul |
| Redbourne | Watford |

Parishes in Buckinghamshire

| | |
|---|---|
| Aston Abbots | Horewood Little |
| Grandborough | Winslow |

*Deanery Jurisdiction of the Diocese of Norwich*

Archdeaconry of Norwich

| | |
|---|---|
| Blofield | Norwich |
| Breckles | Sparham |
| Brisley | Taverham |
| Flegg | Thetford |
| Holt | Toftrees |
| Ingworth | Walsingham |
| Lynn | |

Archdeaconry of Norfolk

| | |
|---|---|
| Brooke | Hingham |
| Burnham | Humbleyard |
| Cranwich | Redenhall |
| Depwade | Repps |
| Fincham | Rockland |
| Heacham | Waxham |

Archdeaconry of Suffolk

| | |
|---|---|
| Bosmere | Loes |
| Carlford | Luthingland |
| Claydon | Orford |
| Colney | Samford |
| Dunwich | South Elmham |
| Hoxne | Wangford |
| Ipswich | Wilford |

Archdeaconry of Sudbury

| | |
|---|---|
| Blackbourne | Stowe |
| Clare | Sudbury |
| Fordham | Thedwastre |
| Hartismere | Thingoe |

# A List of Occupations Encountered in the Wills (Alphabetically, with Computer Code)

### 1. Noncitizens

000 no listing
001 cleric; priest; rector; vicar; bishop; *doctorus thelogicus; capallanus; parsona;* etc.
002 knight; *miles;* gentleman; esquire; squire; duke; earl
003 yeoman
004 husbandman
005 apprentice; servant; *famulus*
006 *advocatus; legum doctorus*
007 baker
008 ballman; bellman
009 barker; tanner
010 barker
082 baxter
201 bedweaver
087 bladesmith
011 bootmaker; laster
012 brazier
013 brewer; *pandoxater*
014 butcher
015 cardmaker
070 carter
016 carpenter
017 caulker; coker

018  chandler
019  chestman; cheseman
072  clothmaker
020  cook
098  cooper
021  cordwainer; corviser; shoemaker; souter
(027  same as above)
(086  same as above)
094  currier
071  cutler
022  doctor [medical]
084  draper
069  dyer
023  fletcher
024  floatman; floater; boatman
025  fisherman
026  fishmonger
028  fuller
030  furrier
031  gardiner
076  glazier; glassmaker
032  glover
033  goldsmith
034  gravedigger
079  grocer
035  haberdasher
036  hayremaker
037  herringman; *allictarvnis*
038  ironmonger; hardwareman
203  hosier
074  labourer
039  leatherdresser; *alictarius*
066  [leprous]
097  lokere; watchman; herdsman
091  lorimer; harnessmaker
040  loder
041  maltman
065  mason
067  mariner
081  mercer
073  merchant
064  miller; molendiman; *molendinarius*

042  millward
043  notary
077  parchmentmaker
078  peynter; painter
093  plumer
044  poulter
045  ragman; rasman
095  reder
068  roper
078  saddler
046  salter
047  scripter
048  shearman; sherman
(055  same as above)
049  shipmaker
050  shipman
051  skinner
052  smith
085  soker; suker
053  spicer
092  sporier; *sportarius;* basketmaker
054  starchmaker
202  strener; maker of strainingcloths (course muslim)
090  senster (fishseller?)
009  tanner
056  tailer; parmenter
(029  same as above)
057  tinker; repairman
058  thatcher; thakker
075  thresher
059  turner
060  tyler; *tegulator; coopertarius*
061  vintner
083  webster
062  weaver
200  wheelwright
096  wiredrawer
099  woodmonger; treemonger
088  woolman
063  worsteadman
080  wright

2. Citizens
- 100 *civis;* burgess; burger
- 101 *civis* and alderman; and gentleman
- 102 aurifaber
- 103 baker
- 104 barber
- 105 bladesmith
- 185 bowyer
- 106 brazier
- 107 brewer; *pandoxater*
- (140 same as above)
- 108 broiderer
- 109 butcher
- 175 carmfex (?)
- (177 same as above)
- 110 carpenter
- 111 chandeler
- 112 chapmaker
- 113 chestman; cheseman
- 114 cordwaner; shoemaker
- 116 *coninicious* (?)
- 117 *cronatus*
- 182 cutler
- (186 same as above)
- 118 draper
- 169 fletcher
- 119 fishmonger; *pistenar;* stockfishmonger
- 120 founder
- 121 fruiterer
- 122 fuller
- 123 furrier
- 124 girdler; *zonarius*
- 125 glazier
- 126 goldsmith
- 127 grocer
- 176 haberdasher
- 173 hosier
- 174 hostler
- 172 husbandman
- 128 ironmonger; hardwareman
- 180 jurisdoctor
- 129 leatherseller
- 130 leatherman
- 131 lester; lyster; salmon seller

132  linendraper
133  marbeler
184  mason
134  merchant
135  mercer
136  notary
(179  same as above)
137  patymaker
138  pasteller
(183  same as above)
139  *pannarius*
141  parchmenmaker
142  *pelliparius;* skinner
143  peuterer
178  plumer
144  poulterer
145  ragman
146  reder
147  salter
148  saddler; sellarius
(115  same as above)
(150  same as above)
149  saffer
151  scripter
152  scissor
153  shearman; sherman
154  sherringgrinder
155  smith
156  spicer
157  stacioner
158  tailer
164  tallowchandeler
159  thatcher; thickwiller
160  timbremonger
161  tinetor
162  tinctor
163  truttor
181  tanner
171  turner
165  upholsterer
166  vintner
167  woodmonger
168  worsteadman
169  yeoman

# APPENDIX C

# *Shrewsbury's* History of the Bubonic Plague

Many of the ideas presented in this thesis run contrary to those expressed by J. F. D. Shrewsbury in his *History of the Bubonic Plague in the British Isles*. [1] Because of this, it was felt essential to discuss his book in some detail, with an emphasis on the fifteenth century. [2] Shrewsbury's main point is the comparative lack of destructiveness of plague. He believes historians have overestimated its frequency and virulence. From 1430 to 1480, he believes there were pestilences only in 1434–1435, 1438–1439, 1444, 1448, 1449–1450, 1454, 1463, 1465, 1471 and 1478, and perhaps in 1472 and 1476, not all of which were plague. [3] Shrewsbury's observations are clearly incomplete; even if some of the local epidemics from 1430 to 1480 had a minimal impact, the national epidemics of 1452, 1457–1459, 1467 and 1473, to name just four, are omitted. [4] Further, he accepts Creighton's dating of the epidemic of 1479–1480 without checking the records himself. [5] Herein lies one of the book's major shortcomings—Shrewsbury's failure to investigate any but printed and easily accessible chronicles and letters. No effort is made to search more obscure printed and manuscript sources; and even when original data are searched, it is done in an extremely uncritical manner. Often, the validity of the records is denied on the basis of uncorroborated value judgements and twentieth century medical information. His misuse of historical records is consistent, if nothing else, as when referring to the Black Death he categorically states ". . . the contemporary records demonstrate conclusively . . . there was no collapse of agriculture, and disruption of the economic life of the nation." [6] Although no footnotes are included, the claim that the paucity of surviving petitions to the king calling for the cessation of taxes makes a great mortality impossible may be quickly dismissed. Without even commenting on the problem of the survival of records, a quick look at the calendar of *Papal Registers* for the fourteenth and fifteenth centuries will show the ecclesiastical side of depopulation.[7]

Shrewsbury does not discuss the existence of endemic areas of plague. He seems to feel that plague had to be continually reintroduced into England in order to exist in epidemic form, and that the necessity of reintroduction prevented it from occurring as frequently as has been claimed.[8] The case presented in this thesis for endemic plague cannot be made as strongly as that for the frequency of epidemic plague. But the evidence of crisis mortality makes the existence of pockets of endemicity tenable, and the contemporary literary evidence which actually describes the virulence and importance of endemic pestilence cannot be denied. Many of Shrewsbury's statements are based on the aetiological character of modern plague. One of his major premises is that epidemic bubonic plague has not changed in character "during the period of recorded history."[9] This is contrary to what other epidemiologists have written.[10]

Shrewsbury diminishes the significance of the effects of pneumonic plague in fifteenth century England, saying it cannot "occur in the absense of the bubonic form."[11] This too seems to run contrary to the evidence. As Shrewsbury acknowledges, many of the probable plague epidemics of the fifteenth century coincided with bad weather; what he does not stress is that in the 1430's, much of this was cold weather. The seasonal patterns of the epidemic of 1433–1435, 1438–1439, and 1479–1480 all hint at the presence of pneumonic plague. Further, William of Worcestre tells us his nephew died two days after contracting the plague in January, 1479–1480, a characteristic sign of pneumonic plague.[12] Although pneumonic plague was not nearly as common as bubonic plague, there is no evidence, either medical or historical, to deny its existence altogether.

There are other questionable points forwarded in the book. There is no fifteenth century evidence, either medical or statistical, indicating that plague struck those aged fifteen to thirty-five most severely.[13] Nor is the Shrewsbury tenet that plague was essentially restricted to areas east and south of a line drawn from Exeter to York entirely feasible.[14] Density of population was important in the dissemination of plague, but *x. cheopis* can survive on rodents other than "domestic" black rats, and even on its own and in animal dung for extended periods of time, and pneumonic plague does not need a base flea or rodent population to spread after its initial penetration, since it is passed on from man to man.[15] Also, interregional travel was far more common in the Middle Ages than Shrewsbury indicates, and was by no means restricted solely to merchants. Thus, both bubonic and pneumonic plague could survive in sparsely populated regions.

The author believes as does Shrewsbury that many diseases other than plague, such as dysentery, influenza and smallpox were present in fifteenth century England. But both fifteenth century quantitative and medical evidence indicate that plague was the primary element controlling mortality in eastern England from 1430 to 1480.

# Notes

1. J. F. D. Shrewsbury, *A History of Bubonic Plague in the British Isles* (Cambridge: Cambridge Univ. Press, 1971).

2. See the excellent review of Christopher Morris, "The Plague in Britain," *Historical Journal*, XIV, 1971.

3. Shrewsbury, *op. cit.*, pp. 141–149.

4. See above, pp. 35–51.

5. Charles Creighton, *A History of Epidemics in Britain* (Cambridge: Cambridge Univ. Press, 1894), I, pp. 231–233.

6. Shrewsbury, *op. cit.*, pp. 123.

7. See above; pp. 35–51.

8. Shrewsbury; *op. cit.*, pp. 1–6.

9. *Ibid.*, p. 29.

10. See above, pp. 58–71.

11. Shrewsbury, *op. cit.*, p. 6.

12. William of Worcestre, *Itineraries*, edited by John Harvey (Oxford:Clarendon Press, 1969), p. 255.

13. Shrewsbury, *op. cit.*, p. 44.

14. *Ibid.*, p. 33.

15. See above, pp. 58–71.

# APPENDIX D

# *Computer Methodology*

Owing to the large number of wills involved in the study, it became apparent quite early that, even for the most elementary calculations, computerization would be necessary. Certain alternations had to be made to prepare the data for this. The original eleven categories were divided into the twenty-three categories discussed in section 1.4. Additionally, a five-digit computer identification number was affixed to each card, making twenty-four computer categories.

The standard eighty column I.B.M. cards were used for punching. The first five columns were given over to the I.D., with the lead zeroes, when necessary, supplied. Columns 6 and 7 were the testator's initials, and column 8 the testator's sex. Columns 9–18 were the literal recordings of the first ten letters of the home village or town, and columns 19–21 the initials of the church in the home parish, if given, being left justified. In this case and in all cases, uncompleted files were left unpunched. Column 22 was the county, using the present delineations with the first initial only.

The occupations were put into a numerical code, as described in section 1.4, in columns 23–25, being right justified with lead zeroes supplied. No listed occupation was left blank. Columns 26–34 and 35–43 respectively were the date the will was made and the date of probate, recorded literally in the fashion described above. Column 44 was season, with 1 being winter, 2 spring, 3 summer, and 4 being autumn.

Column 45 was the number of spouses. If no spouse was mentioned, the column was left blank and reckoned to be zero in all calculations. At times, the blank was made "specific," and at other times a missing data card was supplied. The same method was used for progeny; no reference was left blank and taken to be zero unless specifically mentioned. Column 46 was for dead spouse. Because the number of spouses was rarely greater than

241

1, except among the P.C.C. testators, the alphanumeric "Y" was used rather than a numeric symbol.

Column 45 referred to the number of male progeny. Column 48 represented sons of age, once again using the alphanumeric symbol Y for reasons similar to that of dead spouse. Column 49 was grandsons, also represented as Y. If there were no sons, no sons of age, or no grandsons, all columns were left unpunched and taken to be zero unless specified otherwise. The female categories were punched in precisely the same manner as were the males. Column 50 was number of females; column 51, the daughters of age or married, represented by Y; and column 52, granddaughters, also represented by Y. Column 53 was ascendant generation, represented by 1; column 54, sibling generation, represented by 2; column 55, descendant generation, represented by 3; column 56, servants, represented by 4; and column 57 was godchildren having children, represented by 5.

Columns 58–63 were the literal recordings of bequest to the high altar. Columns 58–60 were right justified with no lead zeroes, and termed "cash." Column 61 was the "unit," with a letter code of "D" being pence, "S" or "/" being shillings, "M" being marks, and "T" being pounds. As stated above, due to a lack of proper conversion factors, those testators who left bequests in kind other than grain, who left no bequests at all, or whose bequests were in obvious disaccord with their testamentary wealth were not included, and were left blank on the computer cards. Because the difficulties involved in calculating the mean of 15,000 pieces of data in different units proved considerable, even for a computer, a new classification for calculating wealth, called conveniently enough, "Wealth," was created. The seven additional, newly created criteria for evaluating it are discussed in depth in Chapter 6. Another new classification, "Age," which has been alluded to, was also created after the original punching scheme had been devised, and has been discussed in detail above.[1] In both the Wealth and Age formats, any blanks or inappropriate data were represented as "99" to prevent the inclusion of misinformation.

A packaged computer program, S.P.S.S., was used to analyze the data, with particular usage being made of the subprograms Codebook, Condescriptive, and Crosstabs.[2] Because of the size of the files, it was not possible to use the Non Parr Corr correlations, and because of the nonparametric nature of the wealth and age data, it was not possible to use the Pearson correlation subprograms. Thus, attempts to ascertain even basic correlations between variables was limited to the bivariate relationships established by the subprogram Crosstabs, a not entirely satisfactory arrangement. The correlation data presented in Chapter 6 are therefore necessarily limited.

The entire sample was divided into groups of thirty separate operations. The divisions were the whole sample, the five decennial splits, and individual runs for the wills from the P.C.C., Norfolk, Suffolk and Hertfordshire. Codebook subprograms, for example, would then be run for such things as spouse, males, females, wealth, age, season, and so forth. The entire operation was then repeated with a variety of limitation factors, such as only males, only females, and so on, programmed in. Subsequent runs were made in an attempt to assess the direct effect of epidemic disease, using especially virulent plague years and plague seasons, such as autumn, 1465, and normal seasons, such as autumn, 1455. Because the 1470's were such an interesting decade—ostensibly one of greater epidemic frequency, yet with a population rise—runs were made for each season in each year—that is, forty individual runs. All of this is discussed as appropriate, in the text.

## NOTES

1. For the age and wealth methodologies, see above, pp. 159–175.
2. The S.P.S.S. program and its relative merits cannot be discussed here. For details of the program, see Norman H. Nie, Dale H. Bent and C. Hadlai Hull, *S.P.S.S.* (Statistical Package for the Social Sciences) (New York: McGraw-Hill, 1970).

# BIBLIOGRAPHY

## A. Primary Sources

### 1. Wills

The wills from the P.C.C., N.C.C. and the archdeaconry courts of Hertfordshire, Norfolk and Suffolk were read on microfilm in the Graduate Library of the University of Michigan. As there were only two untitled reels for the archdeaconry of Suffolk, the names of the first testators are given. Wills from the archdeaconry courts of Norfolk and Sudbury, the peculiar court of Bury St. Edmunds, and the city court of Norwich were read from the original registers in the West Suffolk and Norwich and Norfolk County Record Offices. The jurisdictions are listed alphabetically.

Archdeaconry of Norfolk, 1452–1479

    Grey, 1452–79
    Shaw, 1460–78

Archdeaconry of Norwich, 1469–1480

    Fuller

Archdeaconry of St. Albans, 1430–1480

    Stonham, 1430–70
    Wallingford, 1470–80

Archdeaconry of Sudbury, 1435–1480
  Baldwin, 1439–76
  Hervey, 1476–79
  Fuller, 1642–80

Archdeaconry of Suffolk, 1435–1479
  Richard Dymor; Richard Stewardson

Consistory Court of Norwich, 1430–1480
  Surflete, 1430–36
  Doke, 1436–44
  Wylby, 1444–48
  Aleyn, 1444–48
  Brosyerd, 1454–64
  Neve, 1456–57
  Gilberd, 1472–77
  Betyns, 1457–71
  Jekkys, 1464–72
  Cobald, 1465–68
  Gelour, 1472–79
  Paynot, 1472–73
  Hubert, 1473–91
  Caston, 1479–80

Court of the City of Norwich, 1430–1480
  Wills among enrolled deeds, Rolls 18, 19, 20

Peculiar Court of Bury St. Edmunds, 1430–1480
  Osbourne, 1436–42
  Hawlee, 1443–80
Prerogative Court of Canterbury (P.C.C.), 1430–1480

  Luffenan, 1430–49
  Rous, 1430–52
  Stokton, 1454–62
  Godyn, 1463–68
  Wattys, 1471–80
  Logge, 1479–80

*The Register of Henry Chichele 1430–1447*, (1937), edited by Jacob, E.F., II, Oxford: Univ. Press.

**Indices of Wills.** There are several indices of probated fifteenth century wills. Most of them contain a great many errors, and must be used with extreme caution. When used with care, however, they can be very helpful. Many of the indices seen by the author were privately printed and available only in the local record offices and the Institute of Historical Research in London.

Camp, A. J. (1963), *Wills and Their Whereabouts,* Canterbury: Phillimore.

Crisp, F. A. (1895), *Calendar of Wills . . . at Ipswich,* London: By the Author.

Farrow, M. A. (1942–1945), "Index of Wills Proved at Norwich, 1370–1500," *Norfolk Record Society,* XVI.

Gibson, J. S. W. (1974), *Wills and Where to Find Them,* Chicester, Sussex: Phillimore.

Marshall, G. W. (1895), *A Handbook to the Ancient Courts of Probate and Depositories of Wills,* London: By the Author.

Oswald-Hicks, T. W. (1913), *A Calender of Wills . . . of Suffolk Proved in the P.C.C., 1383–1604,* London: By the Author.

Palgrave-More, Patrick (1971), "Index of Wills Proved in the Norfolk Archdeaconry Court, 1453–1542," *Norfolk Genealogy,* 3.

Redstone, Vincent (1907), *Calendar of Pre-Reformation Wills . . . at Bury St. Edmunds,* Bury St. Edmunds: By the Author.

Smith, J. C. C. (1893–1895), *Prerogative Court of Canterbury Wills 1383–1558,* 10–11, London: British Record Society.

Tymms, Samuel, (1850), *Wills and Inventories from the Registers of the Commissary of Bury St. Edmunds and the Archdeaconry of Sudbury,* XLIX, London: Camden Society.

## 2. Literary Sources

Amundesham, John (1870–1871), *Annales Monasterii S. Albani,* edited by Riley, H. T., 2 vols., London: Longman's.

Arnold, Richard (1811), *Customs of the City of London,* London: F. C. and J. Rivington.

"Brief Notes" (1880), in *Three Fifteenth Century Chronicles,* edited by Gairdner, James, n.s., XXVIII, Westminster: Camden Society.

*The Brut: Chronicles of England* (1960), edited by Brie, F.W.D., II, London: Oxford University Press.

*Canterbury Cathedral Priory Obituary List,* Ms.d 12F.

*Chronicles of the Grey Friars of London* (1827), edited by Nichols, J.G., London: Longmans.

Fabyan, Robert (1811), *New Chronicles of England and France,* edited by Ellis, H., London: F. C. and J. Rivington.

*Great Chronicle of London* (1938), edited by Thomas, A. H., London: G. W. Jones.

Gregory, William (1876), *Chronicle,* in *Historical Collections of a Citizen of London in the Fifteenth Century,* edited by Gairdner, James, n.s., XVII, London: Camden Society.

Herryson, John (1840), *Abbreviata Chronica ab Anno 1377 Usque ad Annum 1469,* Caius College, Cambridge, Ms., edited by Smith, J. J., Cambridge Antiquarian Society: Publications, 1.

———. "Appendix X: Infirmarer's Roll," 37, Henry VI, 1458–59, in Atkinson, T. D., ed. (1933), *An Architectural History of the Benedictine of the Monastery of St. Etheldreda at Ely,* Cambridge: Cambridge Univ. Press.

*Ingulph's Chronicle of the Abbey of Croyland* (1854), edited by Riley, H. T., London: H. G. Bohn.

*Journal D' Un Bourgeois De Paris sous Charles VI et Charles VII* (1929), edited by Mary, André, Paris: Henri Jonquières.

*Paston Letters* (1904), edited by Gairdner, James, I–III, London: Chatto and Windus.

*A Short English Chronicle* (1880), in *Three Fifteenth Century Chronicles,* edited by Gairdner, James, n.s., XXVIII, Westminster: Camden Society.

Stanbridge, John (1956), *A Fifteenth Century Schoolbook,* British Museum, Arundel Ms. 249, edited by Nelson, William, Oxford: Clarendon.

Walsingham, Thomas (1867–1869), *Chronica Monasterii S. Albani,* edited by Riley, H. T., II, p. 285, London: Longmans.

Warkworth, John (1839), *A Chronicle of the First Thirteen Years of the Reign of King Edward the Fourth,* edited by Halliwell, J. O., London: Camden Society.

William of Worcester (1969), *Itinerum,* Corpus Christi College, Cambridge, Unique Ms. 210, edited by Harvey, John, Oxford: Clarendon Press.

Wright, Thomas ed. (1859–1861), *Political Poems and Songs Relating to English History,* London: Longmans.

### 3. Medical Treatises and Recipes

John La Barba, treatise variously titled, with many editions; among them, British Museum, Sloane Ms. 3449, Sloane Ms. 134 (VI), Sloane Ms. 2172, Sloane Ms. 2320, Society of Antiquaries Ms. 101. (All folio pages are cited in Chapter 3.)

John of Bordeaux, treatise variously titled, with many editions; among them, British Museum, Sloane Ms. 706 (VIII), Sloane Ms. 963 (IX), Sloane Ms. 965 (VIII), Sloane Ms. 983 (II), Sloane Ms. 433 (IV), Society of Antiquaries Ms. 101.

British Museum, Sloane Ms. 965 (anonymous).

*For Helthe of Body from Colde,* Society of Antiquaries Ms. 101.

Forestier, Thomas (1490), *Tractus contra pestilentian, thenasmonem et dissenterium,* Rouen. Also, British Museum, Additional Ms. 27582; and British Museum, Arundel Ms. 249.

Knuttson, Bengt (1911), *A Litel Boke . . . for . . . the Pestilence,* edited by Vine, Guthrie, Manchester: John Rylands Library. Also, British Museum, Sloane Ms. 404 and Sloane Ms. 2276.

*A Leechbook or Collection of Medical Recipes of the Fifteenth Century* (1934), edited by Dawson, W. R., London: Macmillan.

*Medica*, LL 1 18, University Library, Cambridge.

"Recipe for Edward IV's Plague Medicine" (1878), *Notes and Queries*, 9.

*Signa Pestilencie*, British Museum, Sloane Ms. 783B.

*Treatise On Sikenese*, Ms. LL 1 18, University Library, Cambridge.

Wymus, John de, *A Regiment Devicyed be Mastur John de Wymus, doctor servant of the Lady Margeret of Borgon*, Society of Antiquaries, Ms. 101.

### 4. Ecclesiastical and Governmental Records, and Treatises of Law

*Calendar of Papal Registers* (1906–1955), edited by Tremlow, J. A., VII–XIII, London: H. M. Stationery Office.

*Calendar of State Papers Relating to Milan (1912)*, edited by Hinds, A. B., London: H. M. Stationery Office.

*Calendar of State Papers and Manuscripts Relating to English Affairs: Venice* (1864), edited by Brown, Rawdon, I, London: H. M. Stationery Office.

Lyndwood, William (1679), *Provinciales seu constitutiones Anglie . . .*, Oxford.

*Proceedings and Ordinances of the Privy Council of England* (1835), edited by Nicholas, N. Harris, IV, London: Eyre and Spottiswoode.

*Register of Edmund Lacy, Bishop of Exeter, 1420–55* (1967), edited by Dunstan, G. R., 5 vols., Torquay: Canterbury and York Society and Devon and Cornwall Society Publications, n.s., 7.

*Rotuli parliamentorum ut et Petiones et Placita in Parliamento* (1761–1783), IV–VI, London.

*Taxatio Ecclesiastica Angliae et Welliae* (1802), London.

*Visitations and Memorials of Southwell Minster* (1891), edited by Leach, A. F., n.s., XLVIII, Westminster: Camden Society.

## B. Selected Secondary Works

Allison, K. J. (1955), "Lost Villages of Norfolk," *Norfolk Archeology*, 31.

Allyn, H. B. (1925), "The Black Death: Its Social and Economic Results," *Annals of Medical History*, VII.

Appleby, Andrew (1973), "Disease or Famine? Mortality in Cumberland and Westmoreland, 1580–1640," *Ec.H.R.*, 2d series, XXIV.

Bailey, N. J. T. (1959), *Mathematical Theory of Epidemics*, London: Hafner Publishing Co.

Baker, A. R. H. (1973), "Changes in the Later Middle Ages," in Darby, H. C., ed., *New Historical Geography of England*, Cambridge: Cambridge University Press.

Baker, A. R. H. and Butlin, R. A., eds. (1973), *Studies of Field Systems in the British Isles*, Cambridge: Cambridge University Press.

Baratier, Edouard (1961), *La Démographie Provençale du XIII<sup>e</sup> au XVI<sup>e</sup> Siècle*, Paris: S.E.V.R.E.N.

Bean, J. M. W. (1962–1963), "Plague, Population, and Economic Decline in England in the Later Middle Ages," *Ec.H.R.*, 2nd series, XV.

Beresford, Maurice (1968), *Deserted Medieval Villages*, London: Lutterworth Press.

———. (1954), *Lost Villages of England*, London: Lutterworth Press.

Biraben, J-N. (1968), "Certain Demographic Characteristics of the Plague Epidemic of 1720–22," *Daedalus*, 97.

———. (1975), *Les hommes et la peste*, The Hague: Mouton.

Boucher, C. E. (1938), "The Black Death in Bristol," *Trans. of the Bristol and Gloucestershire Archeological Society*, 60.

Bridbury, A. R. (1962), *Economic Growth: England in the Later Middle Ages*, London: George Allen and Unwin.

Brownlee, J. (1918), "Certain Aspects of the Theory of Epidemiology in Special Relations to Plague," *Proc. of the Royal Society of Medicine*, II.

Burnet, MacFarlane and White, David (1972), *Natural History of Infectious Disease*, Cambridge: Cambridge University Press.

Campbell, A. M. (1931), *The Black Death and Men of Learning*, New York: Columbia University Press.

Chambers, J. D. (1972), *Population, Economy, and Society in Pre-Industrial England*, Oxford: Oxford University Press.

Clarke, Edwin, ed. (1971), *Modern Methods in the History of Medicine*, London: Athlone.

Clemow, F. G. (1900), "Endemic Centers of Plague," *Journal of Tropical Medicine*, II.

———. (1903), *Geography of Epidemic Disease*, Cambridge: Cambridge University Press.

Coale, A. J. (1971), "Age Patterns at Marriage," *Population Studies*, XXV.

Coale, A. J. and Demeny, P. (1973), *Regional Model Life Tables and Stable Populations*, Princeton: Princeton University Press.

Cornwall, Julian (1962), "English Country Towns in the Fifteen Twenties," *Ec.H.R.*, 2nd series, XV.

———. (1970), "English Population in the Early Sixteenth Century," *Ec.H.R.*, 2nd series; XXIII.

———. (1961–1962), "The People of Rutland in 1522," *Trans. of the Leicestershire Historical Society*, 37.

Crawfurd, R. H. P. (1914), *Plague and Pestilence in Literature and Art*, Oxford: Oxford University Press.

Creighton, Charles (1894), *A History of Epidemics in Britain*, I, Cambridge: Cambridge University Press.

Crosby, A. W. (1972), *The Columbian Exchange*, Westport Conn: Greenwood Press.

Darby, H. C., ed. (1936), *Historical Geography of England before 1800*, Cambridge: Cambridge University Press.

———. (1973), *New Historical Geography of England before 1800*, Cambridge: Cambridge University Press.

Davenport, F. G. (1906), *Economic Development of a Norfolk Manor, 1086–1565*, Cambridge: Cambridge University Press.

D'Irsay, Stephan (1925), "The Black Death and the Medieval Universities," *Annals of Medical History*, VII.

———. (1927), "Defense Reactions During the Black Death," *Annals of Medical History*, IX.

Dulley, A. J. F. (1966), "Four Kentish Towns at the End of the Middle Ages," *Archaeologia Cantiana*, LXXXI.

Ekwall, Eilert (1956), *Studies in the Population of Medieval London*, Stockholm: Almquist and Wiksell.

Fisher, F. J. (1965), "Influenza and Inflation in Tudor England," *Ec.H.R.*, 2nd series, XVIII.

Fisher, J. L. (1943), "The Black Death in Essex," *The Essex Review*, LII.

Forster, Robert and Ranum, Orest, eds. (1975), *Biology of Man in History*, Baltimore: Johns Hopkins University Press.

France, R. S. (1938), "A History of Plague in Lancashire," *Trans. of the Historical Society of Lancashire and Cheshire*, XC.

Gale, A. H. (1959), *Epidemic Diseases*, London: Penguin.

Glass, D. V. and Eversley, D. E. C., eds. (1965), *Population in History*, London: Edward Arnold.

Godfrey-Smith, Tony (1964), "Plague and the Decline of Medieval Europe," *Australian National University Historical Journal*, I.

Goody, Jack (1973), "Strategies of Heirship," *Comparative Studies in Society and History*, 15.

Gottfried, Robert (1976), "Epidemic Disease in Fifteenth Century England," *Journal of Economic History*, XXXVI.

Goubert, Pierre (1960), *Beauvais et le Beauvaisis de 1600 à 1730*, Paris: S.E.V.P.E.N.

———. (1968), "Legitimate Fertility and Infant Mortality in France During the Eighteenth Century," *Daedalus*, 97.

Greenwood, Major (1935), *Epidemics and Crowd Disease*, New York: Macmillan.

———. (1932), *Epidemiology, Historical and Experimental*, London: Oxford University Press.

Guerchberg, S. (1964), "The Controversy Over the Alleged Sowers of the Black Death in the Contemporary Treatises on Plague," in Thrupp, S. L., ed., *Change in Medieval Society*, New York: Appleton-Century-Crofts.

Hajnal, J., "European Marriage Patterns in Perspective," in Glass and Eversley, *Population in History*.

Hallam, H. E. (1961), "Population Density in the Medieval Fenlands," *Ec.H.R.*, 2nd series, XIV.

———. (1965), *Settlement and Society*, Cambridge: Cambridge Univ. Press.

———. (1957–1958), "Some Thirteenth Century Censuses," *Ec.H.R.*, 2nd series, X.

Hare, Ronald (1956), *An Outline of Bacteriology and Immunity*, London: Longmans.

———. (1955), *Pomp and Pestilence*, New York: Philosophical Library.

Harvey, Barbara (1966), "The Population Trend in England Between 1300 and 1348," *T.R.H.S.*, 5th series, XVI.

Henry, Louis (1956), *Anciennes familes genevoises*, Paris: Travaux et Documents de l'I.N.E.D.

Herlihy, David (1965), "Population, Plague and Social Change in Rural Pistoia, 1201–1430," *Ec.H.R.*, 2nd series, XVIII.

Hirst, L. F. (1953), *Conquest of Plague*, Oxford: Oxford Univ. Press.

Hollingsworth, T. H., "British Ducal Families," in Glass and Eversley, *Population in History*.

———. (1965), *Demography of the British Peerage*, supplement to *Population Studies*, XVIII.

———. (1969), *Historical Demography*, Ithaca, N.Y.: Cornell University Press.

Hoskins, W. H. (1956), "English Provincial Towns in the Early Sixteenth Century," *T.R.H.S.*, 5th series, VI.

———. (1957), "The Population of an English Village, 1086–1801," *Leicestershire Archeological and Historical Society*, 33.

Jessopp, A. (1889), "The Black Death in East Anglia" (1889), in his *The Coming of the Friars*, London: T. F. Unwin.

Kingsford, C. L. (1913), *English Historical Literature in the Fifteenth Century*, Oxford: Clarendon Press.

Krause, John (1956–1957), "The Medieval Household: Large or Small," *Ec.H.R.*, 2nd series, IX.

LeBras, Hervé (1973), "Parents, grandparents, bisaïeux," *Population*, 28.

Lee, Ronald (1973), "Population in Pre-Industrial England: An Econometric Analysis," *Quarterly Journal of Economics*, 87.

Leroy Ladurie, Emmanuel (1966), *Les Paysans de Languedoc*, Paris: S.E.V.P.E.N.

———. (1971), *Times of Feast and Times of Famine: A History of Climate Since the Year 1000*, Garden City, N.Y.: Doubleday.

Levett, A. E. (1916), *The Black Death on the Estates of the See of Winchester*, Oxford: Clarendon Press.

———. (1936), *Studies in Manorial History*, Oxford: Clarendon Press.

Listen, W. G. (1924), "The Plague," *British Medical Journal*, 1.

Lunden, Kare (1968), "Four Methods of Estimating the Population of a Norwegian District on the Eve of the Black Death, 1349–1350," *Scandinavian Economic History Review*, XVI.

MacArthur, William (1951–1952), "A Brief Study of English Malaria," *British Medical Bulletin*, 8.

———. (1926), "Old-Time Plague in Britain," *Trans. of the Royal Society of Tropical Medicine and Hygiene*, XIX.

———. (1927), "Old-Time Typhus in Britain," *Trans. of the Royal Society of Tropical Medicine and Hygiene*, XX.

MacFarlane, K. B. (1973), *The Nobility of Later Medival England*, Oxford: Oxford University Press.

McKinley, R. A. (1969), *Norfolk Surnames in the Sixteenth Century*, Leicester: Leicester University Press.

Mode, P. G. (1916), *The Influence of the Black Death on the English Monasteries*, Menasha, Wis.: Geo. Banta Publishing Co.

Morris, Christopher (1971), "The Plague in Britain," *Historical Journal*, XIV.

Mullett, C. F. (1956), *The Bubonic Plague and England*, Lexington, Ky.: University of Kentucky Press.

Neveux, H. (1968), "La Mortalité des Pauvres à Cambrai, 1377–1473," *Annales Demographie Historique*, n.v.

Pickard, R. (1947), *Population and Epidemics of Exeter in Pre-Census Times*, Exeter: By the Author.

Pollitzer, R. (1954), *Plague*, Geneva: W. H. O.

Postan, M. M. (1939), "The Fifteenth Century," *Ec.H.R.*, VIII.

———. (1966), "Medieval Agrarian Society in its Prime: England," in *Cambridge Economic History of Europe*, 2nd ed., I, Cambridge: Cambridge University Press.

———. (1950), "Some Agrarian Evidence of Declining Population in the Later Middle Ages," *Ec.H.R.*, 2nd series, II.

Power, Eileen (1918), "The Effects of the Black Death on Rural Organization in England," *History*, n.s., III.

Rabb, T. K. and Rotberg, R. I., ed. (1971), *The Family in History*, New York: Harper and Row.

Raftis, J. A. (1964), *Tenure and Mobility: Studies in the Social History of the Medieval English Village*, Toronto: Pontifical Institute of Medieval Studies.

Rees, William (1923), "The Black Death in England and Wales as Exhibited in Manorial Documents," *Proc. of the Royal Society of Medicine*, 6.

Ritchie, J. (1958), "Rule of Pestilence," *Medical History*, 2.

Robbins, Helen (1928), "A Comparison of the Effects of the Black Death on the Economic Organization of France and England," *Journal of Political Economy*, XXXVI.

Roberts, D. S. (1966), "Place of Plague in English History," *Proc. of the Royal Society of Medicine*, 59.

Robinson, W. C. (1959–1960), "Money, Population, and Economic Change in Late Medieval Europe," *Ec.H.R.*, 2nd series, XII.

Robo, E. (1929), "The Black Death in the Hundred of Farnham," *English Historical Review*, XLIV.

Rosenthal, J. T. (1973), "Medieval Longevity and the Secular Peerage, 1350–1500," *Population Studies*, XXVII.

———. (1972), *Purchase of Paradise*, London: Routledge and Kegan Paul.

Rowe, Joy (1958), "Medieval Hospitals of Bury St. Edmunds," *Medical History*, 2.

Russell, J. C. (1948), *British Medieval Population*, Albuquerque: Univ. of New Mexico Press.

———. (1966), "Effects of Pestilence and Plague, 1315–1385," *Comparative Studies in Society and History*, 7.

———. (1968), "That Earlier Plague," *Demography*, 5.

Saltmarsh, John (1941), "Plague and Economic Decline in England in the Later Middle Ages," *Cambridge Historical Journal*, 7.

Schofield, R. S. (1972), "Crisis Mortality," *Local Population Studies,* 9.

———. (1965), "Geographical Distribution of Wealth in England, 1334–1649," *Ec.H.R..,* 2nd series, XVIII.

Sheehan, Michael (1963), "The Influence of Canon Law on the Property Rights of Married Women in England," *Medieval Studies,* XXV.

———. (1963), *The Will in Medieval England,* Toronto: Pontifical Institute of Medieval Studies.

Shrewsbury, J. F. D. (1971), *A History of Bubonic Plague in the British Isles,* Cambridge: Cambridge University Press.

———. (1964), *Plague of the Philistines,* London: V. Gollancz.

Sigerist, H. E. (1970), *Civilization and Disease,* 3rd ed., Chicago: University of Chicago Press.

Singer, D. W. (1916), "Some Plague Tractates in the Fourteenth and Fifteenth Centuries," *Proc. of the Royal Society of Medicine,* 92.

Slack, Paul (1972), "Some Aspects of Epidemics in England," D. Phil. thesis, Oxford Univ.

Taylor, M. A. (1935), "Great Epidemics of the Middle Ages: Norwich and Norfolk," *Journal of State Medicine,* 1.

Thompson, A. Hamilton (1914), "The Pestilences of the Fourteenth Century in the Diocese of York," *Archeological Journal,* LXXI.

———. (1911), "The Registers of John Gynewell, Bishop of Lincoln, 1349–50," *Archeological Journal,* LXVIII.

Thrupp, S. L. (1948), *The Merchant Class of Medieval London,* Chicago: University of Chicago Press.

———. (1966), "Plague Effects in Medieval Europe ," *Comparative Studies in Society and History,* VIII.

———. (1965), "Problem of Replacement Ratios in Late Medieval English Population," *Ec.H.R.,* 2nd series, XVIII.

Titow, J. Z. (1969), *English Rural Society,* London: George Allen and Unwin.

———. (1961–1962), "Some Evidence of Thirteenth Century Population Increases," *Ec.H.R.,* 2nd series, XIV.

Tucker, G. S. L. (1963), "English Pre-Industrial Population Trends," *Ec.H.R.,* 2nd series, XVI.

Watts, D. G. (1967), "A Model for the Early Fourteenth Century," *Ec.H.R.,* 2nd series, XX.

Williamson, Raymond (1957), "The Plague in Cambridgeshire," *Medical History,* 1.

Winslow, C-E. A. (1943), *The Conquest of Epidemic Disease,* Princeton: Princeton University Press.

Wrigley, E. A. (1966), "Family Limitation in Pre-Industrial England," *Ec.H.R.,* 2nd series, XIX.

———. (forthcoming), "Fertility Strategy for the Individual and the Group," in Charles Tilly, ed., *Historical Studies of Changing Fertility.*

———. (1968), "Mortality in Pre-Industrial England: The Example of Colyton, Devon, over Three Centuries," *Daedalus,* 97.

———. (1969), *Population and History,* New York: McGraw-Hill.

Wu Lien Teh *et al.,* (1926), *A Treatise on Pneumonic Plague,* Geneva: W.H.O.

# INDEX

DEMCO